Near Birth

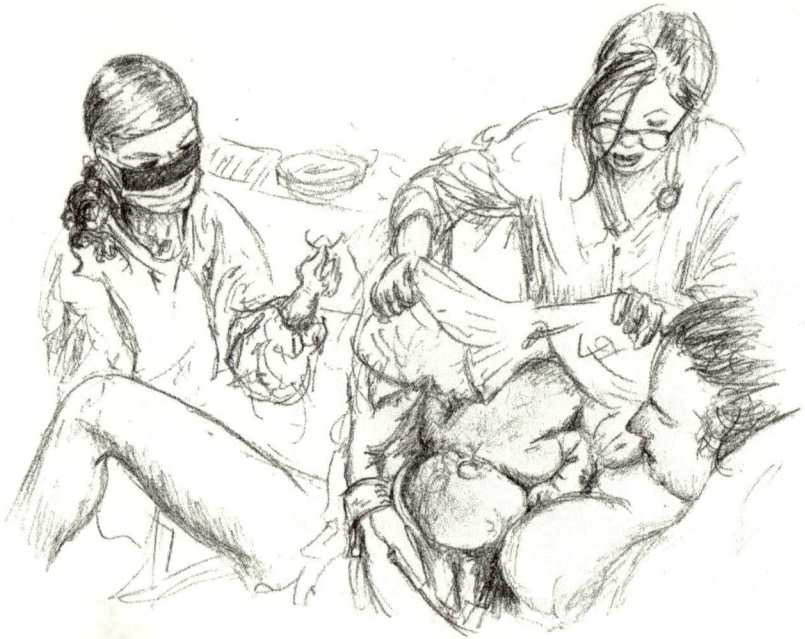

Near Birth

CONTESTED VALUES AND
THE WORK OF DOULAS

Andrea Ford

UNIVERSITY OF CALIFORNIA PRESS

University of California Press
Oakland, California

Cataloging-in-Publication Data is on file at the Library of Congress.

ISBN 978-0-520-41290-3 (cloth)
ISBN 978-0-520-41291-0 (pbk.)
ISBN 978-0-520-41292-7 (ebook)

34 33 32 31 30 29 28 27 26 25
10 9 8 7 6 5 4 3 2 1

CONTENTS

ACKNOWLEDGMENTS

Comparisons between childbearing and other creative processes abound, and for good reason. Conceiving, gestating, birthing, midwifing—the labors of creation are both productive and reproductive. They generate something new, and all new things consist of what came before. This book has been over a decade in the making. Like all books (and all children), this book is composed of what surrounded and composed its creator. It certainly would not exist without the support, insight, and encouragement of many people across California, and in Chicago, Edinburgh, and dotted elsewhere throughout the world. It is my reinterpretation and recombination of rich legacies of scholarship and "everyday theorizing" generated through the lived experiences of other creators. It is grown out of what nourished me.

Infinite thanks are due to Judy Farquhar, Joe Masco, Julie Chu, and Susan Gal for their guidance and inspiration at the University of Chicago Department of Anthropology as my PhD committee and postdoctoral supervisors, with a special nod to Julie for the title! To my wonderful Chicago colleagues who made the PhD and postdoc experience one of support, comradeship, and kindness, who read early drafts and continue to provide an academic community and circles of friendship: Matthew Beeber, Nicholas Carby-Denning, Hannah Chazin, Molly Cunningham, Nate Ela, Ali Feser, Karma Frierson, Matthew Furlong, Colin Halverson, Eric Hirsch, Jenny Miao Hua, Bill Hutchison, Anna Jabloner, Mallory James, Becca Journey, Hiroko Kumaki, Averill Leslie, Amy McLachlan, Erin Moore, Meghan Morris, Victoria Nguyen, Stephanie Palazzo, Alicia Riley, Jeremy Siegman, Joey Weiss, and many others. The University of Chicago's interdisciplinary workshops, particularly U.S. Locations and Medicine and Its Objects, facilitated invaluable stimulating and critical conversations. During fieldwork, the anthropology department at UC Santa Cruz extended a warm welcome. I am particularly grateful to Megan Moodie and Nancy Chen, and to Donna Haraway for a memorable brunch. Kali Rubaii, Alix Johnson, and Rebecca Feinberg invited me into grad student life and the writing community there.

Inevitably, my thinking changed in substantial ways since I handed in my PhD dissertation, as I figured out what kind of scholar and writer I would like to be. This was influenced in large part by new colleagues at the University of Edinburgh, where I have been immersed in the interdisciplinary Centre for Biomedicine, Self and Society (CBSS) within the medical school and thereby exposed to different ways of doing research and considering what kind of work is valuable. Martyn Pickersgill has been the most supportive advisor possible, and thanks are due to those who welcomed me into the wonderful CBSS community: Sarah Cunningham-Burley, Steve Sturdy, Ingrid Young, Giulia De Togni, Julia Swallow, Marlee Tichenor, Jaime Garcia Iglesias, Karissa Patton, Matthew Cull, and many others. Lucy Lowe built a bridge connecting me with the Edinburgh Centre for Medical Anthropology, and Şebnem Susam-Saraeva brought me into new kinds of academic-doula collaborations. My "hormones hub" colleagues have been so much fun to work with on ever-proliferating projects: Sone Erikainen, Roslyn Malcolm, Lisa Raeder, and Celia Roberts.

Grant funding makes research go round, and work on this book was generously supported by the Harper Fellowship and Watkins Fellowship at the University of Chicago, and by the Center for Biomedicine, Self and Society Wellcome Trust grant (209519/Z/17/Z). Numerous conferences and workshops have contributed to my thinking, and thanks are due to the organizers who often also facilitated my attendance. To name only a few: the Chemical Entanglements conference at the UCLA Center for the Study of Women, the Multi-Sighted/Sited/Cited U.S. Locations conference at the University of Chicago, the (In)tangible Technology and Data conference at the University of Helsinki, and the 20th Anniversary Symposium "Testing Women, Testing the Fetus" at the University of Edinburgh. The peripatetic life of academics has made it possible for me to have innumerable conversations with scholars and activists I admire deeply, and from whom I always learn more than I can properly acknowledge.

A few portions of this book are extended in articles and other forums, and I am grateful for the thoughtful suggestions made by the editors and anonymous reviewers of those publications: From chapter 2, the argument on evidence is elaborated in *Medicine Anthropology Theory,* and the argument on hormonal cascades is developed in *Hormonal Theory: A Rebellious Glossary.* Portions of chapter 3 on attuned consent are developed in *Frontiers: A Journal of Woman Studies,* and chapter 5's argument about self-making was formulated in *Cultural Anthropology* with thanks to Heather Paxson for her brilliant editorial work. Chapter 6 includes materials from an article on toxicity/purity in *Catalyst: Feminism, Theory, Technoscience.* The manuscript benefited substantially from the comments of the two UC Press reviewers, and this book would not exist were it not for many years of support, insight, and encouragement from editor Kate Marshall.

The point of ethnography is to learn how to think about a situation together with people for whom it matters. Whether they are understood as informants, interlocutors, colleagues, co-conspirators, or friends, the work hinges on their generosity. To the many people who agreed to talk and work with me across my research sites, I am immensely grateful. For those who invited me to bear witness to them in their birthing vulnerability, I hope what service I gave brought comfort, and I stand in awe of the privilege. To protect privacy, most individual names in the book are pseudonyms. The exceptions are public figures, including activists, scientists, and others who offer their views in public spaces, to whom it seemed disrespectful to omit their names. Since I cannot name people individually, I will share thanks for the Bay Area Doula Project, Santa Cruz Doula Salon, Chicago Volunteer Doulas, and Scottish Doula Network, as well as the facilitators and parents in the childbirth classes I attended and the community centers where we gathered.

Conventionally, the author's own family and friends are mentioned last—reflecting the dual nature of their importance and invisibility in a book like this. Thanks to Ashley, the family friend training to be a labor and delivery nurse, whose enthusiasm sparked my interest in this work ages ago. For supporting me throughout the long process of creating this work, and for making life enjoyable and sustaining, thanks go to my partners: Neil, Karim, and Tom; to my animal companions: Mayflower, Juniper, Djamila, Bayoon, Shanghai, Ivanna, Illian, and Ailsa; and to my beloved friends who have stood the test of time: Nicole, Andréa, Kim, Alisha, and Denia. To my brothers, Dan and Brian, my ancestors, especially Aunt Norma and Grandpa Ralph, and my sprawling and devoted family: our ties give me sustenance and inspire me to create ties ever more widely. And to Mom and Dad, Bev and Ken—you are my roots and my refuge. You set me in motion, and I am grateful.

Introduction

ON BECOMING AN INDIVIDUAL

THE BABY HAS JUST BEEN BORN, has been laid on her mother's flushed and sweaty breast. The baby is bluish and waxy, delicate, alien with her stuttering movements and unfocused eyes. There is an indented ring around the crown of her head, which is bizarrely elongated from the vacuum's grip. As her mother coos at her, her skin takes on the pink cast of a warm-blooded creature, infinitesimally small hairs rising to warm her body as she dries. The doctor is still focused on the pelvis, waiting for the placenta, massaging the fundus—the boggy, soft mound of the uterus that minutes before was taut and straining. She catches the meaty blob in a pink plastic tray, and her blue-gloved hand is slippery with blood as she turns it over under the powerful spotlight, her efficient eyes stroking its surface to make sure it is whole. I, the doula and anthropologist, am standing between worlds, observing on my right the gaze developing between mother and infant, exhausted and enraptured, and on my left the surgeon's concentration as she sews up the mangled perineum with her curving steel needle. Both are intensely focused as they go about their care work. For the first time in hours my own focus softens, a respite from the labor of caring.

This book, and the research on which it is based, is an exercise in standing between worlds. Since 2012 I have been paying attention to birth-related activities and information, including conducting roughly three years of ethnographic fieldwork in the California Bay Area.[1] This included training and practicing as a doula, a nonmedical birth attendant who provides physical, emotional, and informational support for people before, during, and after a birth.[2] Doulas are a relatively new phenomenon, though they take up legacies of midwifery activism. Depending on how you tell the story, the difference between a doula and a midwife is a technicality. In the United States over the past century, midwives have represented devalorized modes of care and taken responsibility for communities excluded from professional medical spaces; the degree of professionalization and bureaucracy in which midwives are enmeshed still varies widely. This underdog identity shapes contemporary doula movements. Doulas are expensive when privately hired, but many also identify as activists and volunteer their labor for those who cannot pay, or work on a sliding scale. People tend to seek out doulas when they are paying particular attention to *how* they want to bring a new life into being. As such, becoming a doula allowed me to delve into the passions and opinions that can make giving birth feel so fraught in this part of the world.

At present, a doula is a trained layperson, whereas a midwife is a medical professional with decision-making power and concomitant liability (until 2021, California hospital midwives were required to practice under a physician with ultimate legal liability).[3] The two are often confused by those outside the birth community, likely because both professions—or "callings," as many are wont to call them—are part of a vibrant set of lifestyle practices, conceptions of health and the body, and ideas about women, family, and community that exceed conventional medical protocols. Childbearing itself exceeds a conventionally defined medical event. It is not a disease or a disorder, but it can be dangerous, and its medical management is deeply entrenched in contemporary America. So as an anthropologist curious about childbearing, I immersed myself in spaces where medicine is interwoven with community, with the personal, with the "alternative." These are spaces where parents, practitioners, infants, activists, media, and technologies interact in efforts to shape what childbearing is, how it's done, and what it means. I call them *birth worlds*.

I paid attention to birth worlds before and after the California fieldwork, as a researcher living in Accra, Chicago, Edinburgh, and throughout my global travels. But California is where I am from, and despite the (deserved) stereotype of anthropologists seeking out far-flung lands from the perspective of their Euro-American universe, I was drawn to the complexities, absurdities, and magic of the place and people I call home. The colonial history of anthropology is rapidly changing, though not quickly enough. If anthropology is at heart about making the strange familiar and the familiar strange, about seeing things differently, then any type of person can do ethnography about any type of place, and its strangeness or familiarity will depend less on the audience's perspective than on the researcher's skill. I was drawn to researching birth after talking with a family friend passionately studying to become a labor and delivery nurse. Bodies and their variability had always been fascinating to me, as had gender and feminism, and the way they were tangled together around birth with such intense anxieties and aspirations made me want to know more. Everyone in my immediate family is a medical professional; I, the ornery one, was drawn to researching medicine as a cultural phenomenon, picking apart why things are done the way they are done and taking nothing for granted. I'm familiar with medicine, but I stand outside it.

Not only is California my home, but I have moral and contractual obligations to the people I work with as a doula. We sometimes also share bonds of friendship. So I am implicated in the worlds I study at the same time as I observe and analyze them. This is always true of ethnographic research (and all research), though to differing degrees. Anthropologists stand between worlds. I stood between practice and analysis, familiar and strange, the perspectives of medical professionals and new parents and activists and researchers . . .

Birthing people stand between worlds too, on the cusp of creative transformation. This book takes all this in-betweenness and uses it to straddle the specificities of births and aspects of American culture at large, aspects that relate to how individuals are valued. Tensions surrounding childbearing make commonsense ideas raw, exposed, and contested. What I came to understand over a decade of paying attention to birth is how births are cultural microcosms. That is, you can use them as lenses to see the way culture works, to see foundational cultural values being worked out in smaller scale. This insight has been a cornerstone of the anthropology of reproduction at least since Brigitte Jordan's 1978 *Birth in Four Cultures*. But cultural values are not static. At any given point they are contested and in flux, and more so in times of upheaval and change. A rich and robust body of scholarly work on new reproductive technologies like IVF and surrogacy delves into how issues in reproduction and kinship are always microcosms of broader cultural values and influence cultural life writ large.[4] The emergence and rise of doulas as birth practitioners throws our current moment of cultural flux into relief and illuminates how efforts to change culture and change birth mirror each other.

This book explores seven American cultural values as seen through the lens of birth. Its chapters dig into progress, experience, autonomy, equality, authenticity, immunity, and redemption. These are *values*, which Hans Joas describes as "emotionally laden notions of that which is desirable."[5] I would add that values are also *problems*. They describe things commonly understood as good, but how they should be achieved and what they look like in practice can be highly variable. Because values are emotionally laden, differences in how they are approached can become fraught with tension. Births are not the only cultural microcosms by any means, but they are particularly interesting ones. Births have long been understood by anthropologists as liminal periods, in-between states where opportunities for rupture come to the fore. That means that whatever aspects of culture are uneasy and unsettled will become even weaker, and the contemporary American moment has plenty of malaise about its values and what kinds of continuity are possible, or not.

The idea that births are microcosms of culture is both a conceptual claim and a methodological one. A microcosm encapsulates in miniature the characteristic qualities of something much larger; it is a cosmos, a world unto itself, yet we can see the macrocosm, the big picture, by looking closely at it. Any contemporary American birth is a microcosm of relationships, not just between different kinds of people, but between bodies, technologies, institutions, and ecologies, between what stimulates desires and what constrains them. That is the conceptual claim; the methodological one is about the way of looking that enables one to see these microcosms. By paying close attention to the specific details of childbearing—the sensory, emotional, contradictory details, which ethnography is so suited for gathering—we can reveal naturalized stories, categories, and values. When something is naturalized, it becomes invisible. It is taken for granted as the only way things could be, the only way they make sense. It becomes a myth. The *sociological imagination* is a way of seeing the social structures that constrain and enable people's possibilities for action: it may seem like losing your job is your fault and your problem, but instead it has far more to do with new city regulations and changing global trade patterns. The *anthropological imagination* is a complementary way of seeing culture, which is how we make meaning through naturalized stories, categories, and values: the way you feel about losing your job stems from how work, worth, and money are culturally equated. It is a way of seeing our myths while they are in action. Once we can see them, we can start to change them, if we want to.

Culture is, in my view and most simply, storytelling. We tell stories to understand why things happen and what we should care about. Stories woven into the fabric of everyday life help us know who belongs where, what to expect, and how to judge good from bad. Stories can be told with words, but also through what is *not* said, with actions, expressions, and touch, in the way spaces are designed and objects are organized, in how money flows and technologies are marketed, in what gets named and what gets abandoned.

"Culture" itself has fallen out of analytical fashion in the past few decades, giving way to what Sherry Ortner calls a "dark" anthropology concerned with politics and injustice.[6] This is understandable given the depressingly entrenched inequalities and exploitation throughout the world, and the climate crises urgently compromising the planet in late capitalism. Yet a return to thinking about culture is not irrelevant in the face of these pressing issues. I am deliberately hearkening back to an older era of scholarship when *culture* was not such a fraught term because I think it is worthwhile to revisit the ideas of storytelling and values after decades of brilliant feminist, Black, Indigenous, and queer critical scholarship, which helps us understand White, middle-class America.[7] Doing so is one experiment among many in locating anthropology's use and purview in a time of overlapping crises and struggles for justice that call into question the entire endeavor.[8] I am attempting to shift the register away from both self-flagellation and the presumption of innocent objectivity, to start from a politically accountable position that does not presume a coherent human subject while examining the forces that make the *idea* of a coherent human subject so enduring. Perhaps it works, perhaps it doesn't; such is the nature of experiments.

In using the blanket term *American culture* I do not mean to lump together and erase the differences between race and class categories and religious, political, and ideological positions; there are infinite cultures intersecting and nested within one another. Households and workplaces have their own cultures, as do immigrant groups, people drawn together by ethnicity, and even those with shared hobbies or aesthetics. What I am examining in this book are values that are part of the American project, problems that are part of the national mythology even if differently situated people within the nation (and outside it) take up different positions vis-à-vis those values. Virtually everyone I encountered during my research engaged with this mythic version of American culture, whether through embracing an American identity or de facto working within American systems and societies. Marilyn Strathern notes that although culture ultimately projects a vision of itself as all-encompassing, "a world-view," something "inevitably inclusive (in the extent to which certain values are shared), or as exclusive (in the extent to which they are not)," it is instead full of layerings, juxtapositions, and differently authoritative voices; culture is a process of struggle to determine meaning by people with unequal access to power.[9]

The kinds of values I am interested in are what Peter Sloterdijk calls "stress concerns," points of contention in a particular society that nonetheless hold it together; he defines a nation as "a collective that succeeds in jointly keeping uncalm."[10] Or, after Bruno Latour's formulation, they are "hybrids" between the ubiquitous dualisms of modernity, allowing us to ignore the contradictions inherent in our most cherished ideas.[11] Lauren Berlant's work elaborates how such shared problems undergird national identity, not so much as conscious decisions we make as compulsions we feel: attachments and identifications, even to what harms us.[12] The seven values in this book—progress, experience, autonomy, equality, authenticity, immunity, and redemption—are not the only American values or the most important ones, but they are the ones that emerged clearly from my research. They are not cleanly divisible, because cultural stories are interwoven with one another. The chapters, therefore, build on and reference each other. They are current problems, sites of upheaval *at this moment* even as they reference longer struggles and instabilities.

What these values have in common is that they all grapple with what it means to be an individual. The individual person is foundational to American ideals of democratic government, personal property ownership, and legal rights. These ideals underpin all liberal societies and are rooted in Enlightenment thought; Louis Dumont describes American individualism as emblematic of "modern ideology."[13] Even the liberal concept of society is predicated on individuals as the basic unit of which society is composed, and the anthropological record (a product of liberal societies) has largely interpreted families, households, communities, tribes, lineages, and dyads in this vein rather than *starting from* relations as much Indigenous and Black scholarship does. The individual has come to be seen as synonymous with the human.[14]

Yet in childbearing the boundaries of the individual are necessarily blurred as one body becomes two. A new person's material and social existence are formulated in conditions of utter dependence: the infant—and, increasingly, the fetus—is the quintessential object of social vulnerability. It is not yet an individual—and neither is a pregnant person. Rights and responsibilities that were conceived to apply to individuals with personal agency become very messy when applied to pregnant, birthing, nursing, fetal, infant, and child people. This is most obvious in debates over abortion, but it also figures into policy issues such as workplace provisions for breastfeeding, maternity/parental leave, and equal pay for women. Such conceptual mess is present in subtle intimacies, like pangs of guilt as a mother checks her breast pump app and sees that she has produced less milk than normal, or a midwife's tense glance at the fetal monitor reading as she wipes the brow of her laboring client. The relationship between these things is what I illustrate throughout this book.

I conducted the bulk of this research in the California Bay Area. California is hardly representative of the nation, and indeed it is exceptional in many ways. But rather than seek out some kind of average place, I was drawn to California as a place of extremes where cherished cultural narratives are pushed to their limits and therefore more easily visible. California is a bellwether for the nation, associated with both utopian and dystopian visions of what America is or could become. From Silicon Valley's reinvention of the world through technology to Hollywood's national storytelling through film, from Disney's fantasyland to San Francisco's communes to LA's metropolitan sprawl, California is a lightning rod for various visions of the future. It is home to experiments in communal and networked ways of living while being characterized by hyperindividualism. It epitomizes the frontier where traditions hold less sway. The major national myth of the American dream is intensified in California, and the California dream has drawn people from every corner of the world since the Gold Rush nearly two centuries ago.[15] This mass migration resulted in a genocide of native peoples alongside an ever-evolving multiculturalism. California can be paradise or hell, but it is always vibrant and dynamic.

Drawn from California's dramatic extremes, this book's insights into taken-for-granted cultural concepts that motivate both regressive and progressive American political positions can, I think, be helpful in reframing approaches to seemingly intractable issues in an increasingly divided nation. White settler nationalism, environmental catastrophes, and gender injustice operate on a different scale than the decisions examined in these pages: whether or not you want a doula, how to feed your baby while needing to work, what can you do about toxic chemicals in your household items while pregnant. Yet moving between these things is what this book does. Taken-for-granted cultural concepts are highlighted in childbearing because they are also destabilized there.

NEAR BIRTH

It might seem odd to some readers that I do not distinguish between home births and hospital births, or unmedicated, medicated, and surgical births. Indeed, in conceiving and conducting this research, I tried to avoid organizing my approach around any particular kinds of actors or ideological orientations. I tried to avoid situating my research within the cultural debates that are, themselves, its object of analysis. The title of this book, *Near Birth,* reflects this. In addition to encompassing pregnancy, birth, and infant care, it invites consideration of a multitude of actors and discourses that are involved in childbearing, including parents and practitioners, technologies and media, and ecologies and activisms. The term *near birth* is a conceptual tool that allows me to avoid separating these things. This means that instead of taking a position amongst the fraught, contradictory, and moralizing cultural stories told about childbearing, which are so overdetermined that they often feel stale, I try to cut things a new way, bringing something else into focus. By playing on the cultural resonance of the term *near death,* which I return to in the conclusion, the term draws attention to the underappreciated cultural weight surrounding beginnings.

"Near birth" refers to what is close to birth both temporally and spatially: ideas about what kinds of people and technologies should be involved, and what potentials and dangers cling nearby. Rather than taking a stance on what constitutes a "good birth" or a "good mother," or describing and contextualizing the competing answers, here I attempt to show the potential futures that hover near birth: will bringing a new person into the world perpetuate the status quo, or will it advance a new way of being and relating? In intellectual theory from Marx through contemporary feminism, reproductive labor refers to maintenance, to keeping humans fed, clothed, housed, and healthy, making new ones and ushering out old ones; it is opposed to the masculine world-building powers of *production.* But a birth is always a beginning, a creation, an opportunity. Reproduction can be about rupture as much as continuity. Ideas about how babies should be born are socially and politically motivated; that is, they naturalize ideas about what kinds of personhood matter, and what ways of doing personhood are valuable. The question "What is the best way to have a baby?" is not only about making a new life, but also about the possibility for making new selves and new worlds.

As I did fieldwork, looking near birth necessarily meant I lacked a clearly defined research object, which made for a messy and sometimes frustrating and discouraging research process. But it gave me plenty of things to pay attention to. I paid attention to ideas about touch and intuition, which are kinds of embodied nearness; they resonate with legacies of thinking about women, femininity, and female sexuality as intrinsically familiar with nearness, as always-already multiple instead of individual.[16] I attended to caregiving relationships, both those caring for the infant and those caring for the childbearing person. Attention to caregiving also included the ways institutions, families, communities, and the state are part of implicit and explicit social contracts about what care is owed, and to whom. I spoke with expectant and recent parents, medical practitioners, community workers, and activists, and I spent time in their homes. I attended social and professional events aimed at these people, including childbirth education classes, fundraisers, salons, conferences, continuing education, volunteer work, and demonstrations. I paid attention to nonhuman entities such as technological objects, consumer goods, microbes, and toxins, and nonphysical entities such as statistics, evidence, and laws. I watched the local and national media for coverage of relevant issues, including the boom in awareness about the United States' abysmal maternal and infant mortality rates and the racial disparities within them, and the increasingly dire and highly politicized situation around abortion access. I participated in media production by writing for Stanford Medicine's blog. And, of course, I got up close and personal with birth through my work as a doula. I take nearness as a methodological challenge to the idea of the researcher as objective bystander, integrating the feminist insight that all knowledge is produced in specific contexts by people who are personally implicated in their work.[17]

That said, I am a White, straight, cisgendered, able-bodied, and middle-class woman, Californian by birth, and I have not borne any children myself. I certainly cannot claim my research evenly encompassed anyone and everyone who gives or attends births in the Bay Area; my aim was to emphasize those who are actively opinionated about childbearing, those who seek to influence it, who are in a sense more near to birth through the attention they pay it. Many, though by no means all, of the people I spoke and worked with were also White, straight, cis, and middle-class. Although I originally intended to distribute my fieldwork more evenly among racially and socioeconomically diverse groups, I encountered a strong bias against doulas volunteering in communities to which they themselves did not demographically belong. This sentiment comes from both a critique of the politics of wealthy White people "saving" people in need and the fact that doula care works much better when doulas and clients share a sociocultural background because it makes it easier for them to feel comfortable with each other. Instead, people who wanted to help and had the means to do so were encouraged to sponsor doulas from underserved communities. I became involved in activist groups and community organizations and gathered secondhand perspectives via friends and acquaintances who were more directly involved in marginalized communities' childbearing.

As such, this project speaks to hegemony, which is the power of what is perceived as normal and unmarked by difference. Hegemony is what is not marginalized. Hegemonic power affects all people's experiences and expectations, though this works differently depending on their personal location in the matrix of intersectionality—that is, the way different aspects of one's identity and demographic situation influence each other.[18] While I discuss race, class, sexual and gender identity, and other ways of being marginalized throughout this book, the experience of marginalized childbearing is not my central concern, nor a project I am best suited to undertake. Other writers have brilliantly delved into this, including Jennifer Nash's *Birthing Black Mothers,* Dána-Ain Davis's *Reproductive Injustice: Racism, Pregnancy, and Premature Birth,* Carolyn Sufrin's *Jailcare: Finding the Safety Net for Women Behind Bars,* and Kelly Ray Knight's *addicted.pregnant.poor.* Also excellent are Gumbs, Martens, and Williams's anthology *Revolutionary Mothering: Love on the Front Lines,* A. K Summers's graphic novel *Pregnant Butch: Nine Long Months Spent in Drag,* and Kath Weston's classic *Families We Choose: Lesbians, Gays, Kinship.* Racial disparities in maternal mortality in the United States, which have recently been receiving long-overdue attention, speak to how different—and differently risky—the experience of childbearing can be for differently situated people.

Somewhat paradoxically, although the demographics most represented in this research had a lot of hegemonic power, the method of looking near birth and practicing as a doula meant that I was engaged with people who fairly explicitly positioned themselves as doing "alternative" things as far as childbearing goes. This positioning often brought people from different demographics together too. So in many ways this book is a study of "fringe" discourses surrounding and talking back to normativity. In the spaces where I spent the most time, there was both power and grappling with the fact that the powerful narratives didn't fit. My aim is to dig into the very concepts that motivate the debates within childbearing. In many ways, the values examined in these chapters, although widely acknowledged as desirable, simply do not fit well with the embodied and social realities of bringing a baby into the world. This book examines both that poor fit and how differently positioned people deal with it. My hope is not just that it presents an unusual take on the drama surrounding birth, nor even that it provides a novel access point for those interested in American cultural "big issues," but that it demonstrates *a method of paying attention* that can be applied elsewhere. This method apprehends immediate details and grandiose potentials as one and the same thing, and in doing so evades some of the categorical traps of the medium layer.

ON LANGUAGE

Although cultural stories are not only or always verbal, they are partially woven out of the words we use, and the words we have at our disposal shape what is thinkable. To destabilize things that seem self-evident and allow other ways of thinking to emerge, I try to play with the language I use. Words are, after all, concepts, and, as Donna Haraway writes in her introduction to *Simians, Cyborgs, and Women,* "Grammar is politics by other means."[19] Over the ten years this book has been in the making, politics have evolved, and choices that were striking in 2013 have come to sound more familiar. I use the term *childbearing* instead of separating the phases of pregnancy, birth, and infant care.[20] Boundaries between mother and infant bodies, or the difference between a fetus and a newborn, may seem self-evident, but they are the sites of much explicit and implicit cultural contestation—all the more so since the repeal of federal abortion rights with the Dobbs decision. I avoid conventional distinctions such as "natural birth" versus "medical birth," or the expertise of healthcare providers versus that of parents, because describing things in these terms reproduces the tensions I am trying to dig beneath.

To loosen the heavily gendered expectations around childbearing, I call someone who bears children a *childbearing person* and only use the terms *mother* and *woman* in specific contexts. This is in solidarity with trans and nonbinary politics, which have become more visible over the past decade, and this choice has theoretical implications as well. *Mother* is connotatively loaded in ways I want to be careful about. It is also imprecise because sometimes different people bear and raise the child, as in the case of adoption. Sometimes a variety of people contribute to bearing the child by providing eggs, wombs, sperm, breast milk, money, and legal lineage, as in the case of IVF, surrogacy, lesbian conception, or milk donation. Using the terms *nursing person, birthing person, pregnant person,* and *caregiver* allows me to separate out childbearing functions, breaking up the idea that one figure, the mother, does all of these things. These terms sounded cumbersome to me at first, but as an American writing about the United States, they allow me to make the familiar strange by unifying what is culturally separated and separating what is culturally unified.

Likewise, the term *woman* evokes a host of loaded feminist and antifeminist rhetoric; *woman* is a category marked as subsidiary to the generic human, presumed to be male. I think using *person* unmarks childbearing as a woman's issue in interesting and productive ways. It posits a quintessentially female experience as the default from which male readers must reconcile their difference, and it invites childbearing to be a human function instead of sequestered as a woman's function. I still use *she* and *her* pronouns whenever I refer to a nonspecific childbearing person because it reinforces the association of femaleness and personhood.

In this vein, I want to destabilize the idea that childbearing is essential to fully realized womanhood or female identity. Not all women bear children, through choice or infertility or unaccommodating circumstances. And women are not the only people who bear children: trans men and other genderqueer folks do too. Being pregnant or nursing is an intensely feminized activity that can be challenging for people who don't identify with outward markers of femininity. While it is true that avoiding the term *woman* obscures the fact of women's categorical repression and limits rallying power around this specific injustice, I believe that restructuring categories themselves is more politically potent than fighting for inclusion or validation. Yet my choices are made in the spirit of experimentation, and I think indeterminacy is something to value highly in both grammatical and political projects. I do use the terms *woman, womanhood, mother,* and *motherhood* when voicing people who use them, or when referring to the way these concepts circulate socially—for example, in rhetoric about the "sanctity of motherhood."

Lastly, two further notes on language. I capitalize Black, White, Indigenous, and other names of racial groups that are culturally and historically contingent in the way they are constituted, as opposed to the natural, biological categories implied by lowercase adjectives.[21] And I do use the term *doula,* which has been critiqued because it is the modern Greek word for (female) slave, and therefore can be offensive and oppressive for multiple reasons, including appropriation, female gendering, and evoking the pain of slavery for both practitioners and recipients of care.[22] I use it because it is what was overwhelmingly used in the communities with which I was connected. The fact that it carries harms within it seems befitting the ambivalent, compromised starting place of, and need for reckoning within, these communities, which is what this book explores.

This book's organization loosely reflects its claim about childbearing being a microcosm: it starts small and scales up. Chapter 1 gives a sense of California as a place and my gravities within it, situating myself as storyteller and locating the stories I tell in a specific part of the world. California is the paradigmatic site of frontier mythology that is oriented around progress, a value that underlies approaches to technology, communities, bodies, spirituality, nature, and moving through space and time, including how to understand history. Chapter 2 develops two distinct ways of understanding the material realities of childbearing bodies—how bodies work—both of which actively circulate in birth worlds; I call them regular and contextual physiology. These are tangled with different legacies of thinking about what experience is, how it can be known, and whose experiences matter. Chapter 3 focuses on immediate relationships near birth, which I describe as negotiations over trust and control that enable people to establish a sense of autonomy, of being the author of their situation as they navigate risk, fear, pain, and power in the birth room. Chapter 4 expands to consider how equality is both essential and impossible in the social arrangements we have established to care for children (and those doing such caring) beyond the labor and birth. These themes have been key issues in critical thought about birth, reproduction, and feminism, and they still resonate.

The later chapters take a broader and more abstract view of what is pertinent to birth. They will be more surprising to readers familiar with scholarship on childbearing. Chapter 5 examines the idea of authenticity, which permeates the supposed binary between nature and culture, between what is intrinsic and what is created. Aspirations to personal authenticity are wound tightly with ideas about the past via stories about evolution and the "primal," as well as with the future via stories about the possibilities for technologically mediated self-design and self-optimization. Chapter 6 explores anxieties about microbes, chemicals, and stress, all of which are understood as toxic in some capacity; immunity is the ability to establish barriers and protect oneself (or one's children), and it persists in being the dominant way people respond to "toxic" situations. Defensive immunity is difficult if not impossible to achieve. Moreover, it eclipses more appropriate, intriguing approaches to our environment that foreground ecology, connections, and relations. Finally, chapter 7 considers activism that aims to create a more just, livable world by changing how birth happens. Different kinds of activism near birth are concerned with redemption, with figuring out what was done wrong and how it can be healed. This requires delving into the ways history is not innocent, and what actual changes we are prepared to make in the present. The questions raised near birth throughout these chapters, from birthing bodies to activist visionaries, are nothing less than what is the future of American society, and what kind of human is being built for it?

Let's swing back from this grandiose statement to that other world, the one where this introduction started. Back in that hospital room—well, family birth center—things are calm. The surgeon has left with smiling congratulations, and the nurse tends to the person who has just birthed a baby, bathing her blood-streaked legs and changing the thick pads she is sitting on. This new mother will use such pads to soak up discharged fluid for weeks afterward, and later she will complain to me that no one prepared her for that. The nurse tucks her in while the janitor mops the floor. The baby has been weighed and injected with vitamin K, and a little striped cap has been snuggled over her cone head. Curled in the hospital bed next to the body she knows from the inside out, she utters soft whimpers, grunts, and snorts. Friends and family have been called—Facebook updated too. A lactation consultant will be in soon, holding the breast like a sandwich as she guides the baby's mouth around the areola, directives that the baby may or may not intuitively understand. Gradually the nurse wraps up her charting, and I say my goodbyes, say I'll be in touch about a postpartum visit, tell them they are both beautiful. I go home, anthropologist and doula, and I write.

ONE

Progress

CALIFORNIA AS BOTH UTOPIA AND DYSTOPIA

WHEN I SHOWED UP AT ROXANNE CUMMINGS'S Victorian farmhouse on Walnut Street in Santa Cruz's westside suburbs, she made me tea with local honey—to support our immunity in the cold season—and sat me down in her warm living room. Pictures of her five children lined bookshelves and an old curio cabinet, and the sofa was adorned with tapestry pillows that caught the colors in the intricate rug underneath our sock-clothed feet. She was probably in her sixties, and her fiery hair was heavily streaked with white above her fine-boned face. She told me how she and her longtime partner in midwifery practice, Kate Bowland, had founded what she called Santa Cruz's "birth culture" in many ways, gesturing at a flagstone path to a door in a building across the lawn that was their office for many years. In thirty years of practice she had been present at more than two thousand births. Among other things, I asked her if she thought that the way babies are born can influence the future. "Oh, goodness yes!" she replied, her face bursting into a smile. Roxanne was among the first people who offered to meet with me during my fieldwork, and I came to know that she was one of the busiest and most established midwives, one of the originals. She and Kate were instrumental in making Santa Cruz a "mecca for Nurse-Midwifery" for the past forty years.[1] But there was no self-importance in her manner. Roxanne invited me to assist at her enormously popular class, Mindfulness-Based Childbirth Education, and that got things rolling for me, the new anthropologist in town. Not long afterward, I learned that she had been diagnosed with terminal cancer.

Two years later I attended a memorial service in honor of her life. One of the speakers uttered a phrase that captured that first meeting: the warm mischief in her eyes made you feel you were a close friend, even if you had just met. Her memorial service was a microcosm of Santa Cruz's birth world culture: old hippies, new idealists, largely unexamined privilege, and a kind of reverence for nature, spirituality, community, and the feminine. Hundreds of people overflowed the community room at the Buddhist-influenced Mount Madonna Center, which had been an important community hub of the home birth movement in the 1970s, to remember Roxanne's life. Having arrived a little late, I added my flip-flops to the massive pile of shoes in the entry hall and snuck around to the side of the auditorium, where I knelt down on the carpet surrounded by people standing or lounging or seated on the floor, babies breastfeeding and toddlers making (and smashing) towers of wooden blocks.

The long service featured many speakers, not just Roxanne's friends and family but also the doctors, midwives, nurses, and parents her work had touched. A reception with cookies and chai made by beloved local businesses followed. Chatting with a few friends, I remembered Roxanne and talked about how the service had reinforced the importance of connecting deeply with people and being a force of love in the world. One friend was a doula with whom I had been thinking of starting a full-spectrum practice, which would have included care for abortion and pregnancy loss alongside birth and infant care.[2] Another was a midwifery student who was moving to Oregon after finishing her long and difficult apprenticeship—difficult due to the precarious nature of direct-entry midwifery, which operates primarily outside formal educational and medical channels. We nibbled gingersnaps and sipped milky spiced tea while leaning over the redwood deck railing, looking out over the forested Santa Cruz Mountains down to the gleaming Monterey Bay.

A GEOGRAPHICAL TOUR—IN A CAR

The Monterey Bay is not the bay referred to by the California Bay Area—that would be the San Francisco Bay, just to the north. I spent time in both places. I began my fieldwork in Berkeley, a notoriously liberal hotspot on the east side of the San Francisco Bay, dominated by the University of California, Berkeley, where I had attended college ten years earlier. I lived at the end of a narrow, winding road up in the hills with a queer Jewish nurse-midwife and her two teenage children, in a house made lively by our combined collection of dogs, cats, and plants. Halfway through I moved from Berkeley to Santa Cruz, where I lived with my then-partner on a sunny hill in the mountains to the northwest of town, a little spot of warmth surrounded by ravines and shady redwood forests. Ferns grew as weeds in my garden. Later I returned to Chicago to finish my PhD, and then I relocated to Scotland, maintaining strong and regular connections to California throughout. Although I formally spent two years in the field, my involvement with birth worlds extended for years before and after. As of this writing, it has spanned well over a decade.

I found Santa Cruz a fascinating bubble of idealistic Whiteness that struck me as narcissistic and self-righteous at times. The Bay Area is far more urban and cosmopolitan than Santa Cruz, and it is much larger, encompassing ethnically diverse communities and vast wealth disparities. Although parts of the Bay Area echo the idealism of Santa Cruz, this is moderated by a kind of gritty social consciousness. The region is increasingly dominated by the power, money, and influence of Silicon Valley and its high-powered tech workers. By contrast, Santa Cruz is a small college town sheltered by a crescent of mountains and abundant parkland, oriented toward the beach and renowned for surf culture; it is a place people go to disconnect from their fast-paced lives. The Bay Area's professional and social networks are spread out, and this applies likewise to birth networks. The Bay itself is a highly salient unit among people who make the area home; individual municipalities have no clear boundaries but are melded by a tissue of suburbs and commuter arteries in a massive sprawl. Midwife friends in the East Bay worked in the North Bay or "the city" (always referring to San Francisco). Parents often worked in San Francisco but lived in Silicon Valley (or vice versa) and so mined multiple cities' shops, classes, and resources. Friends frequently traveled up and down the peninsula for social and professional gatherings. Doulas living in Santa Cruz had many clients in San Jose and Silicon Valley because they were too numerous to be sustained by Santa Cruz's small population, which speaks to Santa Cruz as a kind of mecca of alternative practitioners, and to the frequently acknowledged idea that there was more money "over the hill."

My personal and professional contacts took me throughout the region. I spent a lot of time driving, as did many of the people I interviewed or worked with. Car culture is a thing here, with pop culture representations of people gliding along scenic coastal highways—though, of course, infuriating traffic jams are the more common manifestation of this automotive idyll. Car culture is about freedom, driving off into the future with yourself at the wheel. It is a perfect Californian metaphor. As a mode of getting around, cars prioritize the individual—no working around transit schedules, no sharing space, and you can bring your things with you to be prepared for whatever occurs. The irony happens when all the individuals have to deal with one another. Although Los Angeles has the reputation of being an intensely car-centric metro area, perhaps leading the world in this dubious distinction, the Bay Area is not far behind. Its freeways are crisscrossing concrete parking lots at certain times of day, with bottlenecks at the few bridges that span its namesake body of water, sixteen lanes of thwarted individual mobility. The intimacy of the road trip is far more often a strangely encapsulated alienation, each driver alone in a climate-controlled metal bubble, closed off to the wind that might otherwise blow through one's hair.

The allure of the open road is a quintessential mythology of the West. It speaks to the frontier, a place that is untamed and uninhabited, unlimited and unknown, with no agenda other than scenery for your personal adventure, full of raw material from which to build your life. Historically, American identity is inextricable from Manifest Destiny, the belief that the United States territory should extend from the East Coast to the West, across all three thousand miles of the continent.[3] The mythology of the frontier was both used to further this agenda, and part of why it was so appealing to White settlers in the first place. Myths are stories we tell to make sense of situations. When myths are live, they are understood not as stories but as the truth. And when situations change, as situations always do, the old myths become visible as mere stories, and new ones step into the role of truth. White settlers can now talk about Manifest Destiny, perhaps with an eye roll or chagrined smile, but we take for granted that innovation will solve our new problems. These myths are linked by the value they place on progress. Progress is the idea that we are getting somewhere, that there is a destination that we should be looking toward, someplace that is Not Here, Not Yet.

Like the open road, the ideal of progress can obscure its more complicated, difficult reality. Innovations don't help everyone equally. A moment's consideration of the electronic waste dumps or lithium mines that are the side effect of our now ubiquitous personal electronics will illustrate this. Roadways connect certain places while bypassing others. Like any transit system, roads create disconnection, too. While the open road seems to offer itself up for the taking, it is only open to those with access to cars. The basic infrastructure of movement has been the subject of much controversy in California, including an impassioned fight over a high-speed rail system that would connect Sacramento with Los Angeles, and tech companies' luxury buses for their employees amidst the dearth of decent public transit.[4] So although I drove a lot, this does not mean I evenly absorbed this geographically expansive site. The ways ideas and people circulate are not determined primarily by geographical proximity but by social channels maintained through infrastructure, infrastructure that in turn reflects and reinforces demographic patterns heavily inflected by race and class. I moved along these infrastructural and social channels as a White, educated person with tons of cultural capital if not much money. These channels are evident in the media that composed much of my ethnographic material, as blogs, magazines, books, movies, and advertisements for products and events circulate unevenly, too.

The idea of progress is ubiquitous among Californians, and many are emotionally attached to it as something desirable. It is a value. But that does not mean it looks the same to everyone. As is the case for all the values discussed in this book, the valorization of progress is a problem. The mythos of California as a frontier references the perspective of the East Coast, where the English colonies were located. California was, of course, the traditional home of many Indigenous peoples; it also had its own colonial history entirely independent of the American story. Starting in 1769, the Spanish established Franciscan missions along the Camino Real extending from Baja California in present-day Mexico, up through San Francisco in Alta California. Missions were not beneficent in any current understanding of the word, but California was also not a settler colony in the same way as the United States.[5] Rather than subscribing to a myth of uninhabited land free for the taking, of unlimited fuel for expansion, California's original Europeans operated under a myth of administering to the peoples living there, of integrating them into a pastoral religious imaginary with racialized and gendered hierarchies.[6] After the Spanish colonies gained independence, California was part of Mexico for a while, and indeed, for a brief twenty-five days in 1846, was a nation unto itself, the Bear Flag Republic. Mexican settlers (also known as Californios) and Indigenous people jostled within a caste system.[7] This changed dramatically after the discovery of gold in 1848 and California's precipitous statehood due to a truly massive settler migration (California's nonnative population grew a hundredfold over the following century) and the contemporaneous genocide of Indigenous people.[8]

Northern California is where I grew up. I spent a peaceful childhood in the oak-studded foothills of the Sierras, traditional lands of the Nisenan and Miwok, a few miles from Coloma, the seat of the Gold Rush and its human and ecological devastation. My affection for the land and people I know as home is thoroughly interwoven with my complicity in settler-colonialism and the many ways I've benefited from Whiteness. Choosing to locate my research in Northern California was born from a desire to understand the discontents and aspirations of my own community, a people and place for which I feel a mixture of belonging and distance, tenderness and judgment.

By moving two hours west from the rural Republican Sierra foothills to attend college at UC Berkeley, I became intimately familiar with the ways that progressive and conservative politics are geographically coded. It fascinated me that certain nostalgic and countercultural lifestyle practices, like home birth, homeschooling, and homesteading, were advocated in both rural and urban places by people who would have considered themselves ideologically distinct, to say the least. Progressive and reactionary visions are blurred in such realms; living off the grid is popular in California with both libertarian and socialist sympathizers, and homeschooling is practiced by both those who seek a conservative religious education and those who desire a radically antiauthoritarian education. This seemed to be the case in birth practices as well. If progress is the idea that there is a destination that we should be looking toward that is Not Here, Not Yet, then these alternative approaches to making a life are commenting on where we are now and grappling with where we should be headed. I came to recognize California as a place of extremes that caricature and highlight American culture, and in many ways late liberal society generally. California is in no way *representative* of the nation at large, but it is generative of opinions, ideas, potentials, and imagined futures that have significance far beyond its borders.

PROGRESSING WHERE? UTOPIA AND DYSTOPIA

California exaggerates American ideals and disgraces, from the 1849 Gold Rush that epitomized the American dream of wealth for the taking and entailed a brutal genocide of Native Californians, to the present mythos of prosperity epitomized by the overnight millionaires of the tech world, while urban displacement and homelessness reach crisis levels in California cities. Throughout the twentieth century, the California dream promised a fresh start and new opportunities, both echoing and revising the ideal version of America that was offered to the world.[9] One American in eight now lives in California, and it accounts for an even larger share of the country's output, innovation, job creation, and wealth. With its reputation as a haven for freethinking, it draws people who like to consider themselves iconoclastic and visionary, whether they are libertarian techies, New Age spiritualists, or nostalgic homesteaders; by the end of the twentieth century, this confluence was described as "a heterogeneous orthodoxy for the coming information age: the Californian Ideology."[10] Though California is reliably Democratic in national politics, places like Orange County are foundational to modern conservatism.[11] It has a rich history of civil rights activism, from Cesar Chavez organizing Latinx farmworkers to Angela Davis championing Black women's liberation, from Oakland's Black Panther Party to the Indigenous occupation of Alcatraz Island.[12] Yet civil rights movements tend to disintegrate fairly quickly, a phenomenon I return to in chapter 7. Californian cultural aspirations are somewhat impulsive, at once grandiose and hollow. Joan Didion describes California as "a place in which a boom mentality and a sense of Chekhovian loss meet in uneasy suspension; in which the mind is troubled by some buried but ineradicable suspicion that things better work here, because here, beneath the immense bleached sky, is where we run out of continent."[13]

California epitomizes the frontier, which is key to a settler ideology that values White expansion, including the consumption of natural resources and the elimination of other peoples and ways of being. The logic of the frontier is so ingrained in the "growth of civilization, technological advance, and scientific progress" that it is taken for granted, unworthy of comment, yet Sarah Franklin reminds us that this is a magical logic that is deeply paradoxical, "a mix of historical fact, nationalist fiction, mythic allegory, and colonial propaganda" that leads to mistaking the consequences for the cause.[14] The frontier is the future. It is what's to come, where progress leads, yet it is also an edge or a margin where dominant ideas hold less sway. Entertainment and technology, the primary drivers of California's economic growth, are industries established on the imagination of various futures. The state functions as a national bellwether by setting influential trends, and it acts as a national vanguard: things happen first in California.[15] In particular, California is a vanguard for American conflicts over raced and queer bodies. It is the paradigmatic site of multiple national immigration stereotypes, including both "high-skilled" Asian tech workers feeding Silicon Valley's expanding industries and "low-skilled" Latinx agricultural laborers.[16] In 1994, reactionary anti-immigration laws were passed, to be closely followed by the Rodney King riots and civil rights legislation in 1996. By 1998 White people were a minority in the state, largely due to disparities in fertility rates, making

California the first "majority minority" state.[17] By 2014, Latinx people alone outnumbered White people. The first gay marriage in the country happened in San Francisco in 2004; gay marriage was later banned in 2008, but the ban was challenged in the courts and declared unenforceable in 2013. San Francisco in particular has a longstanding reputation as a haven for gay and lesbian communities,[18] and Los Angeles's Black Cat protest actually preceded New York City's Stonewall Riots, launching the gay rights movement. California's relatively lax laws about IVF and assisted conception have made it an international destination for reproductive tourism and queer family making.

In the wake of the 2016 election of Donald Trump as president and his anti-immigration, White supremacist platform, the state of California aggressively defended immigrants from deportation. Today sanctuary cities abound in California. Yet contemporary politics should be considered alongside a long history of discriminatory legislation, including Japanese internment during World War II and laws prohibiting Asians from owning property, as well as recent outrage over Chinese birth tourism. A 2017 *New York Times* piece titled "Immigrant Shock: Can California Predict the Nation's Future?" claims that California lashes out at diversity before embracing it, and that its demographic change between 1980 and 2000 mirrors the real and projected change in the United States from 2000 until 2050, when Whites are expected to be less than half of the nation's population.[19] It implies that by looking to California, we can see current American politics as a regressive, fearful tantrum that comes before a widespread acceptance of non-White power. Yet California's massive gentrification problem, especially in the San Francisco Bay Area, belies the inclusive rhetoric, as Black and Brown working-class families are tacitly pushed to the margins. California offers final frontiers for both idealists and cynics.

But a utopia from one perspective is a dystopia from another. Consider eugenics. At the turn of the twentieth century, the acceptance of evolutionary theory in biology gave rise to its widespread social application: controlling human evolution to produce better outcomes was a progressive national and international cause in the first half of the twentieth century.[20] Eugenicists wanted to make motherhood an exclusive privilege (and compulsion) rather than an inherent right, to modernize morality through a project linking race, gender, and reproduction. Margaret Sanger, recognized as the founder of Planned Parenthood, promoted a form of elitism that figures poor and colonized women as incapable of restraining themselves, but rather than top-down social engineering she emphasized voluntary cultural checks such as delaying age of marriage (itself a class privilege) and quality over quantity of children. But determining quality is, of course, a way of reproducing existing social hierarchies. Theodore Roosevelt, speaking in 1905 to a national conference of (wealthy, White) mothers, introduced the term *race suicide* to describe self-limiting one's number of children to two. He promoted the idea that not maximally reproducing was betraying the nation, figured as White. This is an example of "positive" eugenics encouraging certain kinds of reproduction, but presidents have engaged in both kinds; during the era just prior, Andrew Jackson issued exhortations to kill Indigenous women and children after battles, as the American settler nation relied not just on military dominance but on the annihilation of the Indigenous population.

Moving into the twentieth century, American eugenics campaigns did not usually center race or ethnicity but were wrapped into issues like class and disability that naturalized what kind of people were seen as responsible and thus fit to reproduce—judgments and categories with direct racial implications, such as the disproportionate institutionalization and sterilization of people of Mexican origin in California state hospitals for the disabled.[21] California sterilized more people than any other U.S. state during this period, one-third of the nation's total. The Sonoma State Home for the Feebleminded, founded in 1884, became the fastest-growing public institution in California by the 1930s and was a nationwide leader in the number of eugenic sterilizations performed.[22] The Human Betterment Foundation (HBF), founded near Los Angeles in 1928, was the primary eugenics institute in the American West, if not the entire United States. It was dissolved during World War II as it was too closely entwined with Nazism; it is historically well supported that Nazis based their science and propaganda on materials from the HBF. From a propaganda perspective, the term *betterment* is brilliant, so seductive and incontrovertible—like *optimization* today.

The problem with utopias, though, is more fundamental than the good and bad effects of a given social experience. It poses a rationalist dilemma: how to make the best plan, how to progress toward the ever-receding ideal, which would have to be static and frozen if it were ever arrived at, since progress would be over. It is a mechanical logic in which the point is the outcome, not the process. But engineering happiness removes personal freedom. Utopia is never inhabitable, for once we arrive we bring with us all of our messiness. Utopia is never here and now; it is always somewhere else. Feminist thinkers have turned this European, masculinist version of utopia on its head. What if utopia *is* here and now? What if instead of the binary either/or switch of a computer chip, the trade-off between freedom and happiness, the linear progress narrative, we go neither forward nor backward but—in Ursula Le Guin's framing—sideways?[23] California is permeated with many versions of utopian sensibility. Call it escapism or idealism, it has been a clarion call for White Americans and a wide swath of others trying to make it in a dissatisfying and hostile world. California is where the future gets dreamed up and test driven, and where it crashes and burns. The outrageous forest fires that have ravaged the state every year since 2017 are the forerunners of a climate disaster that will soon affect every part of the planet. When asked how officials will manage the overlapping crises of heat, fire, and the pandemic all at once, California's governor Gavin Newsom responded, "The future happens here first."[24] Saving the world through technological innovation and Silicon Valley–style enterprise continues to be the dominant route for imagining a way out of this mess, and this obsessive focus on the future and progress is deeply entangled with capitalist, colonial, patriarchal, humanist modes. But California continues to be a space of *difference* as well.

Michel Foucault coined the term *heterotopia* to describe spaces that are somehow "other," worlds within worlds, mirroring and yet upsetting what is outside.[25] Utopia is where everything is good; dystopia is where everything is bad; heterotopia is where things are different. Heterotopias have more layers of meaning than immediately meet the eye. While Foucault discussed ships, cemeteries, bars, brothels, prisons, and public baths as examples of such disturbing, intense, and contradictory places, the concept has been applied to the California missions and could be applied to California itself.[26] Both utopian studies and actual self-described utopian experiments have grown over the past few decades, producing more sophisticated, feminist, and flexible notions of the utopian.[27] This has made room for what Davina Cooper calls "everyday utopias," where conventional activities are enacted in unusual ways, and what Avery Gordon calls "the utopian margins," a zone of exclusion and "fugitive moments of comprehension" as people strive for a livable and humane social existence.[28] These spaces often entail a rejection of individualization as the primary way people understand themselves as having agency and a meaningful existence. They enact utopia as a standpoint in the here and now, not only the future. They are where people "meanwhile carry on," learning from the past and perhaps embracing some kind of spiraling, cyclical "sideways" orientation toward progress.[29]

MOUNT MADONNA AND THE
NATURAL BIRTH MOVEMENT

What does this all have to do with childbearing? It seems we've strayed pretty far from birth. But let's visit two places in the Bay Area that illustrate how Californian "progress" influences birth community and culture. For place is not just a backdrop or a setting but a way of viewing the world, a political orientation that transcends space.[30] These places draw legacies around them that can be spun like a kaleidoscope, morphing through utopian, dystopian, and heterotopian elements. Remember the Mount Madonna Center, where Roxanne's funeral was held? A beautiful Buddhist spiritual retreat high up in the mountains and accessible only by car, it emblematizes the exclusivity I found troubling about Santa Cruz politics, an exclusivity evident in much feminist and environmental activism from this part of the world. Mount Madonna was a hub for the alternative lifestyle movements of the 1960s and '70s, including the natural birth movement. Although civil rights activism was taking place in the same era, the hippie origins of the natural birth movement were overwhelmingly White and middle-class, characterized both by myopic idealism and visionary practical experimentation, and supported by access to social and monetary capital.

Not only was Northern California the national epicenter of "natural" and "alternative" movements for communal living, but it specifically incubated ways of bearing children that would also carry these adjectives for decades.[31] Santa Cruz midwives, including Roxanne's midwifery partner, Kate, were arrested for practicing medicine without a license after starting the first out-of-hospital birth center in 1970. Their rebellious activities centered around ideals of women's self-determination and their connection with their bodies and spiritual power, and they denounced the medicalization of the birth experience for the way it made women passive and mechanical. At a gathering of this elder generation of midwives in 2016, many present spoke fondly of Raven Lang's *Birth Book* from this era and passed around an original copy. Raven was one of the arrested midwives, and she had to self-publish her book because editors in 1972 deemed its many photographs of naked birthing people to be scandalous. The midwives at the gathering were greatly entertained by recounting this—as well as an old joke about eating placentas and considering them the perfect vegan food since no animals were harmed in the process! But these joyfully remembered exploits were clearly threatening to others. Why else would they result in arrests? Liberation from the ways that power is organized can seem dystopian to those currently holding power—in this case, state and medical regulatory authorities.

The natural birth movement has distinguished roots in the Bay Area counterculture beyond Santa Cruz. Ina May Gaskin, often called the mother of modern (White) midwifery, got her start in San Francisco before caravanning to Tennessee and founding The Farm cooperative and birthing center, which is still making national news.[32] She wrote the influential book *Spiritual Midwifery,* which was part personal history of learning to birth babies in the caravan and part collection of rapturous out-of-hospital birth stories; it is still a cultural icon. Berkeley nurse Peggy Vincent catalyzed hospital midwifery, as recounted in her memoir *Baby Catcher;* during my fieldwork I heard her speak at a meeting of the Bay Area Doula Project. Marin-based author and activist Suzanne Arms started a birth center in Palo Alto shortly after the one in Santa Cruz was shut down. A 1975 *New York Times* review of her book, *Immaculate Deception,* states, "Mrs. Arms lives in the notably freethinking San Francisco Bay Area, where preference for home birth has been so marked in recent years that the local obstetrical establishment has been jolted into an uncomfortably defensive posture." In the meantime, "underground" midwives filled the demand for home births on the premise that "pregnant women are not sick, childbirth is not a medical event and all women should have the right to give birth in the circumstances, and with attendants, of their own choosing."[33]

This push for "the natural" was always more political than a rejection of technology itself, emphasizing women's autonomy and solidarity in the face of patriarchal medical institutions. The executive director of the American College of Obstetricians and Gynecologists publicly noted in 1977 the "rising tide of demand for home delivery," describing it as an "anti-intellectual–anti-science revolt," a characterization that reflects dominant ideas about women being less intelligent and rational than men. Yet Gaskin and other midwives leading this movement defied such simplistic categorization.[34] They engaged with local doctors and midwifery manuals, collaborating with and even influencing organized medicine. They did not reject science or technology so much as they demanded that it be integrated with experience, mysticism, feminism, and faith. Their politics could be seen as spiritually and environmentally ahead of their time, or as representing a return to traditional values and a regressive notion of women's role in the community. The movement was not aligned with contemporary feminist groups that fought to legalize abortion and end gendered job discrimination, yet its members had fierce confidence in their own abilities and launched a birthing movement that gained worldwide attention. The birth outcomes they achieved continue to be cited as evidence that home births offer a safe, more humane, and effective alternative to the hospital, and their birth stories inspired many to believe that birth can be something other than a fearful medical event dictated by hospital protocols.

These midwives' embrace of science alongside spirituality and politics is one illustration of how counterculture and cyberculture grew in each other's shadow. In the 1970s, natural living through technology was an aspiration, not a contradiction. Fred Turner shows how a key artifact from this era, the *Whole Earth Catalog,* occupied a common ground between the hippies and the burgeoning tech world. Computers went from symbolizing the despised Cold War military-industrial complex to being tools of a collaborative digital utopia; cybernetics evolved to envision different social and community structures, eventually manifesting in the internet.[35] These visionary movements also shared an influence far beyond their core members. In Ina May Gaskin's words, "It wasn't just a few hippies that were interested in better birth—it was all kinds of people."[36] Like the readers of the *Whole Earth Catalog,* most who read *Spiritual Midwifery* had no intention of giving up their earthly possessions and adopting a communal lifestyle, but the book "allowed them to question the standardized labor and delivery procedures at their local hospital, to consider that birth could be a spiritual as well as physical experience, and to believe that a laboring mother had the right to make informed choices about where and how to give birth."[37]

While birth movements have retained their focus on women's empowerment (controversy over what an empowered woman looks like notwithstanding), the tech world has become notoriously hostile to women, nurturing an exclusive tech bro culture. (Only very recently has FemTech oriented around women's health concerns begun to be recognized as a relevant subgenre of the industry, and it remains to be seen what influence this might have.) As a young adult, I watched Silicon Valley expand and infiltrate the Bay Area, much as the hardware and software it produces have infiltrated daily life. The libertarian-inflected politics of young male millionaires have largely replaced the socialist-leaning politics of the hippies of the prior generation, and "natural" approaches to childbearing are increasingly trendy among the aspirational class who have money and consume heartily, if discriminately.[38] While much of the natural birth movement was led by people who came from an educated, middle-class background, its proponents did not lead affluent lives while they put their activist commitments into practice; by contrast, the Bay Area's current youthful vibrancy is entwined with unbounded capitalist development, entrepreneurship, and an outrageous consumer culture based on luxury items, including ostensibly "green" ones. Consumption has become a primary mode for ethical, aesthetic, and political expression in a frequently self-righteous lifestyle politics that privatizes social commentary. Neoliberal ideologies of individual responsibility underlie gross exaggerations of self-sufficiency, including a not-insignificant movement of Silicon Valley elites preparing to save (only) themselves from impending apocalypse.[39]

I use *Silicon Valley* less as a geographical term than to categorize an aesthetic, moral, and intellectual sensibility tied to this particular place. It is a cultural project, like California, the West, and America itself. Over the past decade or so, the explosion of the tech industry has increased the cultural visibility of the Bay Area as seen from other parts of the country and world, and the Bay Area has supplanted Los Angeles as the dominant Californian metropolitan area. Like California vis-à-vis the nation, the Bay Area and its cultural descendant, Silicon Valley, are not representative but generative, a dynamic cultural project that drives cultural change beyond its physical borders. In J. A. English-Lueck's analysis, immigration, technological saturation, and cultural complexity make Silicon Valley "a microcosm of the social and cultural identities of the future."[40] Silicon Valley is exemplary of privileged, influential lifestyles that are imagined to be countercultural but are fully entwined with neoliberal capital.

Although the neoliberal consumer ethos has intensified, the Bay Area has long combined innovation of both ideological and entrepreneurial sorts into personal development. It is possible to trace the now-ubiquitous idea of self-help to the New Age spirituality emblematized by Mount Madonna, and before that to the manuals that helped settlers on the frontier manage their families' health far from familiar institutions. Personal growth has both a spiritual and an entrepreneurial edge in this individualized version of progress. But like a utopia, the perfect self is always receding. This frame of mind fuels an ever-present anxiety about doing it wrong, or inadequately, or missing opportunities. As Emma Dowling has written, "Where personal growth and wellbeing are mapped onto the logic of capital accumulation, self-realisation means maximising our capacity to be productive, to accrue social, cultural and sexual capital. . . . An ontology of inadequacy follows us around and just won't let us be."[41] This orientation toward progress, now widespread throughout the Western world but catalyzed in California, comes to mean we are never good enough as we are right now (not to mention finding it challenging to gracefully grapple with finitude, as epitomized in tech elites' obsession with longevity and immortality). Approaching the self as a project to be improved and optimized is key to how middle-class doulas operate as a cultural phenomenon.

Silicon Valley haunted all aspects of my fieldwork, but so did the inevitable edges and others of middle-class, heteronormative, White birth. Even though the Bay Area has large numbers of Asian and Latinx people, Black activism frequently came into my ethnographic material as a foil to the often-implicit Whiteness, reflecting race politics in the United States at large, which has been framed predominantly as an issue of Black versus White (though the boundaries of each category have shifted over time). Compared to race issues, which maintained a high profile, issues of class took a back seat. They crept in at the edges. America is notoriously bad at recognizing and talking about class, so this is not surprising, despite class assumptions underpinning nearly everything within hegemonic birth worlds. At the maternity home for vulnerable women where I volunteered, residents (who were mostly White) were more concerned with how they would manage to sustain their own lives than they were with optimizing them or making them look a certain way. Child Protective Services took a lot of the community's attention. So did opioid addiction; methadone, a prescribed medication for childbearing people addicted to opioids, is demonized in policy despite being medically recommended in the circumstances. Custody battles are heartbreaking and reflect a deeply broken approach to drug use, addiction, and poverty. Those giving childbearing advice tend to assume that home is a place of comfort, safety, and autonomy, yet many people cannot take for granted homes in reasonable states of cleanliness and repair, stocked with useful things, and occupied by loving, respectful people. In a childbirth class at a large local hospital, the instructor asked everyone if they had stockpiled various postpartum supplies in their home cabinets; I was accompanying one of the residents, Grecia, who had neither cabinets nor money for supplies, when I was jolted into recognizing how insensitive this standard question was.

As the natural and technological were not opposed in earlier decades, so they are still entwined. People I came across might have gone through several rounds of IVF in order to become pregnant yet be vehemently opposed to drugs during birth. Silicon Valley companies are known for offering egg freezing to employees and tech executives boast of eschewing maternity leave after elective cesareans, yet these wealthy, self-optimizing demographics are also the target audience for privately contracted doulas. I repeatedly found that binary oppositions did not reflect reality. Polarizing language such as "natural" versus "technological" birth, "midwifery" versus "medical" approaches, and "stay at home" versus "career-oriented" mothers felt clichéd and stale, even though these terms persist in both popular and professional spaces. In day-to-day practice, both parents and practitioners shuffle, recombine, and reimagine such categories, balancing ideals with practical possibilities.

Most people I worked with exemplified the pragmatic idealism of Bay Area birth culture by critiquing medically managed birth while taking advantage of its presence. They intended to give birth in a hospital, yet they found natural birth compelling and wanted to make informed decisions about engaging with medical procedures and technologies.[42] In the United States today, the term *natural birth* generally refers to an absence of pain medication. It can also refer more broadly to the absence of medical technology altogether, or simply to vaginal delivery—but it also bears connotations from a rich legacy of activism. Calls to experience one's body deeply, make use of the latest technology, avoid pain, stay safe, respect experts, connect with land and community, or be concerned about the well-being of future generations are resonant for different people in messy and complicated ways. I am fascinated by the alignments that childbearing practices make visible, alignments that do not correspond neatly to other categorizations but which are always influenced by them. Some people practice childbearing similarly but with different reasons or motivations; conversely, it is not uncommon to find individuals who share a background yet have very divergent ideas about childbearing. Within my own family, all of us are healthcare professionals of some sort, yet we have very different ideas about medical care during labor, as well as about gendered caretaking roles. By digging into this tangle, this book explores how tensions near birth in California are symptomatic of competing fantasies of utopian and dystopian American futures, mediated through birthing bodies.

MEDICAL INNOVATION AND THE
MATERNAL HEALTHCARE CRISIS

In her 2020 speech accepting her nomination as vice presidential candidate, Kamala Harris made it known that she was born at Oakland's Kaiser hospital, likely to head off racist accusations of not being American born. This is the second place we'll visit to explore a different aspect of birth worlds. Oakland is home to Kaiser Permanente's national headquarters, and the healthcare giant is the city's largest employer. Kaiser originated in the nearby Richmond shipyards in the 1940s and is the largest managed care organization in the United States. It is an excellent example of California's leadership not just in countercultural approaches to birth, but in birth's medical management and medicine's corporatization. I attended births at several of the Bay Area's Kaiser hospitals, and although the organization has come under some scrutiny recently, its model of coordinating insurance, billing, and all aspects of care delivery (including preventative care) has devoted proponents.

Yet innovations in healthcare delivery don't compensate for the fact that a sizable proportion of Americans do not have health insurance that grants them access to such innovations. More than half of the people who give birth in California are on Medi-Cal, the state's version of Medicaid public insurance. While some parents obsess over the significance and intricacies of childbearing options, contemporary American childbearing has been described as in crisis. Amnesty International's 2010 report "Deadly Delivery: The Maternal Health Care Crisis in the USA" ranks the United States fiftieth in the world for maternal mortality, despite spending twice as much money on maternity healthcare as any country surveyed. There are huge disparities along lines of race and class: Indigenous and Black women are four and eight times more likely to die in birth than White women respectively, and women in poor areas are twice as likely to die as those in wealthy ones. The cesarean rate was 33 percent and steadily rising, more than double the range recommended by the World Health Organization, and in states with a higher-than-average surgical rate, maternal mortality was also significantly higher.

This problem has only recently begun to receive long-overdue attention in the national media, through special reporting by ProPublica and the *New York Times Magazine* in 2017 and 2018, respectively.[43] These reports also drew attention to problems with access to care in rural areas, and how maternal deaths are treated as one-off tragedies as opposed to systemic failures. Maternal disparity statistics are now reported by the Centers for Disease Control and Prevention, which stated in 2019 that Black women are three to four times more likely to die from pregnancy-related causes than White women.[44] In 2021, the American Medical Association described a "culture of disrespect" that marks Black mothers' experiences with conventional medicine, and the Black Maternal Health Momnibus Act of 2021 is working its way through the federal government.[45]

California is hardly exempt from this shameful situation, but it does considerably better than other parts of the United States, largely due to recent efforts by the California Maternal Quality Care Collaborative (CMQCC), founded in 2006 at Stanford's School of Medicine along with the State of California. CMQCC collects statistical data and aims to standardize emergency protocols, similar to how maternity care is managed in countries like the United Kingdom (though the U.K. has its own racial disparities and is far from perfect).[46] California's maternal mortality has decreased by 65 percent over the past decade, while the nation's has grown. Activist groups like Black Women Birthing Justice (BWBJ), based in the East Bay, are working on the issue starting from the standpoint of race. BWBJ's 2016 report *Battling Over Birth: Black Women and the Maternal Health Care Crisis in California* is rich with the perspectives of Black childbearing people.[47] In this vein, the 2018 "Listening to Mothers in California" survey was a sizable piece of research into the issue of poor maternity care and showcases California's efforts to lead on the issue.[48]

Around 99 percent of American births take place in hospitals. Most have adapted significantly to the critiques levied by the natural birth movement. Once-standard procedures such as enemas, pubic shaving, and the use of wheelchairs, which Robbie Davis-Floyd described in the early 1990s as rites of passage that infantilize childbearing women, are rarely practiced. Other objectionable practices such as episiotomies (cutting the perineal tissue between the vagina and anus) and medically inducing labor are less common. Practices that allow for connectivity have also caught on, such as skin-to-skin contact, whereby a newborn is placed on the birthing person's chest immediately after being delivered instead of being cleaned and removed to a nursery, and delayed cord clamping, which allows the placenta's blood to continue pumping into the baby after delivery. Increasing numbers of hospitals promote breastfeeding, sometimes in accordance with the World Health Organization's Baby Friendly Hospital Initiative; unsurprisingly, the vast majority of the American early adopters of this program were located in California. Many wealthier hospitals have changed their branding from "labor and delivery wards" to "family birth centers" and now feature private rooms, double beds, bathtubs or showers, and homey decor that minimizes medical equipment. Yet basic problems with respect persist, such as those that Karen Scott and Dána-Ain Davis theorize as "obstetric racism" and Beatriz Reyes-Foster describes as "maternal vanishing."[49]

American midwives underwent a shift toward working in hospitals in the 1990s in a game-changing (and internally controversial) move toward professionalization. Many lay midwives such as Rox and Kate were opposed to professionalization. They felt that the logistical constraints of hospitals (including liability law, physician supervision, shift scheduling, and the way even the spatial layout foregrounds technological interventions) required too much compromise of the "midwifery model of care" that put women front and center. Yet the potential to make a difference for so many more women by practicing in hospitals tipped the balance at the organizational level.

Doulas evolved in the wake of this professionalization as supplementary providers who act as patient advocates and do the slow, person-oriented care that midwives working in hospitals can no longer do. Although the term *doula,* which troublingly means "female slave" or "servant woman" in modern Greek, was introduced in 1969 by Dana Raphael, a breastfeeding advocate working within the broader natural birth movement, it grew to prominence quite slowly. One of the first professional organizations for doulas, the National Association of Childbirth Assistants, was founded in San Jose in 1984, with the Doulas of North America following in 1992.[50] Doulas increasingly train for and practice postpartum care as well, and they support people through abortion, conception, and pregnancy loss (death doulas are also on the rise). Doulas are becoming increasingly popular; the 2016 "Listening to Mothers" study found that about 10 percent of California births were attended by a doula, with nearly 40 percent of respondents expressing interest in having one, percentages that are likely higher in the Bay Area.[51] Many doulas explicitly conceive of their work as activism, as we will explore in chapter 7.

Doula services are not covered by insurance, and questions of access and oversight are central to deciding what the doula is or should be; these questions are actively being worked out in doula communities. Some public voices have claimed that doulas are the answer to the maternity care crisis, a claim I revisit in chapter 7. Part of the reason doulas are effective is because their loyalties lie only with their client and not with the hospital or insurance systems. Yet the people who stand to benefit most from a doula are usually those without means to pay privately for one. Hiring a doula in the Bay Area can cost between one thousand and four thousand dollars for a standard package of two prenatal meetings and one postpartum, attendance at the delivery, and four weeks of being on-call. Doulas exist as both a niche commodity for bespoke care and an activist platform for birth reform. Put otherwise, they represent both the privatization of health care within neoliberal transformations of public welfare and grassroots activist pushback against an already-privatized, racist, classist, and ineffectual maternity system.

And so it is that many of the ideals of the natural birth movement have yet to be achieved, despite advocacy over the past sixty years. The conversation around birth reform has become far more intersectional, recognizing the many different kinds of oppression and difference that can intersect and compound for a given person. Initiatives led by people of color have risen in visibility, though they are by no means new. Most notably, this includes the powerful reproductive justice framework that encompasses the right to have a child, not have a child, and raise children in a safe and healthy environment, and which centers the perspectives of women of color and poor, queer, and trans folks.[52] A subset of this movement, Birth Justice, has gained prominence alongside outrage about maternal mortality disparities, which has been catalyzed by the Black Lives Matter movement and the difficulties of birthing during the COVID-19 pandemic. The legacy of natural birth has had to grapple with its Whiteness—another topic I revisit in chapter 7.

Activists of color are reclaiming nonmedical birth practices and philosophies as part of their heritage, from midwives who identify as Latinx *parteras*, to pan-Indigenous cradleboard artisans, to the International Center for Traditional Childbearing (ICTC), which changed its name to the National Association to Advance Black Birth (NAABB) in 2018. Racially marked birth practices have been historically marginalized yet have their own vibrant legacies. For example, many histories of American birth state that midwifery was not a recognized profession during the twentieth century with the exception of the Frontier Nursing Service catering to Appalachia, yet California maintained a professional midwifery license from 1917 to 1949. It was largely held by people in the Japanese American community, and its disbanding amidst anti-Japanese sentiment after World War II cannot be coincidental, nor its subsequent relegation to a historical footnote. Much Indigenous discourse about birth and reproductive justice centers the ecological violence of colonial capitalism and the notion of the mother's body as the "first environment," articulating concerns about toxicity decades before they entered White communities' consciousness.[53] Indigenous midwives protesting the Dakota Access pipeline in 2016 articulated their concerns in these ways.[54]

Meanwhile, a medical industrial complex has taken shape as medicine, like the military and prisons, has become dominated by corporate interests and moves further and further away from serving the public good, crumpling under its own weight.[55] Ricki Lake and Abby Epstein's 2008 film, *The Business of Being Born,* is an exposé that touched a public nerve but changed little about childbearing industries. The pharmaceutical industry plays a large role in medicine-as-business, though hospitals themselves are increasingly part of large corporations too. Some, like Kaiser, combine the insurance and hospital industries. Silicon Valley–style health tech companies command billions of venture capital dollars, despite the misleading promises of one such company, Theranos, which became the subject of an explosive scandal. FemTech is a new wave of this hype that proposes to solve women's health issues, including around childbearing. There have been several app-based "postpartum doulas," as well as devices like improved breast pumps, pelvic floor relaxers, and contraction monitors in various stages of development. Progress and profits become entangled, and it simply seems realistic to imagine care near birth in terms of capitalist imperatives. Realism, according to Mark Fisher, is seeing the future as a continuation of the present.[56] By contrast, utopias, dystopias, and heterotopias all involve discontinuity—but to different degrees. Utopian imaginaries necessarily reproduce the status quo to some extent, because the world in which we live conditions what we can imagine as good. By extension, radical critique often takes on a negative dystopian cast because it is so different as to be incomprehensible.

As ever, the Bay Area dramatizes this situation via the coexistence of extremes. Amidst its overflow of unhoused people, it boasts cutting-edge medical institutions with international research reputations, including medical school giants UCSF and Stanford (as well as UCLA in Southern California), which cement California's role as a leader in medical innovation. Part of my fieldwork involved writing for Stanford Medicine's blog bringing research frontiers to a public audience. California historian Kevin Starr elaborates how a leading role in scientific and technological developments has been key to California's utopian pursuit since the transcontinental railroad: "Open, flexible, entrepreneurial, unembarrassed by the profit motive, California emerged as a society friendly to the search for utopia through science and technology." This drive to make the world "a better and more interesting place" can be startlingly myopic.[57] Childbearing practices that were once the province of cultural fringes are becoming widespread as part of a hip, elite parenting culture with access to the best medicine can offer— yet these developments are happening against a late liberal backdrop of rising inequality, divestment from public infrastructure, and a growing gap between those who have access to options and those who do not. In their books *Jailcare* and *addicted.pregnant.poor.,* Carolyn Sufrin and Kelly Ray Knight empathetically detail the current situation of San Francisco's childbearing people who are enmeshed in incarceration, homelessness, prostitution, and drug usage. They are excluded from basic necessities in a way that deeply compromises their reproduction and exposes a hollowness in California's medical glory.

The development of gynecology itself is a key example of medical innovations that require some redemption; J. Marion Sims is usually credited as the father of gynecology for his work developing surgical techniques through forced and unanesthetized experimentation on enslaved women Betsey, Anarcha, and Lucy. He became respected and wealthy by selling these techniques to upper-class White patients.[58] Today, the three women are being recognized as "mothers of gynecology" through a push to correct the historical record; in Alabama, where Sims originally practiced, a large monument to them is "telling their story and shining a light on ongoing racial disparities in the healthcare industry today. [It] stands as a symbol of all of the enslaved women who were experimented upon in the quixotic pursuit of a modern 'science' of gynecology."[59] Californian institutions are, as of very recently, making efforts towards correcting such histories; for example, UCSF's MILK Research Lab is devoted to improving "maternal health outcomes of Black women and birthing people across the life course ... using a Black Feminist approach informed by Life Course Perspective, Reproductive Justice, Racial Equity, and Research Justice."[60] As far as I have seen, it is the first of its kind. We revisit these questions in chapter 7, which considers redemption, a cousin of progress that does not simply blaze forward but takes careful stock of what has been done wrong and how it haunts the present in ways that must be addressed in order to move into just, livable futures. Doulas are central to this work as well.

———

TWO

Experience

WAYS OF KNOWING, BEING, AND
DOING PHYSIOLOGY

"I'M SORRY TO DISTURB YOU, but I'm legally required to let you know that I recommend a cesarean," said the obstetrician. She was addressing Molly, who was squatting on a low chair with a hole cut in its seat, called a birth stool. Molly was flushed and naked and had a trembling, panting glow that was somewhere between triumph and exhaustion. She's a marathon runner, my elderly doula mentor, Anna, proudly explained in our earlier meeting with Molly. She's used to persevering through intense physical situations. Suzanne, the midwife, was kneeling at the base of the stool, fuzzy ponytail brushing the linoleum as she practically laid her head on the hospital room floor, watching Molly's vulva and encouraging her with praise and reports on her progress. Molly had been pushing for over two hours.

This time span—120 minutes—is what precipitated the obstetrician's entrance. I don't know her name, as she didn't spend time in the room with us, but she was tall and poised, the only Black person I saw at the hospital that day. Although I did not record her exact words, the phrase above captures her meaning: she would have been making herself vulnerable to a lawsuit if she did not advise a C-section at this point. It was clear she was making a gesture on principle and didn't really expect Molly to change course. Her effort at persuasion seemed perfunctory, and I found her admission quaint in its frankness—we were at the most natural birth–friendly hospital in the city, after all. Molly did not want medical intervention in the birth, and she had managed without a drop of medication in the twelve hours since we arrived at the hospital. She consulted with Suzanne and Anna and decided she would prefer to keep pushing. We two doulas and Molly's partner, Eric, pressed cold wet cloths against her forehead and neck, offered her water and juice, and shared encouraging platitudes, though she largely found these ministrations annoying and preferred to be undisturbed.

Suzanne, the midwife, watched the baby's descent with her cheek on the floor. She massaged Molly's perineum, the tissue between the vulva and the rectum, oiling it and softening it for the "ring of fire" that would occur when the baby's head emerged. The awkward angle seemed cumbersome but Suzanne was engrossed. Close to hour four, Suzanne set in motion a rapid chain of events. Did she shout something? Call on her pager? Flip a switch on a call box in the room? I didn't register it. But within tens of seconds the obstetrician returned with a flood of people. Molly was lifted bodily onto the hospital bed and laid on her back, and somehow I was stationed by one of her legs and told to raise it to her ear. "Shoulder dystocia," I heard someone say. The obstetrician was manually attempting to loosen the baby while Molly was stretched open like this, and when it didn't work, she cut Molly's perineum with a flash of steel scissors and pulled. In a flush of bloody greenish fluid, the baby was out.

I was struck by Molly's lucidity under the circumstances. She was intent on knowing about her baby's well-being. Aside from the presence in the amniotic fluid of meconium, the fetal feces that is said to indicate distress, the baby was just fine. The nurses (or the pediatrician, I wasn't sure who was who anymore) wiped off the baby, took her Apgar score, and showed her to Molly, who breathlessly coddled her for a few moments. The obstetrician gave Molly a shot of Pitocin to stimulate the uterine contractions that would deliver the placenta and close the uterus's bleeding blood vessels. Soon the doctor explained that although the baby was fine, Molly needed to be taken to surgery, where her perineal damage would be repaired. She had a fourth-degree tear, the highest level, in which the tissue dividing the vagina from the rectum is completely torn. Molly would be put under general anesthesia; when she asked, she was told that the drugs would likely be in her bloodstream when she breastfed her baby for the first time.

Molly was wheeled to surgery on her hospital bed, and a crew of janitors cleaned the room's slippery, spattered floor. They disposed of the delivery table's tools and packaging, which had been set up when Molly was nearing the pushing phase. A new, bigger bed was wheeled in, and under the attention of a nurse, the new baby was settled on her dad's bare chest to sleep.

An hour or so after the birth, which was the second I had ever witnessed, Anna and I went to fetch food for ourselves and Eric. We were all hungry after nearly twenty-four hours of birth support. The two of us debriefed on the bench of a Chipotle. Shoulder dystocia means the shoulder got stuck in the birth canal, essentially. *Why didn't they try the Gaskin maneuver!?* Anna wondered aloud. For years afterward when I retold the story to doulas and midwives, many would indignantly pose this question. I had not yet heard of the Gaskin maneuver, which relieves shoulder dystocia by getting the birthing person onto her hands and knees, thereby slightly altering the shape of the pelvis and allowing the impacted baby to pass through. It is named after Ina May Gaskin, the American midwife with cultlike status introduced in chapter 1, who learned it in Belize from a woman who learned it in Guatemala, where the technique apparently originated—a naming politics some midwives have critiqued as colonial appropriation.

For whatever reasons, the obstetrician did not attempt the Gaskin maneuver, and neither did the midwife.[1] But what struck me most about my conversation with Anna was the ambiguity about the C-section: would it have been better to have gone with it? Fault, blame, and regret were in the air, even though Anna explicitly rejected them, saying we could never know which way would have been better. Was the baby really in distress? Her Apgar was fine, yet there was meconium. Was it really such an urgent situation that it needed to be resolved within seconds? The baby had been compressed with her shoulder for four hours, after all. Maybe the obstetrician's rapid reaction was what saved the baby from harm. Maybe it was hasty and damaging, precipitated by unnecessary panic and a fear-based approach. Did the slower, patient approach facilitated by the midwife fail? It was certainly overwhelmed by the imperative of an "emergency." If protocol had been heeded, would the abdominal trauma of the cesarean have been greater or less than the perineal trauma Molly sustained? Are these even the relevant questions to ask?

WHAT HAPPENS DURING BIRTH?
REGULAR AND CONTEXTUAL BODIES

Situations like Molly's, in which there are many what ifs clinging to the actions of those present, are very common in the birth stories I came across, whether by attending births, talking to people I knew, or reading online forums and blogs. The right course of action for any person present was rarely an accepted thing. Someone usually could have done something different, which might have made for better outcomes, variously defined. Although those involved might not describe it this way, the questions floating around Molly's labor are fundamentally questions about how bodies function—that is, about physiology. Some people currently use the term *physiological birth* to distinguish an approach to birth as a healthy and normal process from an obstetrics approach that generally considers birth a pathological and dangerous process. I am using the term *physiology* somewhat differently, in a way that can encompass both approaches. Basically, I use it to describe ways of knowing what bodies are and how they work. The way we *know* bodies shapes how we *experience* those bodies, both our own and those of others.

Bodily processes are not something that simply exist in the world. They are not natural givens waiting to be discovered, but neither are they something that can be imagined or constructed in any random way. They are both real *and* interpreted, as decades of medical anthropology work shows.[2] Indeed, the way they are interpreted shapes their reality. "Knowing" is a kind of expectation; such expectations shape what happens, and what happens in turn shapes expectations about what will happen next time. If one learns about birth as a dangerous undertaking, one expects an emergency, and bodily signs are interpreted as problems; these problems lead to "emergency situations," reinforcing the idea that birth is dangerous. In philosophical terms, physiology is a co-constituted epistemology and ontology of the body—which is to say, how the body is known (epistemology) and how it exists (ontology) depend upon each other. Such uncertainty about what the body *is* is heightened during birth. Maggie Nelson asks, "Is there something inherently queer about pregnancy itself, insofar as it profoundly alters one's 'normal' state, and occasions a radical intimacy with—and radical alienation from—one's body? How can an experience so profoundly strange and wild and transformative also symbolize or enact the ultimate conformity?"[3] Childbearing pushes the limits of experience, which can be threatening to the status quo—and therefore a target for doubling down on conventional ways of knowing. In Lawrence Kirmayer's words, "The choice of explanations in medicine is always a choice of values."[4]

People in birth worlds have conflicting ways of knowing the body. This is why there is so much contention over how to interpret what happened, and what should be done. I want to describe the physiology of birth. But how to do so? Description cannot be neutral. Even anatomical terms are contested among those I spent time with: fallopian tubes were named after a male anatomist, Gabriele Falloppio, and some people call them ovarian tubes instead. Other substitutions include "rushes" for "contractions" or "due window" for "due date." But let's begin somewhere. During birth, the uterus has to open, the baby has to pass through the vagina, and the placenta has to follow her out. This process can last from a few hours to a few weeks. The cervix, a thick, rubbery donut of muscle, is the gateway to the uterus. During labor, it increases in diameter (dilates), becomes paper-thin (effaces), and tilts upward toward the birthing person's belly to reduce the angle between the uterus and the vagina. Sometimes this is called "ripening." This happens in conjunction with uterine contractions, or the tightening of the muscle at the top of the uterus (the fundus), which stretches open the bottom of the uterus (where the cervix is). The baby descends toward the cervix, easing her way into the pelvis, which is often measured as a transition from a negative to a positive "station."

Usually the back of the baby's head (the occiput) leads the way, which happens when the baby is facing the birthing person's back. Babies in utero can also face the person's belly (occiput posterior, or sunny-side up), be in any degree of rotation between these two positions, or they might extend their neck and exit face-first. A hand or shoulder might descend next to the head (a nuchal hand and shoulder dystocia, respectively). Alternatively, the part that descends could be the baby's bottom or feet (a frank/complete breech and footling breech, respectively). If there are two or more babies, one will descend into the pelvis first and the others will follow. At some point the birthing person will push and the baby will rotate through the tight channel of the pelvis, stretching the perineal tissue as it emerges (crowning). Because the infant is connected to the placenta via the umbilical cord during this process, all her basic functions are still provided for. At various points she will begin to breathe, expel waste (meconium), and gather nutrients (generally by drinking colostrum, the first and especially rich breast milk). The uterus will contract again, detaching the placenta from the uterine wall and expelling it through the vagina. The blood vessels that previously supplied the placenta will stop bleeding. Slowly, the uterus will recover its shape and tone, and it will stop leaking (this can take months).

How this all works, exactly, and, by extension, how it can go wrong, are the contested aspects. Let's look more closely at the cervix. People largely agree that the cervix needs to be dilated to around ten centimeters and 100 percent effaced for pushing to begin. Otherwise, an "incomplete" cervix could be damaged by the baby. But there are at least two ways of conceptualizing this. One is the obstetric partogram. The other is the sphincter model. Each is an exaggerated illustration of two more general ways of approaching physiology, which I describe as *regular* and *contextual*. Both are entwined with American ideas about experience.

The obstetric partogram describes a standard rate of progress at which cervical dilation should take place. It was developed in 1954 by Emanuel Friedman, a doctor who conducted a study of one hundred laboring women and found the average rates of dilation along a curve that was slower at the beginning and accelerated in the second half of labor (approximately one centimeter per hour). A normal labor should last around twelve hours, he concluded, noting that time to dilation was a "good measure of the overall efficiency of the machine."[5] The partogram illustrates cervical dilation as something regular—indeed, mechanical—that should happen in the same way for every birthing person and be managed via technological inputs. It imposes a need to "progress" at a certain pace and not follow erratic rhythms. Where the partogram idea holds sway, labor is generally considered a problem only when it is progressing more slowly than average. In a culture that prioritizes speed and efficiency, this might seem unremarkable, yet it is closely related to the way medical language uses factory metaphors to describe women's bodies and reproductive capacities, as Emily Martin detailed thirty years ago in her book *The Woman in the Body*. Mechanical metaphors have been used in maternity hospitals since at least the eighteenth century, while factory metaphors have been more recently adopted, building in the twentieth-century sciences of work productivity, time and motion studies, and scientific management. This way of thinking values products over processes, and so arriving quickly at the end goal of a healthy baby is the priority—not the experience of arriving there.

Desiring a healthy baby is hardly remarkable in itself, and there is a long history of people valuing speedy labors to minimize pain and danger for the person giving birth; what's new here are the power dynamics inherent in both mechanical and factory metaphors. Both superimpose abstract ideas about how women's bodies *should* work and imply that they need an external operator or manager to function properly, an expert who will "deliver" the baby to the woman (obstetric protocols are called *active management* and *expectant management*). Because the cesarean section requires the most management by the doctor and the least labor by the uterus/woman, it became seen as providing the best products, a metaphorical development that correlated with a dramatic increase in surgical births. Focusing on the product ignores what the birthing person may have been equally concerned about: her own experience of the birth. But then again, these metaphors extend far beyond medical contexts and shape the desires and expectations of lots of childbearing people, and indeed how they experience their bodies, so the two are not necessarily at odds.

Alternatively, the cervix can be understood as a sphincter. Gaskin lays out this approach in *Ina May's Guide to Childbirth,* published in 2003, a frequently referenced classic among those sympathetic to natural birth. She claims the cervical sphincter functions like other voluntary sphincters, such as the throat, urethra, and anus; that is, they do not obey orders, they function best in an atmosphere of familiarity and privacy, and they may suddenly close when their owner is startled or frightened.[6] In this physiological understanding, dilation is not in fact regular but involves bouts of rest, preparation, and rapid melting that cannot be predicted. According to this theory, it is easier to open the cervix at home and while no one is watching, just like it is easier for most people to use the toilet at home and while no one is watching. I've frequently heard the birthing person likened to a mama cat seeking a dark corner of the closet, or a mare stepping away from the herd to birth: they want to feel sheltered and private. When new people enter the birthing space, or hands enter the vagina to check dilation, the cervix might react protectively by retreating, contracting.

Gaskin contrasts this "Sphincter Law" with the obstetric "Law of Three P's," which refer to the passenger (baby), passage (pelvis and vagina), and powers (strength of uterine contractions). She claims the latter approach blames the birthing person for "dysfunctional" labors that don't produce a baby in the allotted time by saying she grew too big a baby, has too small a pelvis, or doesn't have contractions that are strong enough. By contrast, the Sphincter Law attributes longer than average birth times as a problem of "lack of privacy, fear, and stimulation of the wrong parts of the laboring woman's brain." In this model, troubleshooting a stalled labor involves thinking about the birthing person's fears and whether any of the relationships in the room are strained. Gaskin suggests that opening other sphincters facilitates cervical opening, which might require breathing deeply, singing, moaning, or grunting (or, in Anne Enright's forthrightly bovine metaphor, "lowing").[7] Rhythmic, deep noises work better than erratic, high-pitched noises. Defecating and vomiting are often signs of labor progressing. Shifting and moving help the sphincter open, but moreover the ability to move freely creates a sense of security for the birthing person. Creating an amenable environment is paramount. This can be as fundamental as having respectful providers, or as superficial as pillows that smell of home. "As above, so below" Gaskin quips; "our bottom parts function best when our top part—our minds—are either grateful or amused at the antics or activities of our bottoms."[8]

What I describe as regular physiology, epitomized by the partogram, is predicated on the idea that bodily processes are universal. That means they are predictable, uniform across persons, and objectively knowable. On the other hand, contextual physiology, epitomized by the sphincter, approaches bodies as constantly in flux and responsive to the surrounding environment. Bodily processes differ from person to person and are subjectively knowable. Whereas regular physiology takes place in all places and at all times, contextual physiology takes place here and now. In one approach, the body is a machine that requires managerial inputs and needs to be externally set in motion (that is, by medically inducing labor). In the other, the body is a site of organic processes by which it sets itself in motion, and birthing is something bodies intrinsically know how to do. Importantly, these are archetypes to which people I encountered refer and allude, not rigid protocols they enact. They are ideals that don't exist in and of themselves, although they shape real experience because they exist in the cultural imagination and provide lenses for apprehending what kinds of experience are desirable and possible.

A similar difference has been described by other theorists. In the early 1980s, Barbara Katz Rothman distinguished between the medical and midwifery models of birth.[9] A decade later, Robbie Davis-Floyd used the terms *technocratic* and *wholistic* and described a "natural" model of birth as an attempt to reconcile the two.[10] There is now more hybridization between these extremes, both in scholarship and in healthcare practice. Birthing people and birth practitioners negotiate ideologies alongside practical matters like insurance, litigation, and scheduling. Remember that Molly's obstetrician's C-section recommendation was based on malpractice liability: what kind of decisions (what kind of physiology) will stand scrutiny in a court?

I like the terms *regular* and *contextual* because they are capacious. They can apply to many different situations and therefore make it easy to draw analogies between birth physiology, ways bodies are experienced more generally, and modes of living in and organizing society. Although each archetype presents different ways of approaching technology or relations or experience, these are not distinguishing factors in themselves; technology *is* the context of contemporary birth, industrial relations are still relations, and abstraction shapes its own kind of experience. By describing a difference in physiology, I want to draw attention to how bodies are known and experienced as distinct from other factors that influence people's decisions and actions near birth.

Let's return to contentions over what happens during birth. The idea that labor should progress in a predictable way has led to dividing it into separate stages and substages, making a direct analogy with factory labor, as Martin points out.[11] When hospitals started advertising themselves to wealthy families as safe and modern places to give birth in the early twentieth century, they organized their space with the logic of an assembly line, including separate rooms for labor, delivery, and recovery, and a nursery.[12] This has changed, but it illustrates a mode of thinking that is still alive. Stages of birth are commonly based on cervical dilation: early labor is zero to four centimeters, active is four to eight, and transition is eight to ten. But the borders are blurry; people disagree about how much variability is acceptable and whether cervical dilation can be measured at all. The same holds true for the division between labor, pushing, and the delivery of the placenta. Who decides when someone is ready to push, and why? Should the cord be immediately cut or stay attached for a while?

Labor starts long before most pregnant people come to the hospital. Many find out at a routine checkup that they are two centimeters dilated or that they've lost their mucus plug, a thick secretion stoppering the cervix. Contrary to popular media depictions, most labors do not start with the rupture of the amniotic sac, which in any case tends to result more in a trickle than a flood. The general rule I repeatedly heard from hospital providers and in my doula training was "4-1-1," that is, call us when your contractions are four minutes apart, lasting for at least one minute, and this pattern has been going on for at least one hour. This supposedly indicates the arrival at active labor, but stories of surprises in which labor takes place much more quickly than expected are ubiquitous in birth media. For example, in one birth story on Twitter a dad describes his son's accidental home birth because they waited to go to the hospital until 4–1-1, but by then the baby was crowning. One of my interviewees recounted being put in a "weird storage room" in the hospital, wondering in confusion whether the hospital was so overbooked she'd give birth there, before realizing it was the triage room where she was being met with skepticism about her readiness:

> "Are you sure you should be here, you're a first timer, how long have you been
> in labor for?" And I remember saying, "Someone give me a trash can!" and I
> puked, and they're like "Okay, maybe we'll take you seriously now." And they

checked me, and they're like "Holy —, you're nine centimeters dilated! Prep a room!!" All this commotion is happening. "Get a room ready! She's going into labor!" She said, "She's almost ready to push," and I remember being like, "So I can't have anything for pain then?" Nope!

Tales about the opposite experience are ubiquitous, too, stories about labor that stalled or wouldn't start, or the person that reached 4–1-1 and arrived at the hospital to be sorely disappointed that she was only two centimeters dilated. It's not uncommon that she be sent home to catch an extra night's sleep, as happened with my client Brynna—though by this point many pregnant people are impatient to get the baby out and getting them to go home can take some convincing! Equally, a person in this situation might be admitted and start attempting to speed up labor, with conventional methods like drugs or less common ones like using breast pumps for nipple stimulation (to release oxytocin). Another of my clients was in this latter situation and giggled as she held the twin canisters suctioned onto her breasts, comparing herself to the Fembots in the Austin Powers movies. Ina May would have been pleased; laughter opens sphincters.

How long a pregnancy can safely persist is hotly debated. The "due date" is forty weeks from conception (though how conception is calculated is also contested and can involve the date of the last menstrual period or ovulation or ultrasounds to size the fetus). Generally, thirty-eight to forty-two weeks of pregnancy is the range in which labor should start; before is considered premature and after overdue. I have heard that "forty-one is the new forty-two" and that babies are being considered overdue at forty weeks, a trend that has been met with hostility from many birth activists. Whether hospital providers will "allow" a pregnant person to go past forty-two weeks (or indeed forty, or thirty-eight, or whatever is determined to be risky) is an issue many birth activists feel strongly about and a key site where physiological approaches clash.

With all this in mind, consider the question, which is often posed by opinionated actors in birth worlds, of whether childbearing falls under medical purview at all. From a contextual perspective, birth is processual and unpredictable, rooted in particular bodies instead of in an ideal standard body, and variation is not only not alarming but to be expected. In a regular framework, the unpredictability of birth makes it seem inherently risky; the body is perceived to be in an abnormal state that warrants treatment as a pathology, and the response to such an irregular event is, of course, to attempt to regularize it. Ironically, then, according to such a view, virtually no birth is "normal."

There is a medical maxim that a birth can only be declared normal in retrospect. By contrast, there are frequent injunctions among midwifery and doula communities to "believe in" and "trust" birth. Though these phrases initially struck me as very strange (*believe* in birth? Like, that it happens?), they illustrate a contextual physiology that has no trouble incorporating unpredictability into normal bodily functioning.

As archetypes, these physiologies are opposed and static, but in practice they are in conversation. Giving a talk at a Bay Area Doula Project meeting, well-known nurse-midwife Peggy Vincent said, "Abnormalities aren't abnormal; everyone has them." She spent most of her career working in hospitals. Harmony, a hospital midwife I knew as both a new mother and provider, joked with me about "the P's," laughing about the fact that Ina May doesn't like them and only uses her Sphincter Law. The P's had been around long enough to make their way into Roxanne Cummings's Mindfulness-Based Childbirth Education class, which we were both involved with, and long enough to multiply, as we could recall at least ten of them: the passenger, pelvis, and powers, mentioned above, but also provider, partner, placenta, pain coping, position (of baby), psyche (of mom), and—last but not least—patience.

EMERGENCIES, INTERVENTIONS, AND HORMONES: A TANGLE OF CAUSE AND EFFECT

A common argument against medical interventions—and, by extension, regular physiology—is that they cause the problems they claim to fix. Usually this argument refers to the cascade of interventions, which centers around hormones. The way people talk about hormones in birth is a kind of bridge across contextual and regular approaches. Hormones are objectively measurable material substances, but they are also entwined with experiential energies like stress or pleasure. They carry the scientific authority of biology but create and respond to subjective experiences. So they are both scientific and subjective, both physical and social.[13] A doula I met at a Bay Area retreat taught her own natural childbirth preparation course called Birth Chemistry, which featured a molecular diagram of oxytocin with a heart as its logo. I saw necklaces fashioned to represent the same molecule, and a popular science/self-help book came out called *Oxytocin: The Biological Guide to Motherhood*. Hormones, and specifically oxytocin, were rapidly developing a bit of a cult following. And like other pushes from the margins, they are becoming (re) integrated into formal medical ways of knowing.[14]

Stories about a cascade of interventions usually feature Pitocin as the villain. Pitocin, a synthetic form of oxytocin, is commonly given as a drug to start labor or hurry it along. Pitocin effectively causes contractions, but they are often more intense and painful than those caused by oxytocin. Oxytocin flows systemically, including into the brain and fetus, and has pain-relieving properties, while Pitocin targets uterine muscles. The intense contractions prompt laboring people to request pain relief. Often this is in the form of a spinal epidural, in which a thin tube is inserted into the spinal column to deliver anesthetic, numbing the patient from the waist down. The pain relief is extremely effective in most cases, but the birthing person cannot stand or walk and so must lie relatively stationary on a hospital bed. This sedentariness can stall labor (and lying-down, or supine, positions make it more difficult for the baby to pass through the pelvis), in which case the Pitocin is increased. But although the birthing person can no longer feel the intense Pitocin-induced contractions, the fetus can, which can lead to fetal distress, meaning a lack of oxygen demonstrated by changes in heart rate. This hypoxia makes delivery seem urgent, which may lead to an emergency cesarean. Once the baby is born, she will have a fair quantity of drugs in her blood stream from the epidural and may not have experienced the preparatory effects of oxytocin or the rush of adrenaline that floods an unmedicated person in transition to the pushing phase, depending on how advanced the labor was prior to intervention. The baby might therefore be dull or agitated, and neither the baby nor the birthing person will have had the natural hormone cocktail that stimulates bonding and breastfeeding. Challenges with bonding and breastfeeding might contribute to postpartum depression.[15] And so the narrative goes.

This cascade story can be tweaked in either direction, the body interpreted as more or less vulnerable to interventions: judiciously modest amounts of Pitocin can be helpful, providing a boost in power without requiring an epidural, while going to the hospital can itself be seen as a disruption. Birth centers exist to provide an intermediary ground between hospital and home, as do "gentle" labor induction methods like cervical softener drugs and even seaweed sticks called laminaria that swell when wet and help open the cervix. A variation on the cascade story focuses on the fight, flight, or freeze hormones, cortisol and adrenaline, instead of the drug Pitocin, as they can likewise interrupt the oxytocin process. Experiencing stress and fear can inhibit birth on a chemical level (and the Sphincter Law can be explained via this chemical rationale). People I spoke with sometimes expressed concern over having the worst of both worlds, a long labor followed by a surgical birth, wondering if they shouldn't just get surgery earlier; but recently I have been learning more about, and sharing, the possible ways that hormone cascades in unmedicated labors prepare and benefit both the infant and childbearing person, regardless of the labor's "success" or "efficacy" according to the factory metaphor.

Currents of regular and contextual thought, then, create contention over whether medical interventions help or hurt, and what constitutes an emergency. Both questions were integral to Molly's birth experience, and to every other birth I attended or heard about. A "sunny-side up" baby, not to mention a breech baby, is cause for an automatic C-section in many hospitals, while the blog *Midwife Thinking* asserts that a baby with the umbilical cord wrapped around her neck is not cause for emergency action. Gaskin's website provides a host of resources for "naturally" dealing with "dangerous" situations thought to require medical intervention, including shoulder dystocias, breech births, and twins. By contrast, the obstetrician blog *Skeptical OB* rails against unnecessary risks taken in the name of picturesque ideologies, particularly home births, that then cause infant deaths.

What caused what? What prevented what? Did contextual attunement to the body fail or did conditions prohibit it from ever being achieved? Maybe the birthing person's fear prevented her oxytocin from working. Maybe the doula wasn't sufficiently confident or reassuring to stave off fear. Maybe labor induction started the cascade of interventions, or maybe it saved the child's life because it might have died if it had stayed in the womb for too long. Maybe the pressure to make progress created anxiety that halted progress. Maybe the intensive technology of the NICU (neonatal intensive care unit) saved the life of the child born too early, or maybe the fact that it was separated from its mother made its recovery far more difficult, as is being shown by the success of "kangaroo care," which mimics marsupial pouches by holding underdeveloped babies against the birthing person's skin. Or perhaps the premature birth was precipitated by internalized chronic stress, which, it is hypothesized, explains racial disparities in preterm births and introduces a whole host of sociological factors into near birth physiology (chapter 6 explores this further).

Ideas about nature and the self, about animals and technology and spirituality, filter through all of this and are the subject of chapter 5. Here, I want to draw attention to a struggle over whether embodied experience is passive or active, innately or externally driven. Where does it *come from?* Both the partogram and the sphincter illustrate the uterus as having its own mechanism. As the instructor at the standard childbearing class at a large county hospital said, uteruses are just like the lungs or heart: they work without being told what to do. But whether the uterus is a machine that needs to be held to certain standards of efficiency or an animal that instinctively retreats to a safe place, what makes it knowable as such? Is it something else as opposed to "us"? Martin points out how women are held to a double standard, being told that labor is involuntary but that they should be able to push or refrain from pushing on command. Fascinatingly, the textbooks and documents she studies from the 1950s (when the partogram was being developed and labor systematized) openly acknowledge that a woman's environment and emotions have a strong influence on labor. These references disappear in later years.[16]

Like cervical dilation, pushing looks quite different from regular and contextual perspectives. Directed pushing is very common even in "natural" labors. Molly was directed to push once she had completely dilated. Suzanne, her midwife, coached her to hold her breath and bear down with all her might for ten seconds, three times per contraction. This was a standard formula I saw repeated at most hospital births. Many birthing people, at least for their first baby, would need to be told which muscles to use (the same ones used when defecating), how hard to push (until you're purple in the face), and when to push (during the contractions indicated on the fetal monitor screen). I frequently heard the truism that pushing is hard, athletic work compared to dilation, which by contrast must be endured or surrendered to. Molly anticipated preferring the activity of pushing to the passivity of dilation when we spoke during a prenatal visit.

The main concern during pushing is that the fetus will develop a slow or erratic heartbeat (the significant gray zone between reassuring and distressing heart tones raises other questions about how monitoring technology can create perceived emergencies, leading some to advocate "intentional nonknowing").[17] Common hospital protocol links distress with pushing for too long, and directed pushing is supposed to make delivery more efficient. But others think that directed pushing can *cause* distress. If the birthing person is deoxygenated because she is holding her breath, might this not cause the baby to become so too? If she was encouraged to push before her body was ready, cervical dilation notwithstanding, did she miss the rest period she and/or her baby needed? In a regular approach, effective pushing is not a given and the birthing person is likely to need coaching, technical assistance via a vacuum or forceps, or, of course, a cesarean. A contextual approach posits that the birthing person will push when she feels the urge, thanks to an attunement to her body and an environment in which she feels safe. Preventing pushing or trying to "correct" her rhythm is then counterproductive because it undermines the person's confidence in herself. The only person I spoke with who recounted an overwhelming and satisfyingly effective urge to push delivered at home, in child's pose on the floor, with only her inexperienced doula and partner present, as the midwife was still on the way.

Molly's baby didn't exhibit enough distress to alarm her midwife, Suzanne, who was deciding how much variation in heartbeat was acceptable.[18] Was she overconfident that Molly's body was doing what was best for the baby and ignoring small decelerations? Should protracted pushing have been read as signaling a problem well before hour four, as the obstetrician interpreted it? Should either Molly or Suzanne have known to switch Molly's position to all fours for the Gaskin maneuver, and would that have resolved the dystocia? Should Molly have been less active and more attuned? Shoulder dystocias are rare and so emergency measures are accepted; how much more ambiguity is attached to less dramatic labor "problems"? I remember a birth I attended during which the hospital staff determined that the birthing person needed an epidural in the middle of pushing, which is very unusual as epidurals aren't generally administered once the birthing person is past seven or eight centimeters of dilation. Supposedly she needed to relax so the baby could descend, but then the baby became distressed and she was told that pushing was harming her baby, so she had to hold her breath and not push, which is very hard, until the baby was vacuumed out. I felt unequipped to participate in this unforeseen medical discussion, but I wondered afterward if I should have done something different, advocated for her or her body better, calmed her more effectively so she could relax her muscles without the epidural ...

Such entangled questions are unanswerable when there is an implicit contention over physiology. It is this unanswerability that precipitated the sense of guilt, blame, and uncertainty amongst the birthing team following Molly's labor. Birthing is a particularly good site to see how inseparable knowledge and being are. It is not only decisions about procedures or techniques that are in question but also the fluid, indeterminate watercolor of feelings and hypothesized possibilities. Between the two extremes of an idealized regularity wherein any deviation can constitute an emergency and a contextual attunement wherein practically nothing does, actions take on ambivalent meanings. Yet as Emilia Sanabria shows in her work on the hormonal body in Brazil, it is inadequate (though common) to evaluate the politics of intervention via a false dichotomy between technological "interventions" and natural "non-interventions."[19] The natural body must be cultivated and acted upon as well. Bodies are not blank canvases. They are always already constituted through habits of being and knowing.

WHAT IS EXPERIENCE AND WHAT HAVE WITCHES GOT TO DO WITH IT?

When I walked into my first Midwives Alliance of North America (MANA) conference in 2012, midwives were still slightly mythical to me and I was overdressed in my business casual skirt suit. I sat in the main hall of the beautiful Asilomar retreat center just south of Monterey, California, and was taken aback to see a fair number of older women—midwives, presumably—wearing pointy black witch hats on top of their gray braids and buns. I looked on, a pair of eyes in the wings, taking in their irreverent humor and deep comfort with each other even while bickering. At the business meeting later, fancy handmade witch hats were raffled off, to my bafflement. It took me a few years to peel the layers of the reference. There are different historical fantasies circulating in birth worlds—all of which draw from fact, and all of which are ideologically embellished. How people understand what has come before shapes their view on what exists at present and what they want for the future. In *Experience and Its Modes,* Michael Oakeshott writes, "History is a world of abstractions. It is a backwater ... a mutilation of present experience."[20] The significance and coherence of historical experience is always a creation of the present, and often a messy one.

There's the familiar "light of progress" version of birth history, according to which scientific and medical knowledge advanced over the centuries, putting an end to the pain, danger, and death inevitably associated with childbearing before the modern era. Major milestones include the invention of obstetric forceps to deliver "stuck" babies (late 1700s), the advent of germ theory and sterilization (late 1800s), the invention of the speculum and fistula repair techniques (also late 1800s), the development of pain relief in labor (early 1900s), and the development of safe cesarean techniques and infant formula (mid-1900s). This is, of course, alongside more general advances in medicine, such as blood transfusions and ultrasound technolo-

gies. Standardized education and credentialing ensured medical professionals were reliable. These and other triumphs form the default cultural narrative about medical progress.

There is also the lesser-known "medical takeover" version of birth history.
According to this story, a vibrant tradition of female healers and midwives
was systematically eradicated to establish the class, gender, and race relations
necessary for capitalism. This began with the witch hunts in fifteenth-century
Western Europe and spread throughout colonial contexts, more recently cul-
minating in the vilification of Black "granny midwives" (increasingly called
grand midwives to reclaim their important work) in the American South in
the first half of the twentieth century. Throughout this process, professional
credentialing made medical knowledge the exclusive property of White
upper-class men. Barbara Ehrenreich and Deirdre English's classic polemical
pamphlet explaining and expressing outrage about this, *Witches, Midwives,
and Nurses: A History of Women Healers,* was written as part of the 1970s
feminist movement, which was closely allied with the natural birth movement. I encountered Marxist feminist Silvia Federici's detailed and passionate
history of the witch hunts, *Caliban and the Witch,* in the exhibition hall of a
midwifery conference. The witch hats began to make more sense. Witches are
a symbol of feminine knowledge and power, as well as defiance of the systems
that oppress and undermine this knowledge and power. It's no coincidence
that witches have gained traction in the past few decades as critiques of medical hegemony and misogyny have become more mainstream.[21]

Of course, careful versions of history weave between these extremes,
pointing out ways that utopia and dystopia are often two sides of the same
coin. As the dominant story, the light of progress version is usually the one
gaining nuance through critical revision. Forceps were pioneered by barber
surgeons who were in competition with midwives. They played a key role in
advancing heroic medicine, a cultural phenomenon alive and well today
in which dramatic cures outweigh patience, prevention, and recovery. Key in
the development of male midwifery and obstetrics was the idea that physicians should not be "inactive spectators," an idea reverberating through current medical malpractice law.[22] Sterile technique significantly improved the
safety of hospitals, which allowed them to be marketed as fashionable spaces
for the wealthy to seek modern treatments instead of being considered places
for the socially marginalized to receive care. The first pain relief for labor was
the drug scopolamine, which caused "twilight sleep." The drug was an amne-
siac, not an anesthetic, which means laboring people, who were often

restrained using fur-lined handcuffs, felt everything but could not remember it afterward. Scopolamine has resurfaced as a date rape drug, which reverberates disturbingly with recent accusations of obstetric abuse and "birth rape."[23] Yet at the time, securing access to twilight sleep was a major feminist cause. Women were pushing against the misogynistic Christian idea that pain and suffering in labor were Eve's punishment for sin, and thus women's burden to bear.

The revision of the light of progress story involves integrating these dark moments into a progressive social history, wherein "we know better now" and more diverse people are included in prestigious, authoritative spaces—Black women can become obstetricians, after all. But inclusivity doesn't really challenge or expand the fundamental ways that bodies and bodily experience are approached, or at least it does so very slowly. To quote Joy Harjo in "Three Generations of Native American Women's Birth Experience," "She saw an obstetrician in town who was reputed to be one of the best. She had the choice of a birthing room. She had the finest care. Despite this, I once again battled with a system in which physicians are taught the art of healing by dissecting cadavers."[24] Contextual physiology is characteristic of many approaches to health and healing that have existed on the margins of modern professional medicine. Women, poor people, and non-White people have by and large been excluded from "respectable" knowledge production and practice, and often also excluded from—or mistreated within—professional medical care. Yet marginalized people have always cared for bodies, including childbearing bodies, in effective and affirming ways.

What is it to have a body, know a body, care for a body, exist in the world as/with/in a body? Bodies are the locus of human experience, the means and medium by which we apprehend things, our fleshly constraints and enablers. Experience is something one has by virtue of existing—or at least this is the surface story. Experience seems self-evident because it is ubiquitous in everyday language, but it has been a vexing philosophical topic for the past few centuries.[25] European philosophers have been concerned with what experience *is*, but more interesting for my purposes is what experience is imagined to be or do. The ways experience becomes valued and, as such, a "problem" near birth are indicative of cultural stories in action.

To get a sense of the messiness of the concept, consider a basic distinction between inner lived experience and outer sensory experience. The former is about interpretation and integration, the latter discrete stimuli and physical sensation. Each has been considered more valuable than the other at different points since the Enlightenment. A dichotomy between subject and object underlies both these modes, relating back to seventeenth-century Cartesian dualism, the mind-body split that René Descartes launched with his infamous "I think, therefore I am." Walter Benjamin sought to conceive of experience in a way that transcended this subject-object dichotomy, referencing a collective subject beyond the damaged, isolated subjects of modern life; he thought of experience as an intergenerational learning process involving tradition and wisdom.[26] Meanwhile, anthropologists interested in how bodies are lived across the world have amassed a wealth of research contextualizing both individualism and mind-body dualism as products of specific historical and political conditions. As Donna Haraway argues, bodies are never natural in the sense of existing outside human labor, yet as a feature of ideology, "the universalized natural body is the gold standard of hegemonic social discourse."[27] In other words, the fact that we take embodied experience as self-evident and universal is a key way that power relations are perpetuated.

At its core, the question of experience is the question of how we know what is real. Just as there is truth in multiple versions of history, both contextual and regular versions of physiology can tell us true things about bodies. What is more interesting is why each holds an appeal, and for whom (which brings us back to witches, for stories about witches are stories about power). Because regular and contextual knowledge are archetypes, actual practices are always hybrids that fall somewhere within a matrix of possibilities. These hybrids illustrate complex desires that respond to people's experiences whether they approach childbearing as a provider or a parent. Medical knowledge and hospital care represent prestige and access to resources, and they are also associated with responsibility and safety. People who have historically been excluded from these spaces or abused within them may see the promise of inclusion in what is socially valued while also feeling intimidated or defensive, sensing hostility. People who take access for granted might be more concerned with the brusque uniformity of standardized care, which they perceive as lacking meaning, intensity, or personalization (perhaps resonating with a lack of these qualities in bourgeois life more broadly). Contextual approaches might be valued romantically or nostalgically, or they might be valued as part of decolonization and reparation, or perhaps both; meanwhile, it takes conviction and courage to push against the powerful inertia of institutional regularity. Practices or mindsets might sound good in theory but feel wrong in the moment. The complexity of actual experience is a far cry from choosing one approach or another: there are power dynamics at play, and there is the unpredictability of bodies.

Gertrude Fraser describes how elders in an African American community in the South understood the transition away from its midwifery tradition and toward hospital birth in terms not of loss or takeover but of a broader transition to modernity, a transition that also included moving away from subsistence farming, herbal medicine, and apprenticeships. Childbearing practices were not options to be chosen so much as pieces that fit into a natural and social order: "In their view, the community has changed corporally as well as socially and economically. Things are of a piece. Home remedies no longer work because bodies are different and illnesses no longer respond to traditional remedies [nor do the right plants grow anymore]. In turn, bodies are different because the community members' relationship to the land and to God has been irretrievably altered, along with previous norms of behavior."[28] Fraser describes a traditional belief that birthing and postpartum spaces needed to be dark, since, among other things, newborn eyes are sensitive to light; this idea fell by the wayside because newborn eyes were understood to have become able to withstand bright hospital lights without damage. Bodies do not exist in a vacuum, nor do desires. As Fraser explains, "Part of the power of the ideology of science rests in its invalidation of other systems of belief and explanation," an invalidation that shapes not just what explanations have authority but what experience is possible.[29]

Rima Apple similarly describes how infant formula and bottles were taken up by "modern" White housewives in the early twentieth century as tokens of a newly scientific world in which breast milk wasn't considered to be adequate food.[30] The development of milk-evaporation machines to produce formula was part of a kaleidoscope of shifts that resulted in people beginning to conceive of their bodies as incapable of breastfeeding. A 1909 women's magazine states that although in more sheltered times women capably nursed as a matter of course, "times have changed, and in *this nervous high strung age* it often happens that a mother is not able to nurse her little ones, or even when she is it is not deemed advisable, for her or the children's health, for her to do so."[31] "Scientific" and "rational" bottle-feeding was vigorously promoted by the medical profession and the burgeoning formula industry as more healthful and hygienic, while some early feminists championed it as liberating.[32] But it is a different kind of historical empathy to recognize that women began to apprehend the resonance between their bodies and their surroundings as having changed over a generation, such that their milk would no longer nourish a baby to thrive.

In contemporary hospital births, the weight of protocols and doctors' cultural authority makes it hard not only to pursue a different course but even to *want* to pursue a different course. Even people who have a clear idea of what they would like to happen when entering a hospital for birth often accept that their choices and plans are simply no longer feasible when a doctor makes a declaration about clinical circumstances, even about something as benign as "slow progress."[33] How much truer this is in a situation declared an emergency! It takes a fierce commitment to a near birth world to act against medical recommendations, not so much because of the interpersonal power dynamics (though certainly they matter) but because of the way embodied reality can seem tenuous, susceptible to external definition. *Is* there a problem? As midwife Peggy Vincent put it in her provocative question at the Bay Area Doula Project meeting, is it a "big deal" or not to be in labor?

Regular physiology promotes a bird's-eye view of the situation, a view from outside and above: comprehensive, rigid, orderly, predictable, immutable. By contrast, approaching the body contextually is like being on the street: it is flexible, surprising, partial, idiosyncratic, fleeting, and interactive. Here I am borrowing Michel de Certeau's analogy of the difference between looking at a topographical map of a city and actually walking through that city, which he uses to describe the difference between "strategies" and "tactics" in *The Practice of Everyday Life*.[34] Strategies are organized, top-down approaches to social management by those in power, derived from a totalizing view from above. Professional Euro-American medicine has a long history of attempting to regulate unruly bodies, foremost those of women. By contrast, tactics are practices of resistance and life making that are diffuse and sporadic among those with less power. Thinking about power is highly relevant to thinking about knowledge, as the kinds of knowledge that are considered authoritative and acceptable are by and large produced by those with social power. And what is known influences what can be experienced.

The natural birth movement and its aftereffects pushed a version of contextual physiology into mainstream awareness. Women with racial and class power advanced a way of being and knowing that was not abstract or standardized but deeply enmeshed in the surroundings: not the topographical map, but the walk on the street. Evidence and intuition exemplify this turn toward lived experience in contemporary birth worlds: evidence recruits empirical, generalizable experience, and intuition subjective, situated experience. In either form, experience is different from abstract theory. Empiricism is the belief that valid knowledge arises from the senses as opposed to the supernatural, religion, or tradition. Martin Jay claims that American science is underlaid by a "cult of experience" because it is emphatically empirical. Being empirical is something intuition and evidence have in common, but ironically, in birth worlds both are applied in opposition to science, as least as science is institutionally practiced. Evidence and intuition challenge what counts as "fact." Scientific ideology has valued objectivity wherein the knower—the sensor—is in the background or erased altogether; the more theoretical and abstract the knowledge could be, the more trustworthy and valuable it was considered.[35] Intuition and evidence, however, are tactical, not strategic. They re-center the knower and the perspective on the street.

INTUITION AND EVIDENCE:
TWO MODES OF EXPERIENCE

In a nondescript 1980s office building, I gathered with a handful of other women for a meeting of the Santa Cruz Doula Salon, a smaller and somewhat tamer version of the Bay Area Doula Project. This meeting was organized around a speaker sharing her experience with Montessori philosophy on infancy; the talk was interesting, but what I remember most from the meeting was another attendee joking that "do-las" should instead be called "be-las," a quip I heard subsequently in several different contexts. All the attendees agreed that "what [mothers] need is less distraction." Doulas should just "witness" and be "inversely obtrusive" instead of taking action, as too much interference is negatively stimulating and can "stall progress." This is in direct contrast with the historical injunction that physicians should not be inactive spectators. Those at the salon insisted that birthing people require a stable environment to tune into their bodies. Doulas, through their own attunement to the situation, facilitate such an environment.[36] Is the birthing person's attunement with her world so delicate, then, I wondered?

The role of a doula, along with that of a home birth midwife, is often said to be "holding space" for the birthing person. In this protected space, the birthing person is supposedly able to tune into her surroundings, feelings, body, and baby. But the person holding space also needs to know when to step in and coach, when to step back and allow the hospital staff to do their thing, and when to intervene on behalf of her client. Will conflict protect the client's interests or be detrimental by creating bad relationships and a stressed atmosphere? There is no precise formula for such decisions. Rather, it requires intuition. Doula work is an attuned interaction not just with the other human actors but also with the circulating affects and material surroundings. Will turning the lights down help? Does she appreciate this cold washcloth on the back of her neck, or is she too distracted to tell me off? How can I ask her mother to stop talking? By navigating this scene skillfully, the doula can also (the story goes) create conditions in which the birthing person's intuition can flourish. Of course, this is often done clumsily or inexpertly, and there may be no "best" option.

In some ways intuition is deeply practical, almost utilitarian; in others, it takes on a spiritual cast. I attended a singing circle for birth workers and mothers (including aspiring ones) called Wombsong, and a frequent favorite of the group was a song about embodied knowing. The lyrics, repeated in a round, were, "Your body knows the way, heiey / And your mother, and her mother, and her mother before you / Bringing new life to be born." The advice to a childbearing person that she will "just know" what is happening or what to do is both underwhelming and overwhelming. "Just" implies passivity, but for all that the doula salon advocated "being" over "doing," intuition is an active mode. It requires a sensory attunement, which is to say becoming actively attentive to one's immediate experience, even if "doing" nothing. It comes from familiarity, or experience over time. Intuition is learned. Martin Jay claims that a tension between passive and active concepts of experience has been a theme of Euro-American epistemology—which is to say that the role of the knower in making legitimate knowledge has been a tricky issue.[37] I conceive of intuition as situated knowledge drawn from an embodied, sensory relation to the world that emphasizes the connections between things. It involves both personal and collective memory. And it is a learned skill, not an inherent ability.

The problem with the way intuition circulates in birth worlds is that the ability to practice intuitive knowing is often attributed to mothers *as a category*. Discourses around intuition are full of assumptions about gender difference and biology, including a belief that women have an intrinsic ability to connect with others that men don't, or that some kind of feminine instinct knows how to bear and rear children. As Miriam Zoila Pérez states, feminine instinct discourse is a response to the sexism of obstetrics, but it leads to fighting gender essentialism with more gender essentialism.[38] In a personal conversation, Barbara Katz Rothman proposed using the term *tacit knowledge* instead of intuition to avoid these gendered connotations. Anyone can intuit, though it might require varying degrees of effort, talent, or inclination. A carpenter can intuit how wood will behave after decades of working with it. A baker can intuit what dough needs under which conditions. People who become mothers may or may not have been inclined to practice this way of knowing/being prior to having children. Intuitive knowing/being happens in relationships other than the mother-baby one—though being co-embodied during pregnancy does start things off on intimate footing. The idea that mothers are supposed to intuitively know their bodies and their babies' bodies without any instruction or practice can quickly become oppressive or call their aptitude for motherhood into question. When intuition becomes prescriptive it constrains experience rather than encouraging attentiveness to one's experience.

Intuition figured implicitly and explicitly in the birth worlds where I spent time, but it was no one straightforward thing. I will come back to intuition's various guises, from trust in chapter 3 to instinct in chapter 5. Robbie Davis-Floyd and Elizabeth Davis analyzed intuition as authoritative knowledge in alternative birth communities nearly three decades ago. They were both in the audience when Barbara Katz Rothman gave a speech to MANA, the Midwives' Alliance of North America, in New York City in 1992, and they used this speech as a starting point for their analysis. In Rothman's words, "The history of Western obstetrics is the history of technologies of separation. We've separated milk from breasts, mothers from babies, fetuses from pregnancies, sexuality from procreation, pregnancy from motherhood. . . . It is very, very hard to conceptually put back together that which medicine has rendered asunder."[39] She continued by asserting that she has an increasingly difficult time making the meaning of connection, let alone the value of connection, understood. Davis and Davis-Floyd write that for the midwives present at the conference, this ubiquitous drive toward separation crystallized their aloneness in the world of medicine. Intuition is a way of knowing that foregrounds connection instead of separation, predicated on nearness, not distance.

Thomas Csordas likewise thinks of intuition as "embodied knowledge" and argues that healers and their patients share "a highly organized set of bodily dispositions" from which they draw sensory intuitions.[40] Intuition pertains to the present situation, not to predictive power oriented toward outcomes. In other words, it is not instrumental; it is about process more than product. Intuitive bodily knowledge can't be anticipated, even if it is anticipatory. Like contextual physiology, it is necessarily particular and internally derived, so it can't be standardized, institutionalized, or replicated, which delegitimates it in the abstracted, externalized, reproducible knowledge that characterizes what I have called regular physiology and consequently much of medical practice. Although intuition is particular to the person intuiting, it can be transpersonal: a practitioner may know her patient via her own sensorium, and a new parent may intuit her newborn's wants or needs. One can "intuit oneself" because one's self is always immersed in and constituted by what is other than oneself. Intuition is a form of paying attention to the world.

This attention is not passive or disinterested, unlike the "unbiased" or "objective" scientific gaze. I put these in quotes because scientists, of course, are active participants in gathering knowledge in ways specific to them and their field (and many have developed keen intuition for their practice). But the *idea* of what good science is has historically emphasized that the knower needs to disappear. By contrast, intuition has no pretensions against bias. Its sensibility is not about perceiving and assessing the world unidirectionally (hearing, seeing, touching) via measurable qualities (loudness, brightness, temperature); rather, it involves an interaction via the senses: hearing and making noise, looking and being observed, touching and being touched. Intuition is not tactile but haptic; it is what happens between things. Whereas anyone with the required sensory capacity can perceive, intuiting requires a degree of receptivity, a willingness to be altered and surprised. The difference between perception and intuition is in some ways analogous to that between emotion and affect. Emotion is something one person feels (or "has"), while affect is something shared between people, including publics and collectives. Just as relatively standard, clear language can be used to describe perceptions, emotion is mediated by recognizable linguistic and cultural categories; intuitions are more complicated to convey in words, as affect is hard to articulate and own.

Affects are a significant part of intuitive sensibility. William Mazzarella writes that affect implies a way of apprehending social life that does not start with the bounded, intentional subject, yet foregrounds embodiment and sensuous experience.[41] He describes how Brian Massumi "asks us to imagine social life in two simultaneous registers: on the one hand, a register of affective, embodied intensity, and on the other, a register of symbolic mediation and discursive elaboration."[42] Mediation is an interruption, an interpretation, a buffer, where meaning is conveyed through symbols and language that organize "raw" intensity. One way of describing experience is the relationship between affective and mediated registers; although experience is often mobilized as something people "have" and consider their own, it is shaped by factors external to the individual and is in many senses collective. The relation between these registers, Mazzarella writes, is one not of conformity or correspondence but of resonance, interference, amplification, and dampening.[43] Intuition's role near birth might likewise be said to resonate or interfere with more mediated ways of knowing, which in turn might amplify or dampen one's intuitive sense.

Intuition is practical, grounded in the real, but it nonetheless introduces a kind of magic into knowing. Max Weber advanced the term *disenchantment* in 1918 to describe how Enlightenment science and bureaucratic rationality superseded a worldview dominated by superstition, religion, and magic. He found science an inadequate substitute for religion since it cannot fulfill the human desire for communal belonging and transcendent values. It—not scientific knowledge per se but the culture surrounding it—leaches mystery and richness from a world it renders transparent and predictable. Disenchantment is the alienating flip side of scientific progress, he thought. He did not advocate a nostalgic return to pre-Enlightenment "enchantment" but considered the inadequacy of both science and religion to be a fundamental impasse in modern society. Marxist theorists connect this sense of alienation to the success of capitalism. Silvia Federici, mentioned above, positions the witch hunts as a crucial link between the destruction of enchanted thinking and the rise of a patriarchal, class-stratified, imperialist system.[44] Hannah Arendt linked alienation with the rise of totalitarian governments in the twentieth century. The Frankfurt School thinkers in the 1930s lamented the "destruction of experience" in the standardized, modern world. Martin Heidegger viewed modernity as the "age of the world picture" in which the experience of existing in the world is actually one of seeing the world from outside itself: god's perspective, the view from nowhere.[45] De Certeau's distinction between tactics and strategies is another version of this tension between experience and abstraction. The valorization of intuition near birth is not so much a (re)turn to the experiential, then, as a romancing of a certain idea of experience as not alienated and alienating.

. . .

Although a scientific perspective has become quasi-synonymous with the view from nowhere, its empirical roots were all about sense-data, finding truth in our physical surroundings. The complex history of ideas that shaped the culture and practice of science since the Enlightenment has profoundly shaped modern medicine; evidence figured prominently in this history and in current struggles over what counts as knowledge. Medical decision-making might seem self-evidently related to the use of evidence—good care is evidence based, while practices not based on evidence may be harmful or unnecessary, stemming from authoritative traditions rather than what is optimal for the patient. Evidence-based medicine (often abbreviated EBM) has become a dominant, if not yet fully realized, organizing paradigm for healthcare and medicine in the Western world over the past two decades. However, activists I met near birth also use evidence as a rallying point to challenge the medical community about what is optimal, and who gets to decide. Evidence is not as straightforward as it seems.

In 2008, obstetrician-anthropologist Claire Wendland argued that evidence-based obstetrics undermines beneficial care for birthing women by bypassing their experience, and that of the clinician, in favor of aggregated trial-based data that reproduces ideological biases and justifies increases in cesarean sections. In contrast, people I worked with marshaled evidence to oppose obstetric conventions around medicalized birth, such as those Wendland criticizes.[46] These reformists included parents, doulas, midwives, obstetricians, nurses, scientists, and activists—labels that are not mutually exclusive. They use the idea of evidence to push back against hospital interventions, from surgery to pharmaceuticals to monitoring, arguing that existing medical practice is based on litigation, profit, and outdated social conventions, not science. Reformists are in effect claiming that what is needed is not a different epistemology but better science on its own terms. The idea of evidence-based medicine can be appropriated to different ends, and in variable relation to the power dynamics in maternity care.

Being poorly defined yet taken for granted makes evidence both confusing and powerful. In this sense, it is a boundary object—something used in different ways by different communities, "a sort of arrangement that allows different groups to work together without consensus."[47] Boundary objects allow people to think they are talking about the same thing while often talking past each other. Evidence is responsible for conflict between biomedical and reformist orientations toward obstetrics because these communities don't necessarily mean the same thing when they use the term, but evidence can also enable cooperation, especially among reformists. To be clear, there is a robust discussion of different kinds and qualities of evidence among medical researchers (with a small but growing role for qualitative studies). But there is a more fundamental question about the role of experience in producing authoritative knowledge: does evidence mean patient outcomes, or being able to prove the cause of those outcomes? Biomedical evidence is based on experiments used to produce explanations that efface the experience of the knower: this evidence *proves cause,* especially in the case of randomized controlled trials, which are considered the gold standard of evidence-based medicine. By contrast, those who would reform obstetrics use evidence to foreground *patient outcomes,* in which the experience of the birthing person is paramount; this evidence involves getting results and effecting cures, which speak for themselves without needing to be explained.

Is evidence about explanation or efficacy? Isabelle Stengers says this has historically been the distinction between doctors, charlatans, and curers.[48] She traces how contemporary understandings of evidence came into being through social processes of consolidating authority, namely distinguishing "real" doctors from charlatans who merely pretend to be scientific, and certainly from curers who are not interested in authority but only with getting results. Authoritative evidence came to mean evidence that could be used in service of an abstract theory, an explanation. Simply effecting a cure could be due to randomness, the placebo effect, luck, or skill—none of which are scientific. And medicine, as the least scientific of the sciences since it is dependent on the messy and fluctuating human body, has historically been concerned with demonstrating its scientific legitimacy. Without being able to offer an explanatory rationale, evidence is just experience.

Since empirical science came into being, experimentation, objectivity, and recordkeeping have been important factors shaping whose experience counts as evidence.[49] Experimentation developed as part of an elitist gentleman's club that functioned as the earliest scientific gatekeeping, determining who could be a reliable witness to experimental results. And objectivity was part of a movement to distinguish between artistic and scientific truth, which prior to the Enlightenment had been quite aligned (think of Leonardo da Vinci); scientific truth erased the knower and sought a generalized view from nowhere, while artistic truth foregrounded the knower and came to be seen as personal expression. Recordkeeping began as bookkeeping, a way of proving what happened in increasingly complex merchant accounts, which became seen as a type of fact belonging to economics and business, not science proper, because science uses records in service of testing and proving hypotheses. Records are rational but not scientific.

A regular feature of MANA conferences is an update on the MANA Stats Project. Melissa Cheyney, an anthropologist as well as home birth midwife, began the project and urges members to keep records (which most do anyway) and submit them to be aggregated in the database. MANA's collection of statistics starts in 2004 and numbered over a hundred thousand cases by 2016. The point of the project is to use data to show that home birth and midwifery care are safe and beneficial when rates of various mortalities and morbidities are compared with hospital/obstetric care. At the 2012 MANA conference, Cheyney exclaimed that "midwifery is the only intervention ever proven to reduce prematurity!" It's a strange way to phrase it. Since then, I began noticing the ubiquitous term *evidence-based* used to challenge hospital protocols, justify controversial decisions, consolidate surety, and persuade. It sometimes seems an almost requisite language with which to discuss decisions and preferences. This trend revives the practical empiricism of midwives who operated without formal training or protocols, learning instead through hands-on methods like apprenticeships. Such midwives necessarily do much of their work by observing what practices generate which outcomes—that is, they are empiricists, and indeed recordkeeping has long been a cornerstone of home birth midwifery. It seems to me that one could generally substitute "outcomes-based" for "evidence-based" in reformist discourse. Reformist appeals to evidence, including MANA stats, are claims to rationality as opposed to superstition, magic, emotional intelligence, faith/belief, or other kinds of nonauthoritative knowing often associated with midwifery, especially historically.

Reformist activism is beginning to redirect the focus of "good research" onto the patient's perspective. To the extent that maternal satisfaction and postpartum well-being are becoming counted as outcomes, instead of outcomes being limited to standard mortality/morbidity rates, the potential to challenge "regular" protocols using empirical evidence grows. At the end of her piece, Stengers calls for a re-valorization of curers and the nonrational, incorporating their contributions alongside those of doctors. This is what is taking shape in contemporary Bay Area maternity care, when obstetricians join midwives in seeking empirically good outcomes no matter their rationale—though it is not always palatable to the obstetric system. Curers "are not haunted by the idea of being able to disqualify others" but have cultivated an "influencing practice."[50] Stengers asks if modern medicine does not indeed have something to learn from them. One of the older midwives I spoke with explained to me that "pre-stats" she and her cohort just had a feeling that home birth was okay. They didn't feel the need to prove it, nor to consolidate a best practice, as "the nature of midwifery appeals to independent minds, and there will be diverse opinions. . . . We practice from our own innate wisdom, not protocols." Such wisdom is a type of influencing practice, which is its own kind of expertise.

Demanding evidence-based practices is a relatively palatable way to reconcile contextual and relational physiology. Empirical outcomes are at least theoretically important in both frameworks, and no one is against evidence. This is where the term's power comes from. Yet it is being used to subtly undermine medical institutions as they are currently organized—sometimes through deliberate curation and selection of evidence, but often through a genuinely alternative understanding of it. Proponents of activism via evidence are, in effect, using one of medicine's totems against itself, challenging it on what they perceive to be its own terms. This activism gets drawn into social politics, as well—how could it not? When evidence-based care gets conflated with being the decision maker about one's body, as it often does, we are talking about autonomy.

———

THREE

Autonomy

NEGOTIATING TRUST AND CONTROL
IN THE BIRTH ROOM

DANI HAD JUST RETURNED FROM WORK in Santa Cruz when I met her to chat about the birth of her baby, Serena. She showed me around her two-acre farm with its yurt and leafy outdoor bathroom while we waited for Jonah, her husband, to join us. He had picked up two-month-old Serena from his parents' house on his way home from teaching at UC Santa Cruz. We talked in their orchard at dusk, under the fruiting avocado trees and next to blackberry brambles that had just passed their season. Leaves crunched underfoot as we shifted from hammock to chair and back again. The baby gurgled and cooed. When the sun had set completely, we made our way into the yurt, its angle-less interior warmed by a yellow light that was bewitchingly cozy. I was not aware of this idyllic agricultural lane where they made their home, merely a few hundred yards from Highway 17 and its notorious narrow curves, reckless drivers, and traffic jams of pleasure seekers.

Dani and Jonah introduced their birth by saying they "went the traditional medical Western route, although in Santa Cruz that's pretty different." Indeed. Dani was attended by a nurse midwife and had a vaginal birth despite her baby being breech (feet first). She had had a successful external cephalic version, a rare practice in which a practitioner manually rotates the baby in the womb by pressing from outside.[1] She was unmedicated throughout the entire labor and birth (with the exception of Cervidil, a vaginally inserted cervical softener that is a "gentle induction" alternative to Pitocin), and she breastfeeds exclusively. Yet compared to their friends Kim and Paul, whom I had interviewed earlier, her experience was conventional:

JONAH: We [and our friends] have these insanely parallel lives: mirrored partner roles, professional interests, got pregnant and had babies the same weeks, but they chose to go like total hippie style. They never had a sonogram, basically didn't enter a Western medical facility *at all*—

DANI: And we were having sonograms like every three weeks, nonstress tests, low fluids . . .

JONAH: First she was breech, but [home birth] midwives can figure that out. They would've known, it wasn't like they were clueless, but there's a lot that will not be known if you don't take blood samples and, you know, do sonograms. There's a whole lot of risk involved there, and [our friends] just were like, psssh.

DANI: We wanted to know. I wanted to know *everything*. I got all the blood tests, I wanted to know if my kid was gonna have Down's syndrome, and yes, I would have aborted. . . . I wanted to know, so I could make those informed decisions.

JONAH: Risk management was basically in my mind.

Dani and Jonah were making decisions about bodily management based on assessments of how, what, and whom to trust, and what kind and amount of control is agreeable. Kim and Paul, who had a home birth, were making the same assessments but came to different conclusions. Dani and Jonah collected external knowledge via medical testing in order to manage risk and make informed decisions. Kim and Paul trusted that by turning their attention inward they could learn all they needed about their pregnancy, bodies, and child, and they were frustrated when friends and family called the validity of this kind of knowledge into question. You will see the continuity here with regular and contextual ways of approaching physiology; implicit beliefs about physiology influence what it seems reasonable to want to trust or control, and considerations of trust and control influence what conceptions of physiology make sense and feel comfortable. Whether deciding where to birth, which professionals to have nearby, how their partner will be involved, or which procedures to undergo, trust and control are key. Trust and control are, in my analysis, inverses: trust requires relinquishing control, and control comes from mastering that which is not trustworthy. Being able to make such decisions is deeply entwined with the value of autonomy.

Autonomy literally means self-naming. Authoring one's own story, giving oneself a chosen identity, and shaping one's own destiny are key to American culture. Study after study show that people are satisfied with their births when they feel they have been respected during the process, and the key to feeling respected is feeling consulted and acknowledged, and thus able to participate actively in the experience. It matters far less what the actual procedures or outcomes are. People want a healthy baby, of course, but this insight about respect separates process from product, evaluating process on its own terms instead of subordinating it to the medical liability mindset that process can control products. Childbearing people make efforts to author their experience by determining how to trust, and how to control (or retrospectively interpret their experiences using these lenses). This is how they navigate the inevitable themes of risk, pain, fear, and power near birth.

I met Dani, Jonah, Kim, and Paul in the Mindfulness-Based Childbirth Education class taught by Roxanne, the celebrated midwife mentioned in chapter 1. One of the first questions she asked the class was "Who likes to be in control and fix things? What are you like when you're not in control, when things don't go your way?" She explained that many people, particularly those socialized as men, want to fix problems, but that the birth process requires letting go of that desire and simply bearing mindful witness to a strange and intense situation. Roxanne asserted that different personalities are differently suited to the inherent nature of labor; or rather, they have more or less work to do to accept that labor cannot be controlled. "The only way out is through" was a common refrain that I encountered throughout fieldwork, a phrase that invokes surrender, acceptance, and, perhaps paradoxically, the power and will to continue on. In later classes, Roxanne discussed the sorts of available medical interventions and their uses and benefits, and we practiced coping with discomfort by having the pregnant person hold her hand in ice water and try various things to help her accept the sensation: breathing intentionally, receiving massage or affirming words, or practicing a kind of dissociated awareness or nonattachment. In other words, we practiced ways to trust the body that require control of one's anxieties and doubts, and ways to exert control over the body that require trust in medical systems. The class was, in some ways, a preparation for developing tactics of trust and control—that is, tactics of autonomy.

Throughout this book I am interested in how critiques developed on the cultural fringes speak back to dominant interpretations of cultural values, so in this chapter I focus on how people implement contextual understandings of physiology and assert divergence from the inertia of medically managed childbearing. I compare three Santa Cruz couples, all of whom were deeply committed to lifestyles and childbearing decisions they saw as an alternative to conventional practice. The third couple is Sarah and Roger, who birthed at home, like Kim and Paul, but had the experience closest to an unassisted birth of all the people I came across. Free birth, as unassisted birth is often called, is extremely uncommon (though its proponents are disproportionately vocal). I interviewed each couple at different points in their childbearing process—Kim and Paul before the birth, Dani and Jonah shortly after, and Sarah and Roger when their baby was toddling around—and our lives were somewhat entwined in the local community. They were all White and middle-class, with access to family resources even if they did not have much money themselves. They each crafted an approach to their own bodies (and those of their babies) that managed risk, handled pain, confronted fear, and sought power.

RISK: AUTONOMY AS DELIBERATIVE

Kim described to me how she was challenged about her decision to forgo the medical testing Dani sought out and instead trust her intuition. She and Paul met with me in their bungalow a few blocks from the beach, welcoming me on the wide front porch with a summer concoction of blended juices and herbs. Kim was late in her pregnancy but didn't look too uncomfortable in her sundress and sandals as we sat down at the backyard table, their wire-haired dog making his bed at our feet. They were planning a home birth and really excited about it. Much of our discussion revolved around their pride, pleasure, and determination to look inward for all aspects of the pregnancy and birth, and how they negotiated the backlash that their stance caused among their friends and family, who found such trust risky. Kim described how her intuition enabled her to know the baby's position and her belief that she didn't need technological confirmation of the fact.

> I feel like I have been operating on intuition the whole pregnancy because I've really been, like we have done very few tests. And you know, that's been something I've really had to check in with . . . trusting that everything's okay, and that I would know if it's not okay, you know? And that hasn't always been easy. . . . I was like, "I really feel I know the position of this baby, being head down. I'm very clear on that." And people were being like, "You should confirm the position with an ultrasound, be 100 percent," and I'm like, "Well, I've had five midwives palpate my stomach, acupuncturists . . . and I just *know*. I can close my eyes and visualize the baby, and I have the confidence to just trust that." And it's like, "What if it's breech, or what if it's this and that."

She also shared how well-meaning friends' insistence that intuitive knowledge is not enough caused her insecurity and doubt:

With the gestational diabetes, [my midwife friend says,] "I see women every day who are completely healthy, eat this and that, everything's normal in their pregnancy, and they come out with gestational diabetes. It's just something you *wouldn't* intuit" . . . and it gets in my head, and there's definitely been a lot of things I've been challenged on.

Kim said that she has never thought of herself as a radical but has simply decided "as things have arisen" that she doesn't find procedures necessary because she feels "good and confident." That feeling has in turn "boosted" her intuition and confidence. Nonetheless, she said she would feel validated in trusting those instincts after having a "good birth and a healthy baby," because "it haunts you" to think about having possibly been able to prevent something if only a test had been done. But, she said, "I haven't really let that seep in."

Kim and Paul were pressed to provide reasons and engage with statistics about their decision to birth at home, even by supportive friends. It was not so much that Kim and Paul were uninterested in information as that they found different kinds of information relevant and compelling, information that they sourced via attunement and inward attention. Yet in a world where risk is paramount and only certain kinds of information have authority, they had to be translators. When I asked Kim how she had explained her intuition to people, she said that she didn't use that language with everyone and had to justify herself with numbers and "hands-on" information instead.

> KIM: I don't live in a world that's completely, where I'm interacting with only, like, spiritual people who live in that reality. I feel like most people in my life are very practical minded, very scientific minded, so . . . I feel like I've had to, you know, back up some of those decisions. . . . "We've done these kinds of measurements," there's a lot of like hands-on things.
>
> PAUL: We've heard the heartbeat.
>
> KIM: Yeah, "We've listened to the heart tones, we get all the same information that you would get with an ultrasound without doing the ultrasound." Just kinda like have to put it more in that language. But some people really understand the intuition piece, and other people just think it's really bogus if you're like, "I just *feel* like it's a boy." They're like, "That means nothing." So I'd say it's a full spectrum, and I'd say in this town you certainly do have a lot of people that speak that language of intuition. So I just kind of gauge it.

Because medical control is hegemonic in most childbearing situations in the United States, it requires a fair amount of active cultivation to make space for intuition. Kim "gauged" whom she was talking to and how they might react. Some non-intervention childbirth preparation courses teach childbearing people how to deal with those who approach birth with risk at the forefront: the Bradley Method, more popular in past decades, encourages a very defensive and almost aggressive stance on the part of parents entering a hospital, while hypnobirthing, a more recent method for which I sat in on a series of courses, encourages parents to keep a bubble around themselves throughout the pregnancy where no negative stories or critical questions are tolerated. It would have recommended shutting down or leaving social situations like the ones Kim was describing, a tactic that Kim herself eventually came to embrace. Kim grew up in the Midwest, where most of her family still lived, and she said that there, home birth is very uncommon.

> Their initial reactions, my parents were very like, "It seems like an unnecessary risk. It seems selfish, like you're making it all about the mother when it should be about the baby." All these things which did make me feel very defensive. And my mother had two C-sections, [and] her own birth she was born premature, so all her experiences have been birth as a medical emergency, not birth as a natural nonmedical experience. So she had all her fears and anxieties. That was hard for me because I felt like, you know, at first I was wanting to educate my family, sending them materials, then that started to really feel draining to me and put me on the defense a lot, and so I was really more just like, "I'm very confident in this decision, I don't want to discuss it anymore, I want support, and if not then keep your mouth shut."

Going home to a baby shower made her anxious because she knew everyone was curious, and "even when it's genuine curiosity, not criticism, I still felt like I had to be defensive." She tried to ask people to do their own research because the pressure was exhausting: "I had to be this expert.... Of course you go through waves of having fears or anxieties of your own, and I felt I couldn't express those fears or anxieties. I felt like I just had to project pure confidence, and be like everything's great, fine, perfect, smooth."

Kim said that communicating with her family had been a process, "something I had to work on and heal," but that they were now more supportive and understood the situation better. She laughed and said, "It's not like a little old lady showing up with a towel!" She elaborated that home birth midwives have "more experience with birth than any obstetrician" because obstetricians don't learn about natural birth anymore. "[Midwives] show up with equipment. We live two blocks from the hospital. Most things you can detect pretty early on if there's issues." Kim didn't deny that there was an element of risk; she just had decided that she was managing it appropriately.

Risk and safety were evoked by Kim's parents and friends in a coercive way, though not malevolently. They referenced common cultural discourses of risk, which are loaded with worst-case scenarios and moral judgments of self-centeredness.

Discourses of risk are ubiquitous in and around medical settings. In the past fifty years, monitoring, imaging, and testing technologies have majorly changed the landscape of risk around childbearing by providing more forms of standardized knowledge. This includes things like fetal monitors during labor, ultrasounds of the fetus, and amniocentesis screenings for genetic disorders. The widespread embrace of these technologies is partially a continuation of the "light of progress" historical fantasy, whereby technology, professionalism, and medical institutions increase safety and improve outcomes on a unidirectional track. Discourses of risk are compelling, easily capitalized upon, and hard for the consumer/patient to disregard. Diagnostic tests, monitoring, and prescription drugs are used based on how they fit into calculations of risk, not how they alleviate present complaints. Increasingly, health itself is understood as the mitigation of risk, measured via the likelihood of potential problems instead of an actual state of well-being.

Risk-oriented technologies also change the experience of personhood and expertise. Margarete Sandelowski discusses how fetal monitors direct nurses to pay attention to machines instead of patients and orient their expertise around doctors. Nurses become technicians, and the monitor readouts prime evidence of liability.[2] A range of work across the sociology and philosophy of science discusses how ultrasounds and their ubiquitous first photographs make the fetus exist in public, undermining the pregnant person's exclusive relationship and contributing to trends to see the fetus as a separate patient.[3]

Rima Apple chronicles how the aspiration to be a perfect mother has guided American childbearing through all its transitions over the twentieth century, though this aspiration has entailed different things in different decades. In earlier decades, submitting to expert authority and scientific management was paramount, yet the most recent period is characterized by the idea that science and medicine should be used to guide, not dictate, what one does as a mother, highlighting the increasing importance placed on deliberative autonomy.[4] Emily Martin clearly lays out how "it is because the [laboring] woman is really thought of as someone to control that scientific management strategies are thought to be appropriate."[5] Physicians built up a set of practices around the idea that they should not be inactive spectators, and in so doing made childbearing people into inactive spectators—an idea whose time has faded away. Yet navigating still requires a guide, and risk is one of its key principles. When risk seems murky, both evidence and intuition are ways that childbearing people find their way. *What does the evidence say? What does my gut tell me?* Claiming the authority to navigate one's path starts to be its own advice, its own compulsion. It is not simply about choice, because choice is passive in its own way; rather, autonomy in childbearing is about *the process by which one chooses.*

Ivan Illich claims that past a certain threshold, technological advances cease to be useful and indeed change from serving human needs to causing humans to orient around the technology.[6] Consider transportation: the railroads were explosively useful, yet the personal automobile dominates our lives. Or medicine: penicillin, sterile techniques, and blood transfusions have been phenomenally helpful, but many newer drugs, tests, and technologies dominate the clinical encounter and obscure the foundational aspects of health and healing. Illich also writes about iatrogenic illnesses, those that originate from medicine itself, a significant issue with birth interventions.[7] Tech past a certain point mostly offers an illusion of control; consider the proliferating prenatal genetic testing options, which, for one thing, don't necessarily follow through on their hyped-up claims (and are concerning from a disability justice standpoint), but moreover distract from environmental toxins that damage sperm and egg quality in the first place, or the social conditions that encourage delayed childbearing. Writing about amniocentesis and other prenatal genetic testing, Rayna Rapp shows how it's not always clear what purpose such information serves (for example, women are given tests even if they would do nothing differently based on the result), and it can introduce more worries than it assuages.[8] Whereas genetic testing information was useful for Dani (who would have aborted), Kim found it burdensome: "I don't even want that information, because I don't know what I would really do with it."

Trusting in the efficacy of technological management was a primary draw to hospitals among those I spoke with, even for those hoping to birth without interventions, most of whom could have afforded a home birth if they had wished. The ubiquitous idea that the hospital is the safest place to give birth is predicated on access to emergency equipment and procedures. "What if something goes wrong?" was a common phrase I heard. But, given that most births are not emergencies, routine care in the hospital was subject to negotiation. This often pitted childbearing people against hospital staff and protocols. Who allows whom? Which party has a preference instead of a requirement? Who can force the other to comply? These struggles do not necessarily mean either party is acting without the best intentions (though the history of medical racism and misogyny means that sometimes they are).[9] Rather, these confrontations can stem from different attitudes toward risk, which stem from different orientations toward trust and control, which stem from different conceptions of physiology.

The confrontations are also practical: hospital staff are not usually trained in how *not* to use technology. For example, despite there being scant evidence about any benefit in outcomes from continuous fetal monitoring, electric heart rate monitors belted around laboring bellies are ubiquitous, and many nurses' workflow revolves around watching monitor readouts from another room. Vanishingly few practitioners know how to use a fetoscope, a kind of funnel used to manually hear the fetal heartbeat (the tool Kim and Paul's home birth midwife used). Not coincidentally, fetoscopes are much cheaper than monitoring systems, just as home births are much cheaper than hospital births and external versions are a much cheaper way to handle a breech baby than surgery—but in a privatized medical system oriented around profits for medical industries, cost-effectiveness is not actually a virtue. To return to the point, hospital staff often believe that technological risk management is the best form of care and may not be able to operate outside set protocols that foreground technology, whether because of limited knowledge or legal constraints. This is slowly changing. Intermittent monitoring is often an option for low-risk births, and some medical professionals are deliberately avoiding continuous fetal monitoring because excessive medical surveillance actually increases medical risk; Kellie Owens calls this approach a "risk counterculture."[10]

In contrast to Kim and Paul, Dani and Jonah pushed against technological interventions from within the hospital. A little after Dani's due date, one of her nonstress tests came back with alarming results. For their midwife, Alix, who was generally amenable to natural birth, there were too many concerning factors suggesting the need for intervention: being past forty-two weeks, having low amniotic fluid, the fact that the baby had been breech before being turned, and the presence of a large cyst on Dani's placenta throughout the pregnancy, the likes of which no one had seen before. The test result tipped the scale and Alix told Dani that she needed to be induced immediately. But Dani, who had been having these tests done every week for months, felt sure that the test was run improperly. In Jonah's paraphrase of her reaction, "Your person just [messed] up, the kid was asleep, they put the things on me wrong . . . you've gotta redo it." Furthermore, the smaller, more intimate, and low-intervention hospital where Dani and Jonah had been receiving care was full at that time, and they hated the idea that they would have to be induced at the higher-intervention, more mainstream hospital down the road. So the test was rerun at Dani's insistence and it came back with "totally reassuring results." Jonah explained that Dani "had the confidence to basically push back on what allopathic medicine is most known for, which is being like, 'The numbers told us this! And we have to avoid lawsuits immediately.' . . . Most people don't advocate for themselves or have the confidence that something else is possible or probable." Indeed, Dani had cultivated her intuition through months of experience and was able to assert it and be taken seriously (something enabled by her several kinds of privilege).

Dani and Jonah negotiated with medical insistence on technological risk control. They were committed to not having unnecessary interventions, as are many people, but they actively negotiated with their provider about what counted as necessary. They agreed to be induced because of the list of risk factors, but only when they could get into the smaller hospital a day or so later and using a cervical softening method that was gentler than the use of Pitocin. They recognized that providers are not the voice of infallible authority but negotiating their own values and structural constraints. In his retelling, Jonah recognized Alix as doing a balancing act; he thought she was "obviously a wonderful person," but "Western medicine's very litigiously minded and risk averse. . . . They're dealing with trade-offs." According to his impression, medical providers have to compromise on what they think might be the best course of action because they are vulnerable to lawsuits; this undermined Jonah's trust in their expertise. His and Dani's strategy was to filter their interactions with this in mind.

In medical law, although providers are more likely to be punished for intervening too much during pregnancy (causing a miscarriage, for example), they are also often punished for intervening too little during birth (remember, physicians should not be inactive spectators). From a patient perspective, trusting medical institutions is different from trusting a particular medical professional. You may like your own doctor, but she may not be able to act outside the institution that constrains her (for better or worse). Trusting medically managed childbearing involves both the idea that a large-scale institution with a standardized and regularized practice is the best source of guidance (or at least a reliable one), and a faith in science as a method of knowing. It becomes complicated when the science contradicts the institutional imperatives, a tangle that evidence is being used to sort through, as discussed above.

FEAR: AUTONOMY AS COURAGEOUS

Sarah and Roger, the third couple in this chapter, didn't bother with such negotiation over risk. They cultivated an experiential reality in which inwardly sourced qualitative information was all that mattered and they put no stock in external, professional, or technological expertise. They lived in a small studio in the mountains with their son, Gabriel, who was eight months old when I interviewed them. Their humble house was in disarray and they were full of laughter as we talked and made pancakes, the rosy, chubby Gabriel amusing himself under their attentive watch. During the two and a half hours that we chatted, and as I got to know them better in the following months, it became clear that their attention and priorities, particularly Sarah's, revolved around Gabriel. The structure of their work and home lives was the least conventional and stable of the three couples, and their rejection of medical management the most complete. Sarah had been raised in a family that embraced Waldorf/Steiner philosophy and eschewed institutionalized medicine entirely, and Roger worked teaching survival skills and nature connection to groups of kids, college students, and adults. It was beyond obvious to them that they wanted to birth at home, and Sarah was effusive about how wonderful it had been.

After showing me a photo album of Gabriel's first six months, and after I had washed some dishes and rinsed the cast-iron pan, Sarah talked about her midwife, Marion. "She's really carrying the old lineage of looking at birth, and I don't know that anyone else in the area is really doing what she's doing anymore." When I asked what that meant, she said, "She looks at birth as a rite of passage for the mother and father. . . . She wasn't coming as a doctor, she was coming as a witness to the process of transformation we were going through." This orientation is very different from that of most midwives—or even doulas—and contributes to me viewing Sarah and Roger's birth as practically unassisted despite the presence of a midwife. Marion's approach involved lots and lots of listening, they said, and sharing exercises to develop Sarah and Roger's imagination and awareness about what the transformation would have in store for them and how they felt about it.

She was completely, um, aware. Of what a big transformation [birth is] on all levels of the human being, the body, the whole emotional life, your identity as a person, and that felt amazing; it didn't feel like having a doctor coming to check on you. She would do the little things of feeling where everything was at, weighing, you know, the basics of checking on the process, and that was it. . . . We entered this relationship from the beginning that would then be the basis for the birth experience. It was incredible, totally incredible. It felt like someone was taking our hands and slowly guiding us toward this transformative experience.

Only a few weeks before the due date, Marion brought information in the form of a "beautiful, simple birth preparation presentation," Ina May Gaskin's book *Spiritual Midwifery,* which she recommended for its birth stories, as well as some videos that her daughter had taken at births Marion had attended as a midwife. Sarah explained, "She really focused on the fact that each birth is a unique experience for the parents, and not to get a lot of ideas about what it is, or what you're going to 'do' during it." It turned out that Gabriel was born sunny-side up, meaning rotated backward, and Marion didn't even notice until watching the video footage later. Clearly, it was not an issue for anyone present, which, when Sarah told me about it, was precisely her point. Marion gave them practically no preparation for what to expect as a physiological or medical process, no counseling on choices, no discussions of possible outcomes, yet Sarah and Roger both emphasized how prepared they felt. I was surprised at their assertion that their neighbors, who birthed at the small, well-loved progressive hospital with a doula, seemed shockingly unprepared by contrast. Roger said, "Our neighbors were saying all the information they were getting was all the scary things that could go wrong," to which Sarah added, "and all the opinions that are just the current medical opinion on what you're supposed to do for this and that, which—is irrelevant."

Sarah's indifference to medical opinion was bolstered by talking about infant care with others, notably her friend who had been a lactation consultant for decades at the large hospital in town, who told her about current opinions but followed up with, "You know, we actually don't know a lot about milk, and about the relationship between mother and baby," which Sarah said "felt so honest and true." She also talked with a few mothers she respected, each with four or five children, who emphasized that each child had completely different needs around sleep, nursing, birthing, and other activities. Marion responded to her questions about breastfeeding with,

"I hear that you're asking the question, and that's what's important. You're in a relationship with your baby. . . . Try asking your baby." Sarah said Marion never told her she was doing something wrong or advised her what she should do instead, but rather said, "I celebrate and honor you for being in the question. Search toward that." When I commented that that sounded empowering because it didn't suggest that there was an ideal that she was failing to achieve, Sarah exclaimed her agreement. "Yeah! Because what I found out from talking to all those people is that there is no one right way."

Marion's nonanswer helped Sarah feel that instead of going to a doctor, she was "going to an elder, who's celebrating the process I'm in, and helping guide me toward health through that process." To find out what Gabriel needed, Sarah in effect conducted her own empirical experiments. She talked a lot about how important tracking is, seeing what factors get what results. Through guessing and checking, she and Roger learned how to intuit their baby's needs, which was evident during our breakfast. They also talked at length about how Gabriel learned about his world through observation, experimentation, and attentiveness by doing his own tracking of patterns and results. They elaborated on how this is a natural behavior of all children if they are not stifled by overmediating caretakers. They were both very attentive to him, though they largely didn't play with or talk to him; at one point Sarah looked over at him and said, "You're pooping. That's good." I was intrigued and asked her how she knew, and she imitated the telltale grimace for me. They rejected the idea that infant behavior is ever "just what happens." She said, "If you ask your question and you get a really cookie-cutter answer, you get a skinny, crying baby."

They explicitly stated that they had a lot more trust than most people; they embraced it as a general attitude.

ROGER: We realized who [Marion] was used to dealing with: people who just don't understand how to tune into babies or tune into the learning process and grow.

SARAH: And to trust life. We just live our lives out of a lot of trust rather than out of a lot of fear and control. And so we were approaching birth completely from that perspective. Wow, this is crazy and big and I fully trust this process.

As Sarah and Roger readily noted, their attitude toward trust is uncommon. Partially, this rarity is due to the ubiquity and power of risk rhetoric. Hearing someone say—or even imply—that your baby is at risk is immensely persuasive because of the fear it stimulates, and this is all the more true if it is said by someone with cultural authority, like a doctor. Fear is closely related to guilt and shame, which abound near birth, especially regarding mothers' choices and abilities.[11] Rejecting fear does not prevent it, of course, but it frees one to use other considerations as guides for action. To the extent that fear-based decisions are an unspoken default in contemporary American culture, particularly around parenting, it requires intentional self-positioning around alternative values and affects.[12]

Childbearing involves a fear of the unknown since it is treated so privately. In much of America it is an isolated experience; many people have not seen a birth or breastfeeding or cared for infants until they have their own. I usually asked clients or childbearing interviewees if they had ever seen a birth before, even of an animal, and the vast majority said no. In my experience, although I had seen cats, cattle, and horses give birth, the first time I attended a human birth (as a doula) was nonetheless striking. Media representations of birth are often sensationalizing and inaccurate and emphasize pain and panic. The lack of knowledge or experience around what to expect or what is even possible creates a vulnerability to fear. When coupled with the way risk dominates medical approaches, this fear becomes immanent, and thus something people have to negotiate quite actively. People who have had children before but had a negative experience may be fearful of repeating it. Fear is not only a factor for childbearing people; providers are likely afraid of lawsuits but perhaps also of feeling out of control or responsible for negative outcomes. Particularly for doctors, who are socialized to be experts and saviors, fear is an inappropriate emotion usually alleviated through technocratic management.

Preparing a birth plan has become a trend and trope among middle-class birthing people. In creating a birth plan, pregnant people (sometimes with the input of partners, doulas, or family members) come up with a list of instructions about procedures they do or do not want done, and under what circumstances. Learning about what to expect and developing a sense of agency allows people to feel more in control, and thereby manage fear differently than by cultivating trust. But planning the experience is difficult, both because there are so many factors in the hospital environment that are outside one's control and because birthing bodies are unpredictable. The idea that emotions have a strong impact on physiology, or that childbearing embodiment can be naturally intuited, can lead to blaming oneself if one's physiology appears to malfunction (tying in with broader cultural mother blame): one didn't trust enough or wasn't able to subdue fear.

There has been a movement for doulas to use the term *birth wishes* or *birth intentions* instead of birth plan to mark this inability to maintain control and to avoid setting someone up for failure. The phrasing is a concession to bodily unpredictability but also to the hospital environment, where experts often refuse to be controlled by a patient. It accedes to a power hierarchy from the get-go, whereby patients have wishes but staff are responsible for needs. The idea that there might be an explicit struggle for control is common in birth worlds—birthing people are told they might need to stand up to the hospital staff and defend their rights, and providers talk disparagingly about combative patients—but in practice, the confrontations I experienced were much more subdued. There were tensions, but they were undergirded by exhaustion and uncertainty. What does it look like to stand up for yourself when you want a good outcome but you're not sure how to achieve it and you've also been awake and in pain for the past thirty hours? Giving consent is crucial for feeling a sense of autonomy, yet the birth room is a very difficult environment in which to do so because of the power dynamics and physiological intensity. I've described doula work as facilitating *attuned consent*, which acknowledges ambiguity and complexity, pays close attention to nonverbal communication while being highly embodied, and is noncoercive without presuming equality—an aspirational ideal for doulas and many who would like to see better births.[13]

Doula circles I was familiar with prioritized good relationships with hospital staff, which partially has to do with contextual physiology ideas about how the birthing body responds to surrounding emotional tensions. In turn, the hospitals I experienced were trying to be more accommodating of patients with opinions, who were in any case becoming more common, in a kind of give-and-take dialectic over control. In practice, the birth plan seemed to indicate a general approach more than any specific set of procedural preferences. There was a standard set of requests: no induction, no epidural, not to be offered pain medication or be asked about pain level, minimal cervical checks, having mobile or intermittent monitoring, skin-to-skin contact after birth, not offering the baby any bottles, formula, or sugar water, not bathing the baby, leaving the waxy vernix, and waiting to do vitamin K shots and eye cream, among others. Indeed, many of these preferences have recently become supported by evidence and have become part of many hospitals' new standard protocols.

Medical providers also are called upon to balance trust and control in the power relationships around birth. One hospital midwife explained that when she teaches childbirth education, she shows the expectant parents the giant epidural needle and all manner of medical implements and fully discloses their side effects, such as that an epidural can lead to lifelong lower back pain. She said, "Ignorance is bliss. The moms won't even see the needle go in; do they really need to know what it looks like? But knowledge is power. I walk that line in teaching." She explained how her training at UCSF emphasized ethics, particularly for underserved populations, and mused about the possibility of truly informed consent, or fully unbiased presentation of facts; she was comfortable admitting that neither ever happen in a medical setting, "but you have to think about it." She felt she was helping childbearing people by familiarizing them with the complexity of the situation: the sight of the tools, the feel of the plastic, the potentials that cling to them for relief and damage.

In doula training we were encouraged not only to give information about procedures and options, but also to cultivate a conversation about hopes and fears, including about parenting, one's own childhood, experiences with trauma or abuse, and the relationship with one's partner. These conversations could become pretty intimate but were considered necessary to help people make decisions and enter into the birth experience with a sense of autonomy. Sometimes, people had hopes or fears that foreclosed certain kinds of conversations and information, as was the case for Sarah and Roger. They described feeling fear and repulsion about hospitals and rigorously protected a bubble around Sarah where no fearful or negative language was welcome, even from Marion, because she felt "so open right now." She quite literally felt that fear-inducing information would compromise her and her baby's safety.

Birth plans are a rational tool, and as much as they might incorporate hopes and fears in their design, they are ineffective at preparing people for the affects that have such sway in the birth room. Hospitals are spaces of surveillance and hierarchy, no matter how empathetic individual providers might be. For most people hospitals are unfamiliar and disorienting if not alarming on a sensory level. Once fear is invoked, usually through language about risk and brusque, authoritative manners, it is almost impossible to resist the flow of interventions. A doula colleague said she can't work in hospitals anymore because she just sees them as sites of abuse; hospital births become a no-exit situation where consent is at best perfunctory and at worst actually impossible.

Programs like hypnobirthing, which I was surprised to find is fairly popular despite it initially sounding improbable to me, help a childbearing person develop the ability to tune out external information. As I learned through assisting with an eight-week course, students of hypnobirthing learn to associate a relaxed and disconnected mental state with certain triggers like audio recordings, smells, or visualizations, often pertaining to a favorite place, so they can call that mental state into being at will. This basic technique is used more widely than hypnobirthing programs, too. This cultivated mental state is a buffer between the person and the hospital (doulas can also serve as such a buffer). These programs usually recommend keeping a negativity-free bubble around the parents, as Sarah and Roger did for themselves. Both are tactics to stave off fear.

Doula work is often promoted with language about a nonfearful way of relating. For example, an email targeted at doulas from the Wisdom Way Institute asked if its reader was "looking for a career grounded in love and compassion?" and described a way of being with another person wherein "I'm not pulling away from you, manipulating you, or shielding myself from you. I'm not fearful, I'm not averse, I'm willing to meet you." In my own experience and that of others I spoke with, this work of "meeting" required a tricky relationship to one's own ego. There is something selfless about bearing witness to another, but it requires a confident solidity that comes from comfort with oneself, and no need to either self-negate or self-aggrandize. Knowing yourself allows you to know if the all-important fit is right with a potential client, which many doulas discussed in terms of intuition.

Sarah and Roger's home birth midwife, Marion, was like a doula in this respect. She had to meet them where they were while also setting her own boundaries. When they were talking about potentially needing to transfer to the hospital because they were a good half hour away by car, Sarah and Roger said they had friends who lived right next to the hospital and they could stay there if anything seemed concerning. In Sarah's words, Marion "knew I would only agree to go to hospital under the most dire circumstances, so she was afraid I would resist going, and if I really needed to go it would get into a too-late situation." Marion did agree that the majority of conditions leading to transfers don't really require hospitals, like "failure to progress" (which I've increasingly heard called "failure to wait") or a baby being "too big"—which Roger explained was perceived to be an issue during his sister's birth, a hospital birth that he and his family found horrible. But Marion's boundary was that they would have to go to the hospital if the baby weren't born within twenty-four hours after Sarah's water broke. Sarah recounted, "That's the line, so she got a little testy with me, 'There's a point where you're really gonna need to just trust me!' She could see who she's dealing with, someone who's more fearful of going to the hospital than having a home birth." When I asked about that fear, Roger said it was more of a repulsion and that he just didn't believe the hospital model was helpful. A hospital birth would have been disappointing since he "wanted Gabriel to be born in a nurturing loving space," which is difficult to create in a hospital. "For me, I put a lot of significance in his beginning in the world. . . . I think it affects you for the rest of your life." This is a different way of framing what the risks are, and what there is to be afraid of in birth, yet navigating risk and fear is still key.

PAIN: AUTONOMY AS AWARENESS

Birth, especially unmedicated birth, is an intense experience. Yet the sensations of labor—that is, the pain itself—was rarely the focus of people I talked to about their births. It was often present in oblique ways, an elephant in the room. Pain was mediated via stories about its purpose and effects, about eluding it or controlling it. People who experienced unanesthetized labor often emphasized that it was painful or very uncomfortable, but this was not the center of the story. Pain is neither straightforward nor—I came to realize—necessarily significant. A widely referenced adage in Bay Area birth worlds is that pain is not the same as suffering. Suffering comes from resisting pain; suffering is a choice. Suffering, according to this adage, is a second-order experience, a mediated experience. Many in the natural birth movement of the 1970s used the words "rushes" or "surges" instead of contractions, and they talked about "intensity" or "sensations" instead of pain. Some, including some medical doctors, claim that ecstatic or orgasmic birth is possible when pain is embraced as intensity instead of something that signals a problem.[14] Ina May Gaskin claims more than 20 percent of people she spoke with experienced orgasms during birth (though I didn't hear stories of any!). Ecstasy, or *ecstasis*, means outside the normal, and some type of otherworldly feeling did dominate stories of unmedicated labor. Dani did not consider labor painful but described it as a decidedly unpleasant experience. She actually likened it to hell (but we'll come back to that in chapter 5).

> DANI: I wouldn't call labor pain. I would call it, like, a deep physical sensation that is *not* comfortable.
>
> ME: Intense?

DANI: Uncomfortable.

JONAH: Uncomfortable.

DANI: But it's so different from cutting your finger or breaking your arm, that's why I don't call it pain. . . . I mean, I definitely didn't have an ecstatic birth, it was *hella uncomfortable.*

JONAH: Orgasms—

DANI: And there were *no* orgasms involved. But I wouldn't call it, definitely not pleasurable, but I wouldn't call it pain just because pain is something different; it just has a different category in my brain.

Kim's midwestern friends were genuinely baffled about her decision to eschew pain medication: "They're like . . . 'I just don't get it. . . . Why would you want to experience pain?'" She found it really exhausting to keep explaining herself. Her explanation would have had to introduce an entirely different outlook on bodies, on experience. Although it would have been possible to say something about the narcotics in epidurals being bad for babies, which would have fit into more common frames of reference like the health of the baby being paramount, this was not actually Kim's reason. The baby's health was not a reason I encountered frequently for forgoing epidurals. The looming question, then, is what kind of society interprets pain so obviously and immediately as suffering?

Bay Area filmmaker and academic Irene Lusztig directed *The Motherhood Archives,* a film about the lessons childbearing women were given over the past century regarding what they should want and feel. She claims that contemporary birth is suspended between two ideas: it is both natural and pathological. The medical explanation of pain as a pathological symptom of a disease is inadequate, yet valorizing pain evokes a misogynistic Christian heritage wherein labor pain is God's punishment of Eve. Lusztig marvels at the irony in the redeployment of past misogyny within contemporary feminism: "That it's empowering and self-actualizing for a woman to be fully present in that experience of pain, that that's a really desirable state—to me that's really problematic."[15] Grantly Dick-Read, the British obstetrician who coined the term *natural childbirth* and wrote the first books about it, made an explicitly Christian appeal to the experience of being inside pain as a form of spirituality. That history has been erased, along with an argument formerly used to support women's access to twilight sleep in the early twentieth century, namely that humans experiencing intense, abject pain are suffering and have a right to relief. This could be considered an earlier iteration of discourses about human rights in childbirth, though today such claims often insist that women have the right to not have their bodies interfered with against their will. This is no coincidence: the right to relieve pain and the right to experience it are both about self-determination.

I don't find the idea of desirable pain inherently problematic, as Lusztig does, though it's important not to erase the misogynistic history of this idea. There is a weird misogyny in embracing labor pain, but also a feminized and often spiritualized form of power; they are two sides of the same coin. This dilemma echoes a central dilemma of feminism: whether to disavow the "feminine" qualities and activities that are devalued in a patriarchy in favor of attaining those "masculine" ones that are valued, or instead to embrace what has been coded feminine and seek to revalue it (or, equally problematically, to do both and have it all). In mediating pain through the stories one tells about it, one has some amount of control, and therefore power. Both refusing and embracing pain medication, and the stories one tells about why one has done so, are about crafting the experience—which is an act of autonomy. Virtually no one I worked or spoke with wanted pain-relieving drugs as soon and as much as possible; they wanted to decide based on how they were feeling, a far more common approach than a hard line either for or against pain-reducing technology.

In and of itself, experiencing pain (or not) is not significant in this context. *Choosing* to experience pain, versus being told one *should* or *must* experience pain, is significant. The value placed on experience, discussed in the prior chapter, suggests there is something preferable about being aware versus numb. Anesthetizing, removing the capacity to sense, seems contrary to being actively involved in the experience. But then again, deciding what one *wants* to sense or not is also a form of active involvement. Pain is not simply pathological or natural; it's moral and spiritual, as is the relief of pain. Do people want to experience pain because it is "intensity" and not suffering, or because it *is* suffering and suffering is good? The idea that experiencing pain is somehow noble and a sign of one's moral standing is also a very American way of thinking, resonant with the Protestant work ethic and the frontier mentality that embraces roughing it. It is called *labor* after all, and suffering through work is widely accepted as good. In American medical history there was even a cultural debate about anesthesia in surgery based upon the idea that pain was the moral work of the surgery process. Current ideals of convenience, efficiency, and even "self-care" push against the nobility of suffering and work. That one can and should decide for oneself which ideals to valorize is what came forward in my discussions with people more clearly than any particular narrative.

Sarah explained that due to her family's Waldorf-based beliefs about illness and injury, she had never voluntarily used pain medication for anything, including intense menstrual cramps and dental procedures. She had a best friend who underwent twelve leg surgeries with no anesthesia. Even though she didn't do any preparation for birth-specific pain management, she recognized that she had been preparing techniques for coping with pain her entire life. "I just knew pain is something we can have a relationship with," she said. Marion told her that "pain during birth stands for purposeful, anticipated, intermittent, and necessary . . . something you're expecting, that is completely natural, and not saying something is wrong, but that your body is opening." I had earlier asked Sarah if she would call labor painful, and she said, "Oh goodness, yeah, definitely! I knew that the pain was asking me to open more and more rather than contract, which is the natural gesture toward pain, to contract, withdraw. And I knew that in birth you need to do the other gesture." A Gaskin book she had read prepared her with this philosophy, and when the pain grew to more than she could handle alone, she grabbed onto Roger and "looked in his eyes to ground myself."

> It got to a place where I, within my own abilities, I couldn't continue to stay open to the pain. It was beyond what I could alone move, and you have to somehow move that energy rather than have that reaction and get stuck. So then I remembered she said look into the eyes of someone who trusts and knows that you can do it. So for an hour, [Roger] also just said I was squeezing his hand with more strength than he knew I had! It kept the energy moving. . . . The pushing was really very painful.

For Sarah, pain was anything but pathological. Even illness was not pathological to her but an indication of an emotional root cause she sought to remedy whenever she displayed symptoms.

An aside: Sarah chose to have a relationship with the intense pain of labor, but what she described as *suffering* was the work of attending to Gabriel intensively during his first year. She expressed no doubts that this suffering would be worth it, but that did not make her intensive approach to infant care easy. The pain of labor is brief compared to the sleepless months, raw and inflamed nipples, aching back, and isolation that accompany infancy for many. We'll return to infant care and mothers' suffering in chapter 4, but note that the navigation between pushing through and giving in reappears—

without many technological fixes on offer. There is a bigger-picture question about what kinds of pain and suffering are seen, cared about, and considered problems worth solving. The power to navigate pain comes partially from the presence of possible solutions, which exceeds autonomy.

Most people do not have Sarah's relationship with pain. Many of the clients I worked with as a doula were concerned to know how many pain-relieving items were in my tool kit, and I felt compelled to list possible positions (with rationale for which circumstances they would be useful in) and comfort measures like heat and coolness, scents, visualization, breathing patterns, affirmations, TENS electrical stimulation units, and water immersion. These are measures to manage pain, whether by mitigating it, distracting someone from it, or allowing someone to encounter it in a mindful way. There is a widely circulating idea that a birthing person will feel more comfortable and empowered if she can move around freely. One doula collective described one of its members as the "ninja doula" for positioning; if they suspected a positioning issue at a long labor, they would call her in to work her magic. Further, there is the idea that an unmedicated person will move her body to where it needs to be physiologically—hunched forward for occiput posterior babies that induce back pain, leaning back to relieve a pinched cervix if the baby descends before full dilation, or on her hands and knees or squatting to deliver using gravity.

Often my doula clients appreciated being massaged during labor. I used a lot of pressure in massages, and when someone's partner or mom wanted to help, I often demonstrated how to touch the birthing person firmly and solidly instead of using the gentle, tickly caresses they tended to find annoying. A staple of my tool kit is counterpressure during a contraction, which entails pressing as hard as possible on the coccyx or squeezing the hip bones together from behind. Dani's explanation of her sensations during labor involved movement and pressure. She said, "I was just trying to get into the most comfy position, which is hilarious because there *is* no comfy position!" She described "yoga stretching mode" using balls and mats. When I mentioned pressure, she shared that her midwife said she once saw a laboring goat that just wanted to ram its head up against a wall. "That was me. I just wanted someone to push my head really hard."

Pain is sensorially and emotionally demanding. There is something appealing about this embodied intensity that draws people over and above the idea that birthing without medication is healthier for the baby. Such intensity appeals to a wholly different sensibility than one of convenience or ease. Contextual understandings of bodies are appealing in part because they feed a desire for intensity. The kinds of rhetoric surrounding unmedicated labor in doula training, childbirth education, and more broadly in the community included truisms like "the only way out is through," transcending "the point where you literally can't go on," and that being exhausted and hopeless "means you are nearly there." Yet as desperate as this could be for people, including people as determined as Sarah, the surrender to intensity was often shrouded in beautiful aesthetics. Consider the lyrics of another Wombsong favorite: "I'm opening, I'm oh-oh-pening / I'm opening up in sweet surrender to the luminous love-light of my babe." This is not only about cultivating a mental state of trust and opening instead of fear and tightening but also suggests that laboring will be light and sweet. Perhaps this counteracts the fearful drama surrounding birth; perhaps it prepares people poorly for how difficult unmedicated labor can be; perhaps both. The desire for intensity can be a romantic and nostalgic sensibility predicated on White middle-class experience, situated in a life where convenience, ease, and safety are taken for granted (consider the typical audience for camping, hiking, and extreme sports). People operating from Black, Brown, and Indigenous perspectives may embrace challenge for different reasons, such as a desire to decolonize embodied experience as an act of racial autonomy from White-dominant culture.

There is a pervasive racist idea that White women are fragile and Black bodies are hardy, "thick-skinned," and insensitive to pain. Laura Briggs has detailed how historical racism in gynecology and obstetrics manifested in ideas about Black "savagery" and White "over-civilization," rendering some women hysterical and others subhuman. Dána-Ain Davis writes about contemporary obstetric racism, manifesting (among other ways) in how Black-bodied people are less likely to receive epidurals when they've requested them (White people often get epidurals despite requesting *not* to have them) and even in how considerately IV lines are inserted. Many who are distrusting and suspicious of institutional medical authority are responding to long intergenerational histories of abuse, of not being empowered to assert basic autonomy in those relationships.[16] Technology is often seen as an effortless transcendence of material constraints and specificity: part of its mythology is that it works the same everywhere and for everyone, but this obscures crucial questions of access and history.

Childbirth transgresses the boundary between illness and health via pain. Birth is not an illness, as activists are quick to point out, but it's culturally strange to think of the body in pain as something good and natural. On the other hand, the idea that birth should be a joyful experience is intensively promoted within Bay Area birth worlds. There is a pervasive aestheticization of (White, middle-class) birth, babies, and motherhood. Media images that have become ubiquitous in natural birth communities present a kind of in-your-face insistence that birth isn't messy or painful, that it's nothing to be afraid of. These push against the fearmongering and sensationalizing portrayals in mainstream media while producing a set of expectations and desires that don't mesh neatly with birth realities. Fears are always twinned with hopes, and managing one entails managing the other. Having the ability to decide whether, when, and how to receive medical pain relief provides the birthing person an important sense of control, coupled with respect. Although this ability is imperfectly available, the desire for it indicates a desire for autonomy.

POWER: AUTONOMY AS SELF-ACTUALIZATION

In the words of Barbara Katz Rothman, "Birth is not only about making babies. Birth is about making mothers—strong, competent, capable mothers who trust themselves and know their inner strength."[17] Stories of "bad births" overwhelmingly feature talk of feeling disempowered, whether because the birthing person was manipulated, ignored, bewildered, disrespected, or outright abused by authority figures, relatively independently of what actual procedures were or weren't done. Ilona, a new mother I interviewed, had a fourth-degree perineal tear after her baby's birth, which she certainly wouldn't have chosen had she had perfect control of her bodily processes, but she was overall quite pleased with the birth experience because she felt in control of the social dynamics and the decisions being made throughout, including the choice to have an episiotomy, which undoubtedly contributed to the tearing but also allowed her baby's "unusually large" head to emerge after a period of fruitless pushing. Chelsea, a doula client of mine, was comfortable deciding when she had had enough of the physical sensations of labor and wanted her epidural put in. For a few reasons, including a progressive/permissive suburban hospital, the presence of a doula, class/race privilege, and self-education, she was able to do just that and felt quite satisfied.

Feeling autonomous and feeling empowered are closely linked. Part of why autonomy is compelling is because it feels powerful, and vice versa. But the term *empowerment* is often used in an aggressively individualizing way, which obscures how isolating autonomy can be, and how powerful collectives can be. The dance between embracing and rejecting biomedical knowledge, intuition, technical expertise, institutional structures, and ideas about risk, fear, and pain is a negotiation of feelings and experiences of power. For many people I worked and spoke with, the quintessential form of empowerment was personal power—the ability not only to chart one's own course but to become the best version of oneself. Both trust and control were approached in service of current ideals around optimization, authenticity, and ultimately self-actualization. Finding self-actualization in the process of bringing another being into existence is a shift away from reproduction becoming meaningful in a gendered matrix of responsibilities to others. Yet the attitude of "I did it for myself" nonetheless reinforces the linkage between female fulfillment and bearing children (inevitably, paradoxically).

Empowerment has many faces. Being able to decide is clearly important to feeling empowered and autonomous. Using evidence to assess risks has become a quintessential sign of responsible self-education, a precursor to charting one's own course and developing a birth plan. The popularity of the website EvidenceBasedBirth.com, started by a PhD-level nurse who curates reports on hot-topic issues and promotes them through separate sections of her website for parents and providers, evidences this. Information is power in the midst of the contemporary cultural pressure to manage risks that both come from, and are mitigated by, hospitals and medical providers. More fundamental than having information and the power to decide is having options from which to choose. Christa Craven writes about the struggle for legalization of home birth and home birth midwives, noting that while such options are important, they are still framed in a consumer model of choice, which does little for people who are not empowered to be consumers.[18] Reproductive justice movements have long pursued a more transformative vision of good options that don't depend on one's buying power, but rather draw from mutual aid and political action that supports the well-being of people who are Black and Brown, poor, disabled, trans, and queer.

Various kinds of privilege and power are entwined with the ability to trust and control. Practices of trusting one's body are complicated for people who have negative relationships with their bodies because they've experienced abuse. Asserting oneself is harder for those who don't have support from their family, partner, or doula/midwife during their childbearing process, or who don't have easy access to the internet or a library as sources of information and perspectives. Trusting hospitals and doctors is much easier when you can assume that hospital staff have the best intentions for you, and that your interests are protected by the law, which has not been true for women generally and especially not for those at the intersections of race, class, disability, and heteronormative discrimination.[19] The idea that childbearing people should be able to make all decisions about their care, their bodies, and their children's bodies has long been a feminist stance, though dominant versions of White feminism have elaborated this in terms of choice without insisting that people also have good options from which to choose. Asserting that women themselves—not politicians, doctors, husbands, or institutions—should be in control of their fertility, motherhood, and bodies implies that women should be trusted to make such decisions. More profound critiques, such as those within reproductive justice movements, assert that women should furthermore have access to the means that enable them to be trustworthy, such as the material resources for raising a family, access to education, good mental health, communities safe from crime and police brutality, and healthcare provision of whatever form they are comfortable with. There will be more on this in chapters 4 and 7.

But there is something else that resonates with the drive to feel powerful for many I encountered: experiencing intensity, which goes beyond mere intellectual control and enables and embraces a raw kind of physical and emotional power. Tones of spirituality often accompanied discourse about the power of the (specifically female) body, of trusting oneself and one's intuition, and even one's baby. In this way the female body sometimes became a spiritualized form of truth and power (we'll revisit this in chapter 5). Recall the shirt designed and sold by MANA, emblazoned with the word "Believe" followed by "women, babies, birth, midwives." I interpret this message as belief in intuition as a mode of relating to the world, promoting the idea that medical interference undermines women, babies, birth, and midwives by disrupting their self-derived embodied knowledge—and their concomitant power. As a parent in birth class reported, his wife "looked like a warrior" when she was in labor. American ideals of self-reliance uphold a kind of toughness or determination, an empowering suffering. While some valorizations of suffering evoke self-transcendence, the power in an intuitive, contextual body might be called *immanence*—here and now; physical and visceral and utterly gripping.

Dealing with the intensity around birth, both the pain and the power, is mediated by variously inflected desires for autonomy, to *own* one's experience. But one never owns one's experience. There is an indeterminate matrix of how intensity resonates. It can yield birth trauma, postpartum depression, a backlash against the trusted body failing to deliver, or technology's side effects. There is a rhythm of amplification and dampening between immanence and transcendence. A contextual understanding of bodies is hard to ever fully enact because people who find it compelling still struggle with the inherent unpredictability of childbearing. Whatever the appeal of intensity and connection, they nonetheless want regularity in the outcome, not shoulder dystocia, not death.

The discourse of risk flags these possibilities and makes them difficult to balance against other possibilities that are not articulated via percentages. Enacting contextual physiology relinquishes control in a way that is jarring to many people. In my initial reading of Ina May Gaskin's *Spiritual Midwifery,* I was enraptured by the approach; upon dipping into it again over the course of fieldwork, with more experience, I became bewildered by how casual they were, giving birth in vans with no trained person present! This casual receptivity is both appealing and horrifying. In a culture so steeped in maternal shame, the guilt over having taken "risks" would be hard to stave off if anything negative happened.

A few of my doula clients wanted a home birth or else an elective cesarean, rejecting that intermediate ground of trying for a natural birth amidst the cascade of induction technologies and hospital environments. While this was an uncommon position that was often inflected by their specific histories, it made sense to me and many of the birth professionals I spoke with. It was fairly obvious to them that the trauma often came from the indeterminate matrix of intensity amplifying and dampening, the stew of not knowing what mode to be in, what type of risks and hopes to attend to, how to bridge physiological understandings while in the midst of intense discomfort. Better to be clear one way or the other.

In *A Paradise Built in Hell,* Rebecca Solnit argues that our present social structures prevent deep social ties and meaningful work from being achieved; yet when tragedies or disasters befall, such structures are crushed, and deep ties and meaningful work spring up in their wake.[20] If some births are individual traumas (and many are described this way by those that endure them, even when they have conventional outcomes), and if some people's experiences of childbearing are likewise traumatic (albeit intermixed with joy and love), and even though such traumas are shushed and called normal, perhaps they create individual hells from which phoenixes might rise. In a world in which reproductive work is sequestered to domestic, private realms, perhaps the personal trauma is what generates transformative power. A friend in Chicago described her home birth rapturously as what "reconnected her with her feminism." So many say they became a doula or an activist after giving birth and finding it . . . surprising. Intense. Transformative.

FOUR

Equality

SOCIAL REPRODUCTION AND
GENDERED RESPONSIBILITY

I WAS IN THE KITCHEN chopping yellow tomatoes for a chutney. "You're *making* chutney?" exclaimed Rachel when she returned from her day of teaching. She was a midwife and nurse practitioner whose Berkeley home I shared, and she had been struggling to get back into practice after taking years off to raise and homeschool her children. She was continually impressed with my cooking endeavors, which was silly as she was an excellent chef herself, often urging her loved ones to eat the bounty of California produce filling the kitchen. Professionally, she was struggling, both with an institution that views competence via a continuous resume and recent experience, and with her personal convictions about proper maternity care. "It's *not* midwifery" she repeatedly said of hospital midwifery practice. There isn't enough time to develop personal connections with her patients, to provide continuous support, to offer the kinds of support she finds valuable. It's too restricted by bureaucracy and protocols, and the staff are spread too thin. Meanwhile, she had been teaching the labor and delivery rotation for nursing students at the nearby state university.

After coming over to sniff the bubbling cinnamon, raisins, and onions, she said she asked her students today what the number one reaction is when people learn they are pregnant. Her students were baffled, or at least divided. Joy? Panic? No, she said, shaking her black curls as she put her arms akimbo. Overwhelmingly, the first reaction to pregnancy is ambivalence—some negotiation between a number of feelings.[1] It doesn't matter if the pregnancy is anticipated or unanticipated; the response is almost never straightforward. And no wonder. The ambivalence attached to any individual pregnancy is hardly surprising in a culture that is itself ambivalent toward pregnancy. Bearing children is romanticized, yet it is unsupported. It is socially necessary, but it is framed as an expression of personal choice. Mothers are celebrated, but simultaneously they are not treated as full persons. Different strands of feminism have long grappled with how to approach childbearing: Embrace it? Renounce it? We have just discussed autonomy. Yet in childbearing the very idea of the self is in question, as one body becomes two, and the newly created people are so achingly dependent that they significantly constrain whoever is charged with caring for them. Sheila Heti parses this in her book about deciding whether or not to have a child: "On the one hand, the joy of children. On the other hand, the misery of them. On the one hand, the freedom of not having children. On the other hand, the loss of never having had them . . . as though a child is something to have, not something to do. The doing is what seems hard. The having seems marvelous. But one doesn't have a child, one does it."[2]

Theorists of reproduction and social justice have used the concept of relational autonomy to acknowledge the ways we are all dependent on each other, especially in reproduction, and how true autonomy requires recognizing this and integrating it into supportive systems that enable self-authorship. Relational autonomy pushes against the "pull yourself up by your bootstraps" American cliché. Yet they sit awkwardly together, autonomy and relations. We want to author our own stories, but we cannot do that alone. And the conditions that enable our choices are far from equal, much as equality might be prized as a constitutional American virtue. Equality was not extended to certain sexes, races, and classes, and it's easy to make the case that humanity was denied to those people as well—yet the idea of the human that was implicit in the founding of the country took for granted the labor and contributions of those excluded. Attempting to include childbearing people in the rights, responsibilities, and prerogatives that make up equal individuals causes us to question the very possibility of equality.

THE MOMMY WARS AND THE WAR ON WOMEN

In January 2015 an ad went viral on social media. The setting is a city park, where a young auburn-haired woman sits on a bench, a baby cozied up to her chest in a padded carrier. Birds chirp. Then pounding music starts as three stroller-pushing women round the bend, heads haughtily raised. Two other baby-wearing mothers appear and sit next to auburn hair, emphatically dropping bulky pastel diaper bags. The ridiculous posturing accelerates! Another trio of mothers descends the park stairs, spraying milk from baby bottles. Yet another trio talks on cell phones while sporting black skirt suits and black bassinets. Next, the camera cuts to a contingent of five baby-holding dudes grilling at their picnic table, and then a queer family sitting on their picnic blanket. A final trio of mothers appear doing the warrior pose on their yoga mats, with babies in slings around their torsos. "Oh look, the breast police have arrived," says one of the bottle-spraying moms, aiming her comment at four women wearing capes to cover what are ostensibly nursing babies. A full-scale war of words breaks out. "Drug-free pool birth, dolphin assisted," says one gloating woman, gesturing inside her blue stroller. A baby-wearing dad mocked by a woman jeering "Mommy's day off?" calls out sexism. In another spat, someone citing the environmental impact of disposable diapers to shame a mother who uses them is counter-insulted by the epithet "crunchy granola mom." In retribution for being called "part-time moms," the skirt-suited ladies accuse the stay-at-home moms of getting mani-pedis all day.

They all move in for the kill, storming the park's play structure, when suddenly someone lets her stroller roll down a hill. The bumping soundtrack goes silent as, in slow motion, everyone leaves the battle to chase the endangered baby. The stroller slows and the baby's mom picks her up, breathlessly reassuring and thanking the crowd. In a communal catharsis, the unharmed baby evokes hugs, tears, and soft piano music, with the words "No matter what our beliefs, we are parents first" fading onto the screen. "Welcome to the Sisterhood of Motherhood." This ad, called "The Mother 'Hood Official Video," was paid for by Similac, one of the two large American formula companies. The final image is the word "Similac" against a black screen. By October of that year, it had received over eight million views on YouTube.

This commercial is old now, but I still find it an excellent caricature of how choices about mothering practices are highly charged with moralizing rhetoric while completely erasing the experience of mothers for whom poverty, racism, and non-normative family making constrain the options from which they might choose. The term *mommy wars* describes cultural tussles over the right way to parent (a pressure that largely falls upon female shoulders). In its narrowest sense, mommy wars oppose stay-at-home and working mothers, though the phenomenon can include several other stereotyped battles over how to birth, feed, transport, and diaper one's baby, and how involved fathers or partners should be. Staged in popular media, the mommy wars are catchy jabs at various parenting practices that impugn mothers' morality and trap them in a variety of catch-22's: damned if you do work, or breastfeed, or have an epidural, and damned if you don't. The phrase originated in the mid-2000s, notably in two nonfiction books, Miriam Peskowitz's *The Truth Behind the Mommy Wars: Who Decides What Makes a Good Mother?* and Leslie Morgan Steiner's *Mommy Wars: Stay-at-Home and Career Moms Face Off about Their Choices, Their Lives, Their Families.* The term was popularized in the *New York Times'* parenting column, Motherlode; although editor Lisa Belkin made a statement about gender inclusivity in her 2008 inaugural post (the column's punning title notwithstanding), its title changed to Well Family in 2016 alongside broader cultural shifts that made these wars less explicit but no less relevant.

These conflicts are highly classed. The figure of the (White) stay-at-home mom carries moral valences that are opposite from those of the (Black) "welfare mother," suggesting that giving up a career in order to mother is noble, while declining to do precarious and poorly paid work for the same reason is lazy or disingenuous. The term *stay-at-home mom* presumes that women do have a choice about working, an assumption that excludes a huge swath of mothers who are poor, lower middle class, and/or single. Stereotyped characters, such as those in the commercial, present parenting practices as choices or identities instead of complex negotiations of situational constraints and desires that are culturally coded and socially enforced. Childbearing decisions have as much to do with material survival as ideology, yet these stereotypes tend to collapse mothers into one dimension, calling into question whether they love their baby enough while erasing the lack of institutional support for parenting, women's aptitudes and desires that don't pertain to mothering, and a culture that devalues reproductive work as well as women's workplace labor.

A sister term, the *opt-out revolution,* which was introduced by Lisa Belkin's controversial *New York Times* article in 2003 and revisited in 2013, describes well-educated professional women opting to stop their careers and focus on reproductive labor while their husbands earn.[3] The class privilege is to the side of her point, which is that feminist women who have achieved the highest echelons of male-like educational and professional success don't actually want to "rule the world." She says that while this "opting out" might look like "a revolution stalled," it indicates that "women are redefining success. And in doing so, they are redefining work." This phenomenon has evolved into the explosive power of "momfluencers" who capitalize on their (usually White, stay-at-home) motherhood by cultivating a social media presence that idealizes and romanticizes their choices, often with a not-terribly-covert ideological position that can range from organic hipster to religious conservative "trad-wife."[4] Judgments have become less warlike and more implicit in the age of Instagram—a topic to which we'll return.

The opposing poles that are constructed in the mommy wars are ideals that are more or less approximated in certain times, places, and persons. They are narratives that are deployed to induce reassurance or guilt, to sell things or persuade, to rationalize decisions or assuage the pain of unpleasant fates. This messy stew was evident in the online backlash about the Similac commercial; emotional rawness, defensiveness, belligerence, and vulnerability ran throughout the cries of agreement about the harmful divisiveness of judgments, the refutations of the ad's sentimental manipulation (they're selling formula after all), and the contention that the mommy wars are good for society because they encourage dialogue and sharing of perspectives. Some refused to consider all choices equal, invoking culturally loaded ideas about science and nature and mother love; others leaned toward a more socially critical position, pointing out the difference between making fully informed choices from among a number of accessible options and choosing the least bad option from a space of constraint or ignorance.

Around the same time, the *war on women* became a common term to describe largely Republican policies attempting to restrict women's rights, particularly their reproductive rights. California Democratic senator Barbara Boxer and Representative Nancy Pelosi actively popularized the term after the 2010 midterm election in which Republicans won a majority of the House, though it originated around a decade earlier with Republican political consultant Tanya Melich's *The Republican War against Women: An Insider's Report from Behind the Lines*. The war encompasses restrictions on contraception and abortion but also the ongoing refusal to establish regulations against sexual violence and workplace discrimination, enacting a view of women's bodies as vehicles for sex and baby making. Many ways of policing childbearing people have been included under this banner, from Purvi Patel's criminalized miscarriage in 2013 to the 2016 FDA ruling that all sexually active women of childbearing age who are not taking birth control should not drink alcohol, regardless of their intent to get pregnant. After the 2016 election in which Trump became president and Republicans took control of the House and Senate, laying the groundwork for their recent Supreme Court majority, the Women's March launched a massive protest against the crass, misogynistic leader—and, more broadly, against the Republican war on women. The 2022 Supreme Court decision to overturn *Roe v. Wade* and remove legal protection for abortion has dramatically intensified the threats to women's reproductive rights, leading to the "West Coast firewall" that California, Oregon, and Washington organized in response to protect abortion access and abortion seekers from elsewhere.

Of course, the war on women is intersectional in that restrictions and punishments are worse for those facing other kinds of discrimination in addition to being female. People who don't have health insurance or family money or pale skin will have more troubles and fewer resources to buffer against them. There is more awareness of intersectionality today, yet still little awareness of the longer history and present manifestations of eugenic thought in the United States.[5] Concerns about women's sexuality and reproduction are deeply entwined with ideas about shaping and managing the population, not just individual choices and freedoms. This legacy echoes through ideas about what kinds of families are acceptable and deserving. In 1965 Senator Daniel Moynihan infamously traced the Black family's "degeneration" to a matriarchal structure in *The Moynihan Report*; the term *welfare mother*, popularized by Ronald Reagan in his 1976 presidential campaign, continues this discriminatory, simplistic, and inaccurate framing. Meanwhile, Black feminists have pointed out that Black family making is deeply shaped by violence against kinship relations during slavery, and that concerns with racial justice over and above the individual family are central to contemporary Black mothering.[6] Indigenous scholars have critiqued the heteronormative nuclear family structure as a tool of settler colonialism.[7] Elite concerns with population growth among poor, non-White, and colonized people echo this agenda, citing the planet's limited resources yet often neglecting to consider the vast disparities in resource use by colonial nations.[8] The availability of expensive assisted reproductive technologies like in vitro fertilization (IVF) and preimplantation genetic testing encourages investment in wealthy, heteronormative American women's fertility while bypassing the reproductive desires of others.[9] Socially disempowered women, from domestic slaves to immigrant nannies, have been, and continue to be, essential service providers facilitating the reproduction of wealthier others.

And so, in ways both intensely personalized and highly politicized, these two wars characterize the landscape of reproductive choice in contemporary America. Choice often implies equality—of options, of resources, of power—but it is abundantly clear that opportunities and power dynamics in U.S.

society are not equal. There is a more fundamental problem: the concept of equality presumes that there are individuals who are separate, able, and basically uniform, erasing care relationships, dependencies, and responsibilities that shift over time. But recognizing these specificities easily slips into deterministic ideas about what different kinds of people can and should do. Endeavors to correct childbearing inequalities often lead to patronizing advocacy initiatives and education programs rather than to critiques of racism, colonialism, capitalism, and ableism. Policies that would go a long way toward improving people's options, like months (or years) of paid parental leave, mandated pumping rooms at work, and universal health care, also require the state to get involved in reproduction, which is unsettling given the many different reasons people have to mistrust the state. Power dynamics keep equality at bay, yet the durable desire for equality serves the ideological function of deflecting attention from these power dynamics. If we could only get equality right, the story goes, we could escape judgment, isolation, overwhelm, coercion, and frustration.

The relationships near birth are where the value of equality is contested. These relationships are both real and imagined: they take place via actual practices while emotion-laden ideas about what they could or should be lead to aspirations and disappointments. They include relationships with the state as both provider and policer, and with practitioners like doctors, midwives, and doulas who are variously positioned in relation to institutions like hospitals and insurance. They include relationships within families and between couples, and among childbearing people themselves. Being equal in these relationships is nigh on impossible, yet people try. These attempts are visible in how care is talked about and practiced. The war on women is a contest over *who* should care, over who should be doing what kind of reproductive labor and making decisions about childbearing, while the mommy wars are contests over *how* women should care, over the proper way to negotiate the demands and expectations related to reproductive labor. To say that women aren't equal slips so easily into saying they don't have individual rights—and you get the war on women. But saying they *are* equal sets them up for failure in a society that doesn't support reproductive work or the different positions people find themselves in—and you get the mommy wars. Care is not only done but deployed; it is talked about and managed in ways that have political motivations and effects, as well as very real consequences for how people feel as they go about the necessary work of care.

One autumn midmorning I was driving my Santa Cruz housemate, Kaylee, and her six-month-old baby, Finn, to an Attachment Parenting International (API) support group. The meeting was held at The Village in Santa Cruz, a community center that hosts various childbearing classes and support groups. Yes, as in "It takes a village to raise a child," which I've been told is an African proverb popularized by Hillary Clinton in her eponymous book about children in America. Once we parked and entered the slightly shabby building, it became clear we were the only ones attending the group. The facilitator, Eva, however, was upbeat about this because of how much attention Kaylee would get. (Later, she bemoaned the fact that API groups in Kansas are packed with people, while on the California coast they are "a dime a dozen.")

Since Kaylee was unfamiliar with attachment parenting, Eva began with some history. She said the philosophy is based on the book *The Continuum Concept* by Jean Liedloff, in which the author goes to the Amazon and hangs out with natives, noticing that their kids are all so content and "grew up to be such *kind* people," in Eva's words. Liedloff "comes back advocating those child-rearing practices." I had heard of this book from a friend in Chicago, who had recently given birth and effusively recommended it. Eva digressed, explaining how some people don't respect the book because Liedloff isn't a trained anthropologist. She protested that there *was* an anthropologist, Meredith Small, who did a cross-cultural comparison study and came to the same conclusions.[10] "People believe the scientific one," Eva scoffed.

Eva explained that "biology hasn't caught up to culture." Babies' biology, she said, "expects certain things that our culture doesn't offer," such as being held 24/7 and being breastfed for four years. API recommends infants and children share a family bed with their parents, distinguishing this from co-sleeping, in which the infant is merely in the same room. Eva told us that health agencies like the American Pediatrics Association advocate co-sleeping but "don't trust people to bed share," and she cited evidence from the University of Notre Dame's Mother-Baby Behavioral Sleep Laboratory to persuade us that co-sleeping is not only safe but ideal. Another tenet of API is positive discipline, which goes against behavioralist ideas of rewarding desired behavior and punishing undesired behavior. Eva said such ideas are "silly, because you expect that by treating a child badly you will get her to be good." Rather, kids need belonging and significance, and if they are acting out it's because they aren't getting this. "Mistaken goals," Eva called these ideas about punishment.

Kaylee gently pushed back on the philosophy Eva was espousing. Kaylee was trained in acupuncture, massage, and traditional Chinese medicine, though she was taking a break from pursuing these professionally while Finn was a baby. She reflected that "attachment" is an "interesting" term, as in Buddhism one is looking to get away from attachment. She asked what the difference is between nurturing and spoiling; should she run to fulfill Finn's every need? She didn't want to be a pushover. The thing is, Eva said, at this age he can't be spoiled because everything he wants is exactly what he needs! When he gets older, he will start having wants as opposed to needs, like adults do. "This stage is about developing trust in you. He won't care what you say when he's older unless he trusts you." However, he had started biting Kaylee during breastfeeding, with apparent glee. This is a problem, Eva acknowledged, and "the first occasion for discipline." Eva suggested Kaylee pry his mouth open with a finger when he does this and make "ouch" sounds to communicate her pain. Kaylee was unsure about "wearing" Finn, a practice in line with the attachment parenting ideal of constant contact instead of transporting babies in a bassinet or stroller. Kaylee had a carrier for the front of her body, but he was so heavy it hurt to use it. Eva suggested she wear him on her back and taught her to do so after class. "How do you even get him in there?" Kaylee asked—it wasn't at all intuitive to her!

Kaylee was actively working out both the boundaries and points of connection between herself and Finn. They were a study in learning how to navigate two bodies that used to be one, or one body that was in the process of becoming two, depending on how you look at it. Intuiting each other took practice and attention, and trial and error. When we were hanging out before the API meeting, Kaylee said Finn knew they were moving house soon because she was stressed about it. She said she could hug him close and know if he wanted breast milk or solid food, and that he uttered a "primal cry" when she left the room for a while, "not like crying, but like, 'Hey mom, I'm over here!'" She was vigilant, keeping a close eye when I held him or when he was set down on a blanket or bed. When he was fussy, she would practice a guess and check method of troubleshooting, offering her breast, sometimes concluding he was tired. When I accompanied her to another appointment, Finn was fussy and she asked him to communicate more clearly, saying, "I don't know what that means" while shaking her head. "What does that mean, Finn?"

The moment in the API meeting that stood out most to me was brief. Amidst all this back and forth, Kaylee asked, "What about *me* taking care of *my* body?" Eva swiftly answered, "Oh yes, it takes a village. We weren't meant to parent alone." I knew Kaylee struggled with the role her partner, Chad, took in raising Finn, both wanting more from him and not feeling comfortable giving over control. They were struggling to find a home and a community in the Bay Area, and indeed a year later moved back to Southern California, where Kaylee's family were. In the meeting, Eva didn't elaborate further on how to create this village. The three of us sat in the empty space, flirting with the possibility of a weekly support group, and the irony hung in the room. We quickly moved on.

· · ·

Learning to navigate life with an infant and, soon enough, a toddler, tested the personal boundaries of everyone I spoke with. In many ways, the childbearing body is still held in common after the birth. Breastfeeding babies not only rely on the nursing person's milk, but her let-down response is stimulated by the baby's cry; people pumping milk often look at a picture of their baby. Breast milk enables them to share an immune system in real time, and the milk's composition changes with the needs and developmental stage of the baby. If the mother and baby sleep near each other, their sleep rhythms synchronize; some claim that this nearness helps the baby learn to regulate its sleep and its temperature, and even that it reduces the risk of sudden infant death syndrome (SIDS). In Bay Area birth worlds I noticed the terms *childbearing year* and *fourth trimester* become increasingly popular to account for how intensive the postbirth period is. Sometimes people, mostly out-of-hospital midwives, used the term *motherbaby* to join the childbearing person and infant into a single unit, a single organism. The way it was used romanticized this bond, but its creepy overtones come from denying individual personhood to the mother. There is a slippery slope between noting unity during a brief period, and in particular ways, and naturalizing it as a woman's purpose and source of meaning!

Many of the contextual physiology practices described in chapter 2 are intended to support the bond between mother and baby, such as preserving the natural hormonal cascades by avoiding drugs during labor, leaving the baby alert and calm instead of dull or agitated, and stimulating milk production. Breastfeeding produces oxytocin in both the nursing person and child, and it is said to increase their bond and reduce the likelihood of postpartum depression. I heard once or twice that a newborn's visual focal range is about the same as the distance from an adult's chest to her eyes, allowing them to lock gazes during nursing. Although you could bottle-feed while holding the baby at your breast, some people advocated using a thin tube attached to the nipple to feed formula or donor milk in a way that most closely approximated the experience of breastfeeding, and sometimes also to train the baby to nurse when milk production was faltering. Nursing is neither self-evident nor easy for many childbearing people and their babies. It is a learned skill, and one that Americans are generally poorly acquainted with, as we don't often witness or ask about it. Problems like inverted nipples and mastitis can make it complicated and extremely painful. As a result, discourse about the inherent rightness of postpartum co-embodiment can be frustrating and insulting.

Despite the intensity of this period, much childbearing discourse focuses on pregnancy and birth, with a bit about breastfeeding thrown in here or there. This lack of conversation contributes to the surprise, bewilderment, or depression many people experience with a new baby. I volunteered in a Birthing from Within childbirth course in which the instructor illustrated childbearing as a labyrinth; birth is the center of the labyrinth and there is a whole journey of arriving there—but not only that, there is an equally long journey afterward. This metaphor was useful to most of the parents I spoke with, and I used it often in my work as a doula. Not only is the postpartum period full of adjustment and learning, but navigating how to be in a relationship with one's baby as they grow is something that continues for a lifetime. Roxanne's Mindfulness-Based Childbirth Education course, mentioned in chapter 1, began with this acknowledgment and made repeated connections to the family life that attendees were creating; they were given a parenting book instead of a birth book to take home. This stood out to me because it was unique among the many courses I sat in on.

A truism across birth classes and doula events was that it is crucial that postpartum time be as peaceful as possible. It was often framed as "an excuse to finally clear your calendar completely!" for perhaps a month, for all parents involved, and not to feel guilty about accepting help or declining to be social. This emphasis pushes against a broader cultural insistence that things get back to normal as soon as possible. Reading things culturally, "normal" means restoring a clear division between subjects, including "getting my body back," establishing the baby's routine, and going back to work. Both the ability to interrupt normal life to integrate a new being, and to function normally soon after doing so, are huge privileges in a society that doesn't make much provision for parental leave or childcare and shames those who receive material support. (Twenty years ago, California became the first state to pass a paid family leave program, which has helped tens of millions of Californians and set the stage for other states' improvement.) It takes significant personal, social, and family resources to deviate from the mold of being a productive individual worker in order to rest and provide care, and it also takes significant resources to outsource the care labor in order to return to the mold. It is as though the work of caring for a child is incompatible with what is expected of citizens, as Sharon Hays posits in a tongue-in-cheek way in her article "Why Can't a Mother Be More Like a Businessman?" Meanwhile, the necessity of care persists.

Care is occupying oneself with the needs of another. It is deeply entwined with vulnerability and responsibility. A newborn baby is perhaps the quintessential object of care in its utter vulnerability, its neediness begging the question "who is responsible for this?" Annemarie Mol contrasts the "logic of care" with the ubiquitous "logic of choice" we have seen illustrated in chapter 3.[11] I follow Mol in saying that care is always reciprocal, often erratic, a process of tinkering and craftwork collaboratively produced by both the givers and recipients. I also emphasize that care is not exclusively human but intimately involves tools and technologies, and that values are central to messy deliberations of what is considered good and bad care.[12] Care is always profoundly interconnected with power and structures, institutions and inequalities, because the questions of who does care work and what resources are available for it are hotly contested.

Mothers are supposed to intuit care, like birth. This manifests as expectations of being naturally or instinctively caring, with heavy overtones of martyrdom. If they fail at this, the law faults them in ways it never would men (or even nonmother women). Anna Tsing describes how the cultural trope of the "monster mother" starts with a failure to nurture, how juries and newscasters wonder, appalled, "How could a *mother* do that?"[13] In the case of antiabortion politics, the language is often about protecting vulnerable fetal life *from* mothers, mothers who fail at this basic nurturance and are shamed for it. Postpartum depression hotlines for new mothers who fantasize about harming their infants reassure them that these intrusive thoughts aren't something they would *actually* do—desire to harm is so incompatible with cultural ideas of motherhood that allowing mother-rage to share a border with mother-love is simply unthinkable.[14] In her classic 1978 book merging psychoanalysis and feminism, *The Reproduction of Mothering*, Nancy Chodorow introduced the now commonplace thesis that women "mother" and men don't because female psychic experience is heavily shaped by the mother-daughter relationship (in a heteronormative nuclear family) in ways that dispose women to prioritize connection and nurturing more than men do, and to source their sense of self-worth from it. Psychic formation and cultural expectation reinforce each other.

In the past few decades, intensive mothering has become a hegemonic ideal. Susan Douglas and Meredith Michaels scathingly call it the "new momism."[15] It extends far beyond mere nurturance to encompass a variety of imperatives, from attachment parenting to professional-quality baking and sewing to organizing a rigorous schedule of enrichment activities for one's children (while documenting it all on social media). This ratcheting up of expectations amidst the disintegration of social welfare supports, the plummeting viability of single-income households, and aggression against reproductive healthcare provision makes for an impossible-feeling set of demands. In this context, mothers in various socioeconomic situations might not be able to meet their infants' needs because they are doing the work of two (or more!) humans, because the "needs" are inflated with affect-ridden hype, because they have any number of other legitimate calls for their attention and resources, and/or because the social context in which they are trying to meet needs is hostile to them. The specter of infant needs not being met is tossed around culturally like a hot potato, moving between mothers, fathers, state programs, personal networks, charities . . . but somehow always landing back in the lap of the mother.

The baby needs care, yes, but what about the mothers? The doula profession has developed to "mother the mother" and attend to her needs. And then doulas host self-care retreats to help themselves heal from the demands of this chain of care work. When I attended such a retreat in a remote spot in the Santa Cruz Mountains, the emotional release was palpable as women accustomed to serving allowed themselves to be cared for (by each other). Fathers, partners, and family members provide childbearing care in kaleidoscopic variations. The role of men has changed enormously over the past century, including an expectation that they not only be present at the birth but also be actively supportive, alongside trends toward more involved dads and more equal sharing of domestic labor. Peggy Simpkin's best-selling doula manual is titled *The Birth Partner: A Complete Guide to Childbirth for Dads,*

Doulas, and Other Labor Companions, and the idea of the husband as birth coach evolved out of Lamaze programs in prior decades. Yet there is a balancing act between implicating men in birth and childbearing responsibilities and inviting them to have control.[16] Doctors, nurses, and midwives are important players in the apparatus of care; so are the janitors and orderlies in hospitals; so are lawyers and policy makers.

The apparatus of care extends beyond people. Tools for caring for the "motherbaby" include established mechanical technologies like fetal monitors, vacuum extractors, and breast pumps, and innovations like mobile apps for monitoring contractions and virtual postpartum doulas. Technologies shape *how* people care, and they are unevenly accessible. Institutions, from charities to governments to hospitals, deal in the practice of care but perhaps more importantly deal in discourse about it, shaping expectations and emotions that are often inconsistent with practical options. State subsidies for food, housing, healthcare, or other basic parenting needs are politically contested at best, yet neither is the state offering to subsidize childcare (and there is an extreme shortage of childcare providers because it's not a financially viable profession). The U.S. Surgeon General issued a statement in support of breastfeeding in 2011, but across the United States employers are not responsible for providing parental leave or lactation facilities. WIC programs exist to provide food for women, infants, and children in need, yet the state has failed to regulate formula marketing to meet World Health Organization standards. Popular media and social media shape perceptions of care; laws surrounding familial obligations, reproductive rights, and medical malpractice are key in assigning responsibility for care. Many care services are not categorizable: diaper laundering, prenatal vitamin manufacturing, maternity clothing resale shops, doulas who volunteer in prisons, centers like The Village. The overlapping matrices of care near birth are dazzling in their complexity, or at least would be dazzling if things womanly, bodily, and mundane were culturally contiguous with splendor.

The ubiquity of "care" near birth can make the term seem both daunting and useless. But care is not only essential to understanding Bay Area birth worlds; birth worlds speak to the logic of care on a far grander scale. The question of care, at base, is the question of the social contract: What is one owed? What does one owe? For all the rhetoric about equality, the social contract is uneven, designed around a supposedly generic individual who at every turn shows himself to be White, wealthy, able-bodied, and male. This person is able to seem autonomous and successful largely because his needs are met by marginalized others, and thereby both his needs and the work done by the others are made invisible—the poorly paid janitor who cleans the office, the Brown woman who prepares the food he purchases, the wife who shops for his toilet paper and gestates his baby and maintains his social connections. Equality has been reframed as equality of opportunity, which would attribute differing outcomes to individual motivation if equality of opportunity existed (it does not). It has been distinguished from equity, which focuses on what is needed to equalize outcomes. (In the classic example, one male and one female toilet is equal, but four female toilets would be equitable as the line outside the female bathroom is four times as long.) But equality requires grappling with the basic logic of the social contract—and how co-embodiment fits, or rather doesn't fit, into it.

CO-EMBODIMENT AND THE SOCIAL CONTRACT

The modern social contract takes us back at least to the eighteenth century, when the liberal democratic social order was coming into being on the heels of the Enlightenment. Rebecca Kukla cites this period as a crucial turning point in Euro-American thought about mothers' bodies.[17] Before this, going back to Hippocrates, medical tracts were emphatic about the ability of the mother to impair her offspring in the womb. A pregnant woman's thoughts, desires, and experiences were understood to cause birthmarks and temperamental characteristics, even the delivery of a "monster" or stillbirth. Women's bodies were seen as highly porous and susceptible to influence, and also dangerous and unpredictable, needing firm direction and protection. These beliefs yielded what Kukla calls the unruly mother archetype. After the eighteenth century, another archetype emerged and coexisted with the unruly mother. In this archetype—the fetish mother—a mother could shape her child through an all-encompassing and flawless exercise of maternal care, with no upward limit on how positive her influence could be. Both archetypes persist to this day. It is not hard to recognize the fetish mother in new momism and intensive mothering, and the unruly mother in the blaming and regulating of monster mothers.

The fetish mother was intimately linked with changes in Euro-American political thought. New civic institutions and democratic governance not only originated a new kind of public sphere, but they also entailed the creation of a shadow private sphere where domestic concerns would take place; the one was the condition for the other. With this new public-private division came a set of gender relations that naturalized women's place in the private and domestic. This followed the separation of productive and reproductive work that accompanied wage labor and the transition to a market economy. Carole Pateman elaborates how, under the aegis of liberty, equality, and individual rights, a social organization based on monarchic patriarchy (hierarchical power) changed to one of democratic fraternity (horizontal power).[18] Men were made equals in a social contract and women became the domestic counterparts to these newly empowered citizens, implicitly written out of political subjecthood themselves and forced into what Pateman calls a "sexual contract," a necessary supporting role.

Entering the nineteenth century, embodied sexual difference became linked not only with economic difference via waged versus reproductive labor, but with political difference via the categorical right of men to access women's bodies and domestic labor and women's categorical exclusion from political life. Pateman argues that subordination is implicit in the idea of contracts (now the primary basis for politics, law, and trade) because they treat people in different social positions and different bodies as if they were equally free with equal options and concerns; such is clearly not the case in the heterosexual marriage contract or the employment contract. The decontextualized, disembodied, contract-making, self-owning individual is "the fulcrum on which the modern patriarchy turns," she writes.[19] It is not possible to simply treat women "the same as men" within this framework, as the framework itself is predicated on the exclusion of domestic life from political life, and women have different stakes in domestic life than men do for historical, cultural, and biological reasons.

There was social unrest about the place of women after these economic and political transformations, broadly glossed as "the woman question" and centered on issues of marriage, women's suffrage, and reproductive, property, legal, and medical rights. Bourgeois women increasingly and unsurprisingly found their political and economic exclusion hypocritical, frustrating, and depressing—they were having nervous breakdowns, unable to either care for their household or enter public life. Jane Addams, Margaret Sanger, and Charlotte Perkins Gilman are famous examples of those who recovered from years or decades of dysphoria, newly motivated to change society. (In Gilman's well-known and haunting short story "The Yellow Wall-Paper," she describes becoming insane due to the "cure" of total intellectual and physical rest prescribed by an eminent physician; she wrote it after divorcing her wealthy husband and taking off with her baby and her pen to California.)[20]

Barbara Ehrenreich claims that there were two approaches to answering the woman question: rationalist and romantic, which were opposed but based on the same set of fundamental assumptions.[21] Within the rationalist approach, if "progress" meant mechanizing and industrializing life's functions, why not include domestic and reproductive tasks? Then women could be included in the workforce just as men were. Much speculative fiction has explored this possibility, for example through ectogenesis (growing babies in artificial wombs) or a class of professional child bearers. Notably, such alternate ways of childbearing are usually considered dystopian. It is no coincidence that the competing romantic approach won out in bourgeois thought. In it, home and women are romanticized via powerful connotations of intimacy, comfort, and nourishment. The domestic realm is naturalized as the site where emotional and biological appetites for food, sex, rest, and beauty are fulfilled, and it is fundamentally opposed to the ugly, brusque, grueling, calculating world of factories and offices. In the romantic view, women are both subordinated and put on a pedestal. Their work is both priceless and worthless. Childhood started being romanticized as a time of innocence and purity; prior, children participated in the work and life of the family to the extent that they were able.[22] This shift in ideas about childhood happened first in wealthy families and gradually expanded through child labor laws and universal education; children's perceived innocence is still coded by class and, importantly, race.

Ehrenreich argues that bourgeois women found this romantic account compelling because it was linked with the idea of science, and therefore with the progressive force that liberated society from the patriarchy of church and king; the title of her polemical history is *For Her Own Good: 150 Years of the Experts' Advice to Women*. The precedent for this was set back in the Enlightenment with Jean-Jacques Rousseau's publication of *Emile*, an influential polemical tract about child rearing. It argued that a new political order required a new kind of person—a citizen—which required a new kind of education, which depended largely on the mother (Emile is a boy; the book's final section discusses Sophie, a daughter, as a sort of afterthought). *Emile* naturalized women as caretakers, upholding their reproductive work as a kind of sacred patriotic duty; it was particularly emphatic about breastfeeding, not for the nutritional reasons much touted today but for emotional and "natural" ones. Londa Schiebinger shows how this era's breastfeeding politics were so important that they influenced the adoption of the term *mammal* in the new taxonomic science, marking mammary glands as the most important shared feature of the group that included humans—establishing breastfeeding as crucial to humans' place in the natural order of things, validated by science.[23]

Social movements tend to focus on helping people access rights and prerogatives from which they have been excluded, whether voting or education or citizenship or bank accounts. But inclusion doesn't change the categories or logics underlying the rights and prerogatives. Not only does this mean change is slow and partial, but in many ways inclusion reinforces oppressive institutions and expectations. Sometimes categories can't expand because they were imagined in relation to an excluded group, an "outside" that gave the category its meaning and provided its conditions of possibility. Property-owning men could be equals in the public sphere only through the shadow personhood of their domestic counterparts; this exclusion is both necessary for the sociopolitical order to function, and entwined with real biological differences in bodies and their capacities. In other words, equality as a foundational value cannot accommodate difference.

From Simone de Beauvoir to Iris Marion Young, female philosophers have claimed that women's embodiment is fundamentally different from that of men because of pregnancy.[24] The pregnant body is both subject and object, self and other, which the modern ideology of the unified and independent subject cannot accommodate. Julia Kristeva develops an analysis of the "abject maternal body" wherein the binary division between self and other has become blurred, framing such a loss of self as repulsive, degrading.[25] It's easy to see why parturition—the moment when the two bodies become separable—has been given such significance. You might even say it is fetishized, given greater importance than it inherently warrants. Consider the American hospital practice of issuing birth certificates very shortly after birth, bureaucratically recognizing the infant as a citizen. Similarly, the baby becomes a separate patient immediately after parturition, under the purview of a separate doctor. But this breaks down sometimes; does the pediatrician have a say when her patient is inside the body of the obstetrician's patient, for example in fetal surgery?[26] Interestingly, lactation falls outside the purview of any medical specialty; neither obstetricians nor pediatricians nor gynecologists are trained to research, diagnose, or treat physiological lactation problems—which, consequently, are poorly understood. Apprehending and caring for the motherbaby falls outside medical specialties, which developed around individual (male) bodies.

There are many pop culture references to pregnancy as an alien invasion: one's body is not one's own anymore. "When did you start feeling like your baby was a separate person?" I would ask people, some with their baby inside the womb, some with her at their breast or sleeping nearby. Many responded that it was when they first felt the baby move inside them, which happens sometime in the second trimester. "Quickening," it used to be called. It used to be a guide for determining when abortion was prudent or possible. Sonora, whom I knew from a birth class and interviewed when her infant was two months old, spoke about how her body was not hers during pregnancy:

> I joked and called it a parasite, which people thought was not funny, but I was dead serious about it because my pregnancy was pretty gnarly.... The first trimester I was on a boat the whole time, you know, just seasick, then in the second I had a hard time managing my blood sugar because she was sucking all of the fat out of me. I was lightheaded and really dizzy and coped by eating an unbelievable amount of ice cream, peanut butter, and salami [laughter]....
> I didn't want to eat them, but if I didn't eat them I was gonna pass out.

Sonora's parasite baby affected her activity—"working too much" was causing her amniotic fluid level to drop. She explained, laughing, "I just had to slow down! Had to do a month of jammie time.... It was amazing. I read trashy novels, sipped Coke, and laid in a hammock. I mean, I was hella pregnant, so it wasn't comfortable. But." It's worth remembering that her social position allowed her to slow down; if it hadn't, perhaps her low fluid levels would have led to an induction or premature birth. Postpartum experiences also push uncomfortably against individual needs and personal boundaries. The Baby-Friendly Hospital Initiative, started by UNICEF and the World Health Organization to support successful breastfeeding, has faced pushback because participating hospitals can be seen as prioritizing the baby's needs over the birthing person's needs; many people struggle to breastfeed or simply do not want to, or they crave restoring a sense of their own edges.

Taken seriously on a phenomenological level, the concept of the motherbaby is jarring for many Americans. How can incomplete (child) persons and overflowing (childbearing) persons be fitted into the mold of autonomous individual persons? In many ways, a child is a person in process. Indeed, many (if not most) societies delay infant personhood and view infants and even children as liminal and incomplete.[27] Yet so much about the way childbearing is approached in the United States involves searching for hard lines between life and nonlife, rights and nonrights, dependence and independence, mother and infant bodies. Fetuses—and even embryos or fertilized eggs—are increasingly recognized in conservative politics as valuable individuals,[28] yet fetal personhood automatically calls into question maternal personhood. The idea of *processual* personhood would allow, for example, the recognition that fetuses can be alive and meaningful without being equal to a fully developed member of the community; that an abortion can be the death of a person while also being right. Or that nursing people and those responsible for a small child need to be physically near their babies while neither being relegated to domestic spheres nor forced into full-time paid work; where might it become normal to see babes in arms? Co-embodiment requires more flexible concepts of personhood that account for various kinds of dependency as well as autonomy, concepts that recognize that people have a variety of needs that do and don't persist. Such a reframing is needed for disability rights, chronic and acute illness, aging, and other forms of social dependency as well—but implementing it is far from straightforward. Childbearing invites reorganizing society around conditions of varying dependence and difference rather than posing a set of contradictions that individuals must absorb through personal trade-offs and sacrifices.

These fundamental issues with the social contract were not resolved when first-wave feminism succeeded in gaining women's suffrage, nor when second-wave feminism denounced how suffocating domesticity was, opening up prestigious economic and political positions to women, nor when third-wave feminism "reclaimed" the feminine and launched a #MeToo reckoning with sexual consent. Activism for gender fluidity and nonbinary social organization is sometimes considered a fourth wave, but even decentering gender as a category system wouldn't resolve the problem with equality, which is deeper than gender. It is an issue of difference and dependence, which bring us back to the question of whether (and in what ways) individuals can exist at all.

Louis Dumont elaborates what happens when individuals are the cornerstone of social organization: it makes equality both desirable and impossible.[29] Such societies recognize a wide freedom of choice, as individuals demand part of the "value-making capacity"; value either attaches to the whole of society and is inscribed in the very system, or it attaches to the individual. For individuals to be autonomous and equal, relations between people must be subordinated and minimized; the person is primarily seen as the navigator of their context, the author of their story, as described in chapter 3. Their successes and failures appear to be due to their own competence and character in the face of "nature," which takes on the guise of the inevitable—as if human context were not largely made by humans and able to be changed by us. By contrast, in societies governed by tradition and hierarchy, it is society that makes sure that ideas and actions are in conformity with the order of the world as it is understood; people are compelled to consciously insert themselves in this order. This minimizes their "freedom." But when individual subjects are expected to establish the relations between social representations and their own actions—to author their story—there is an artificial distance produced between people and the world surrounding them, a world that becomes inert and disenchanted (as do their own bodies). This absolute subject-object divide allows an individual will to be detached from nature and applied to its subjugation, an idea fundamental to the regular physiology described in chapter 2.

In minimizing socially determined values and hierarchies in favor of this man-to-nature relation, people are made equal by not recognizing their difference—by subordinating difference to equality. This seems as though it will erase distinctions in the long term. However, people still want to be recognized, want to think of a world order and a place in it. Dumont claims an "equal" place is a contradiction. "It is only by a perversion or impoverishment of the notion of order that we may believe . . . that equality can by itself constitute an order." To have a place, to belong, difference must be acknowledged. Equality and recognition cannot coexist. Dumont offers a tantalizingly vague "third way" between equality and hierarchy: conflict. Conflict allows for recognition of difference *and* for people to assert their non-subordination. Yet, he notes, "that conflict is inevitable and perhaps necessary is one thing, and to posit it as an ideal . . . is quite another."[30] The mommy wars and war on women are interesting to consider in this light.

Another theorist from the same era, Ivan Illich, controversially writes against gender equality, but he does not advocate for the subordination of either sex.[31] Rather, he argues against universalism and the ideal of a "neutral" sexless person because that epitomizes the decontextualized, interchangeable subjectivity of capitalism: people who are primarily economic subjects: workers and consumers. He extolls, perhaps romantically, situations in which people belong in a particular, contextual "vernacular" instead of a neutral, regular universality, with differences in their roles that give them a sense of belonging, a place in a larger order. It doesn't matter what tasks are attributed to what gender—or, I would elaborate, whether the divisions are along lines of gender or some other social category system. The point is that people are parts in a coherent whole that is larger than themselves.

The question is, can there be difference without hierarchy? Dumont says no (unless there is conflict); Illich seems to suggest the possibility; Jack Halberstam embraces it. In his book *Trans,* Halberstam argues that the meaningful difference between category systems is fixity versus mutability. Is one's belonging in a particular category predetermined, or could it change?[32] Are the boundaries and responsibilities of those categories fixed? He illustrates this using *The Lego Movie,* in which people are happily mixing and matching pieces to create an infinite variety of worlds until this becomes threatened by the glue-wielding villain.[33] What is clear across these works is that an equality worth having has to look like something other than inclusion in a neutral, universal kind of personhood. Childbearing makes us realize that most of us are both less and more than people in this sense.

Thomas Dumm elaborates how loneliness is an inevitable aspect of the modern condition. The word *alone* comes from "all one," the sovereign individual, "floating through undifferentiated space, and yet pregnant with a sense of self."[34] Loneliness is how we come to know, trust, and be ourselves; it is the trade-off of individualism. Hannah Arendt shows how this sense of dislocation lends itself to totalitarianism, which seems worryingly relevant in light of current federal politics.[35] In America in particular, loneliness is stubbornly viewed as a problem of personal circumstance instead of social organization.[36] Looking at Kaylee's challenges with new motherhood in light of this genealogy, she seemed to me profoundly lonely, a condition that has little to do with her social calendar.

DOULAS AS "PAID FAMILY MEMBERS"

I was waiting in line to get into the Bernie Sanders rally in 2016. My friend and fellow doula, Joanie, and I were standing on a bridge over the San Lorenzo River in Santa Cruz, about a quarter mile away from the venue. The line really was that long, and once we got in, the rally was packed. Joanie was chatting with the young woman standing next to us, explaining what a doula is. She rattled off things a doula might do, which ranged from asking a pregnant person about her hopes and fears, to giving a back massage during labor, to folding laundry and cooking dinner in a home with a new infant. She summed it up, "It's like a paid family member. It's what people used to do for each other."

This struck me. *Was* a doula like a paid family member? Since when do people need paid family members? I began to think about the history of paid, and unpaid, and enslaved domestic service work, which has long been a feature of class- and race-stratified American societies. Joanie and the young woman began to chat about nannies, as the young woman said she loves nannying. When Joanie claimed nannies don't do your dishes and laundry, she protested that some do! We discussed how Doulas of North America (DONA) says doula care should stop at twelve weeks postpartum, after which the person providing care is "just a nanny." Joanie protests this, saying a doula does more than a nanny. She is concerned about the mom and not just the baby; she looks for emotional problems and has resources for postpartum depression, breastfeeding, and parenting. The role Joanie is describing sounds like a friend, nurse, counselor, and maid rolled into one.

The term *family member* introduces a kind of intimacy that exceeds, or is at least qualitatively different from, the categories of both medical professional and domestic labor. Doulas challenge the difference between medical and domestic skills, operating in the borderlands where, for example, listening impartially to a person's anxieties and then rocking their newborn while they take a nap reduces the clinical incidence of postpartum depression. This confluence echoes the many ways nurturance, healing, and women's work have overlapped. Another doula collective I encountered was called the Seven Sisters, one of whom would stop by a newly postpartum household every day of the week to provide help and care. The social role of a doula transgresses the boundary between love and money, offering a kind of intimacy that Joanie compared to kinship, yet in a professional context. The 2018 film *Tully* explores the increasingly intimate relationship between a mother of three and her night nanny, who is exposed as a kind of hallucination stemming from the mother's exhaustion (and loneliness); the portrayal showcases the ambiguous power of someone both enmeshed in the heart of the family yet still an outsider during this vulnerable period.

Doulas dabble in multiple categories—medical professional, domestic labor, therapist, and family member—while challenging the boundaries between them. The appeal of the doula is in this idealized crossover: a healthcare provider who has time and patience to listen deeply; a back massage and clean kitchen delivered without having to ask; intimacy without the baggage of a lasting or reciprocal relationship. One of the key questions emerging from this nexus is, what kind of work—what kind of relationships and responsibilities—are valued? This is evident very literally in the question of payment, but money is tied to other recognitions of value, such as what is accorded prestige, and what is made easy versus difficult. As we've seen, the social contract is predicated on distinctions between family relationships and professional relationships, between the public realms of money and exchange and the private realms of love and selfless giving.

Childbearing women are caught in a double bind: On the one hand, if they assert their autonomy as individual contributors to political, economic, and social life (that is, if they claim to be no different than men in this respect), they compromise the support and value they might claim for reproductive work while perpetuating a supposed public life on which private circumstance has no bearing. On the other hand, if they claim that domestic circumstance, childbearing, care work, and reproductive biology require recognition and accommodation in civic life, if they argue for supports that enable them to take on these demands, they risk compromising their professional advancement and their ability to be seen as valuable, serious, and productive. This double bind leads to undervaluing both women's domestic and paid labor. The infamous wage gap is acknowledged to be largely a function of motherhood, whether actual or potential, and a "second shift" of unpaid domestic labor awaits many women at home—plus a "third shift" of the work required to balance and repair the damages caused by being responsible for both paid and domestic labor, and the feeling of doing neither adequately.[37] People of all genders are caught in a similar bind insofar as the individual citizen-worker-consumer—free to engage in or break off commitments, not compelled by obligations to care for others, able to get their own needs met without particular hardship, not defined by their relationships but by their work—remains the unspoken, inherently limiting ideal. But the "paid family member" transgresses this distinction, opening up a new version of the classic problem.

The family, by which I mean the nuclear family household as a social ideal, was both produced by and necessary for the liberal democratic social contract we just explored. Heteronormativity is a way of describing the gendered, sexual, and property relations that underlie this family ideal. LGBTQ practice and activism during the twentieth century disrupted this norm, opening up opportunities for different ways of relating sexually and making families and households, as did technologically enabled reproductive practices like IVF and surrogacy. But heteronormative family ideals often still shape what is desirable, as in gay marriage. Encompassing both heteronormativity and homonormativity, Indigenous scholar Kim TallBear speaks about the nuclear family as part of settler sexuality: ways of relating that enforce monogamy, private property, and a particular kind of recognition by the state, which were imposed on Indigenous peoples and are part of ongoing Indigenous dispossession.[38] Settler sexuality stabilizes and normalizes the colonial state while denigrating other ways of being in relation, including friendships and extended families, nonmonogamy, and relationships with more-than-human life. Marxist feminists have a long history of arguing that the family is exploitative, as represented by the Wages for Housework campaign in the 1970s, which was associated with the international socialist movement, and Sophie Lewis's recent polemic flipping social qualms with paid surrogacy on their head by claiming that unpaid gestation is the real outrage.[39] These are moves to seek social justice by doing away with the division between the public and private spheres.

The romantic "it takes a village to raise a child" discourse bypasses these fundamental problems, vaguely invoking a fallback on friends and family who are themselves not recognized or remunerated for doing care work. Though very wealthy people might be able to pay for all the help they need, and impoverished communities have long communalized all kinds of labor and resources to enable survival, most people rely on a mix of informal and paid support. The cost of childcare varies widely across formal and informal provision, from the exploitation of undocumented immigrants to elite pre-schools with annual tuition in the tens of thousands of dollars, not to mention waiting lists that aspirational families join years in advance (sometimes even before the baby is born). Most day care facilities don't accept infants under one or two years of age, but statutory California maternity leave is six weeks (of "disability" pay), making private arrangements (paid or unpaid) necessary; some people I know share the cost of a nanny with other families with infants. There is a structural lack of childcare workers, who are terribly paid (many leave a profession they love to earn a living wage in retail or hospitality), while the resumes requested of elite nannies show that the age of the teenage babysitter is long gone. Meanwhile, elite employers are ramping up the generosity of their reproductive support to retain talent, from six months of paternity leave to childcare reimbursement, from flexible at-home working to unlimited vacation. A 2022 *New York Times* article titled "It Takes a Village to Care for a Baby. And for a Lucky Few, a Luxury Hotel" describes a "postnatal retreat" charging $1,400 a night.[40] As with so much of social life in the Bay Area and more broadly, deepening inequality is the theme.

Childbearing may well be the first time privileged people encounter a true need for community support: I think of two San Francisco moms looking for parenting communities who, "inspired by the success of dating sites," started a short-lived website called The Village to create in-person connections. While there are now innumerable online parent groups, threads, and accounts, social media can disconnect as much as it connects, and the physicality of child-rearing begs for in-person support. Parenting-oriented community centers, which sell goods and host courses and meetings, fill some of this need; Natural Resources in San Francisco is a longstanding example. Often people stay in touch with their childbirth class cohort of people giving birth around the same time; the increasingly popular Centering Pregnancy curriculum focuses on group prenatal classes for this reason. The ideal of community both exposes and hides the utter vulnerability of "doing it all" and "having it all," the stubbornly persistent aspiration of White, middle-class feminism.

There is an uptick in popular media that discusses chosen family and friendship, creating a "tribe," the social prejudices against single people, and the increasing acceptance of childlessness and single parenting by choice, taking inspiration from communities who have long practiced kinship in less bourgeois ways—Mia Birdsong's *How We Show Up* is a paradigmatic example.[41] In some ways, this echoes California's 1960s legacy of alternative living arrangements like cooperatives and intentional communities, utopian projects that drew White, middle-class people from around the country and often featured shared child-rearing.[42] Recent articles also disentangle people's feelings about their children and their partners: Ayelet Waldman "scandalously" reveals and defends that she loves her husband more than her children, while Honor Jones states, "I could be myself and be a mother. I got divorced because I could not be myself and a wife."[43] This echoes Adrienne Rich's durable distinction between the practice of mothering and the institution of motherhood, the latter being framed by patriarchal nuclear family norms.[44] Increasingly, predetermined family desires and responsibilities are seen as the problem; any number of permutations are possible and potentially good. (Whether institutional inertia can catch up to them is another question, as is the conservative backlash against such explorations.)

Advocates of "natural birth" often look somewhat nostalgically to the pre-1900 tradition of childbearing as communal, domestic, and woman-centric, part of a historical period before the nuclear family became such a rigidly idealized norm. Yet they also encourage a woman's husband or partner to take an active, intimate role, thereby both problematizing and naturalizing the nuclear family.[45] That the partner would be involved in the birth—

or at the very least would be present—was a starting point for most coupled people I encountered, a presumption and a moral compulsion. There was one exception, a case in which a woman's husband declined to be involved (he believed his role as a father was to be supportive in other ways), and she struggled to reconcile herself to this situation—as did most people I mentioned it to! Despite liberal sentiments embracing all ways of making families, and doulas aspiring to honor their client's preferences, a partner declining to be present at the birth pushed the limits of comprehensibility.

Part of a doula's work is facilitating partners' involvement in the birth and infant care in a way that is tailored to the particular individuals; my doula training and many subsequent social encounters emphasized that we should assuage partners' concerns that we might take their place and help them be "useful" during an unfamiliar and potentially upsetting experience. This was something many couples appreciated, in my experience. However, particularly when a concerning medical situation arose, partners could become protective (and scared) and want to follow doctors' orders whether or not they aligned with what their birthing partners wanted. It is complex to navigate such situations as a doula; deferring to the partner is easy to do, and perhaps rightly so, for the doula will not remain part of the family. When I asked an experienced doula if she kept in touch with clients, she said she remained friends with some, but "you have to understand it is a business relationship after all."

Doulas epitomize the desire for a personal relationship in childbearing care, yet by professionalizing such care (and relationship), doula work becomes an institution and, perhaps, an industry. Doulas are not unaware of this. There is contention over certification and standardization. There is a strong preference for birthing people to be served by doulas from their own communities, which certainly helps establish trust and rapport, as I learned from experience, and works to decolonize birth by returning its care to the hands of people from whom it was forcibly removed. Yet underserved and marginalized communities are often those least able to pay high sums for care, however valuable it may be. One Latina doula I spoke with advocated doulas being as community based and unprofessionalized as possible, literally one's friend or family member tagging along and operating on a reciprocal basis—which makes me leap into possible worlds where time is not money and livelihoods are not precarious. Some respected community doula collectives resist inclusion in insurance and certification bureaucracies, saying this would actually reduce access for their communities—more on this in chapter 7.

The question of pay is a thorny one. The doula community is divided over whether the priority should be enabling practitioners to make a living, or getting doula care to any and all people who need it. Often doulas and doula collectives operate for free or reduced cost for some clients, much like pro bono law, effectively using their wealthier clients to subsidize others. Some use a more explicit sliding scale of fees and must decide whether to ask their clients for proof of need or simply trust their honesty (I encountered both models). A different, though not mutually exclusive, approach is arguing that doulas' skilled, difficult work should be valued far more highly; being appropriately paid legitimates it as a profession, raising the value of feminized care work in a masculinist economy. Joanie was passionately among this camp—her web page "What's in a fee?" explains what the hundreds or thousands of dollars charged for birth support goes toward (several hours-long prenatal and postpartum visits, usually in the client's home, four weeks of being on call 24/7, plus in-person support throughout the entire labor, which can last for days, and phone and text support throughout the pregnancy). Doctors spend far less time with a patient than doulas, and their compensation is far greater; it isn't unreasonable they be paid more, but the enormity of this disparity reinforces a skewed idea of what is valuable.

Many doulas discouraged volunteering because it devalues the work and undermines other doulas' ability to make a living; it also tends to reproduce colonial and racist patterns of novices "practicing" on Black, Brown, and poor bodies. Doulas from underserved communities encouraged White doulas who wanted to help to sponsor a doula from the underserved community, to give money instead of time—a gesture toward rectifying a deeper problem of historic and ongoing dispossession. When I volunteered at a home for pregnant people and new mothers, many of whom faced challenges such as domestic violence, drug addiction, or being unhoused, the money relationship came up a few times. Unpaid services tended to be undervalued by residents, the predominantly White, middle-class volunteer doulas felt. An ongoing discussion revolved around how to not be taken for granted while not rubbing the fact of charity in clients' faces, perhaps by being paid a nominal amount or disclosing our usual fees.

The alternative to privatized care is most obviously social welfare programs, though the possibility of them being implemented seems to be diminishing—after all, Bernie Sanders, who supported universal healthcare, did not get elected in 2016. On one level, doulas are part of a neoliberal morality wherein individuals understand themselves as good people because they take care of their families when the state abdicates its responsibility to care. But there is also a valid mistrust of the state's ability to organize what communities—or families—do for each other. Doulas as I came to know them are not nostalgic for an era of social welfare that never fully existed and was never inclusive or equalizing anyway. Access to healthcare doesn't necessarily mean access to supportive, nurturing healthcare, as doulas are well aware. Doula communities seem to be angling at something to the side of easy political narratives.

Doulas' labor calls the paradigm of contract making between equal individuals into question: first, by introducing into the doctor-patient relationship a third party who can facilitate attuned consent in the midst of complex power imbalances (as discussed in chapter 3); and second, by exposing the contradictions of the love-versus-money dichotomy undergirding normative ideas of family, which shape how we understand valuable work. By raising questions about the norm of payment for services in a context of vast wealth disparities, while paradoxically responding to the desire (and need) to access care without the ongoing reciprocity entailed in kinship (because payment cancels the debt), doulas pinpoint a key tension in contemporary life. People are not equal, yet we all need care and to feel a sense of agency and respect, and (in current individualist understandings) this comes from feeling equal. In a system in which equality is impossible, doulas both fill in the gaps and break everything open.

FIVE

Authenticity

TECHNOLOGY, NATURE, AND TIME

MY SOCIAL MEDIA FEED SHOWED ME a friend's post about a doula who offers birth videography, surrounded by exclamations to the effect of "How beautiful!" and "Isn't birth amazing?" The videographer filtered most of her footage using gentle grayscale tones and overlaid it with a soundtrack of acoustic music. A hand bathed a forehead with a cloth alongside smooth flute notes, a hugely pregnant woman swayed on all fours in the birth tub against soft piano chords, and a newborn's face was set to vocals about love. In these personalized videos the birthing body's viscerality is muted: there is no bloody water, flushed and sweat-streaked face, or blotchy purple infant; no vomit or wrenching groans, no smell of feces as the birthing person pushes, mixed with the peppermint oil the midwife matter-of-factly shakes onto the Chux pad to cover the scent and spare her embarrassment. The only vocalizations are rhythmic moaning and gentle encouragements. The montage format gives no sense of duration, effacing tedium and exhaustion.

In these videos, which epitomize an aesthetic that can be found throughout birth-related media, the messiness, pain, and danger near birth are glossed over to make way for an aesthetic proper to an empowering physical accomplishment, a peaceful and intimate moment, or a joyous outpouring of love. This is not a fraud or a farce—there certainly are peaceful and gentle births or rushes of love, and the power of the experience is not diminished by skipping over the feces—but the editing mediates the birthing body, marking out certain aspects as more valuable than others. When producing an alternative aesthetic to rationalized medical control, it is not necessarily any less true to represent the birthing body as serene and powerful instead of highlighting its suffering and embarrassing tendencies. But it is mediation all the same.

Bearing new life is profoundly corporeal. As much as motherhood, parenthood, and reproduction are social, relational, structural, political, and significant (in the sense of signs and symbols), the flesh of the birthing body pulls and pushes as a new body exits it. Tissues tear. Tissues are compressed and cut and exhausted. This opening of the flesh can be empowering, cathartic, violent, triumphant, traumatic, groggy, numbed, frightening, peaceful, orgasmic. It can be many things, highlighting how our bodies exceed our control. The term *visceral* refers to the viscera, the gut, not the head or heart, not the intellect or emotions. It is outside the mediation of thinking and feeling. This is both deeply appealing and abhorrent: the appeal of some kind of universal and involuntary truth, and the horror of slipping into anonymous, abject flesh. The unmediated body promises insight into our truest selves and threatens our social and subjective identities. Seeking something raw, real, and unmediated is a quest for the authentic.

Authenticity has become a ubiquitous component of taste, consumption, and the hipster aesthetic of late capitalism—a reaction against mass-produced, overly industrialized materials of daily life.[1] But this drive has a deeper history stretching back to the Enlightenment, manifesting in protests against a version of progress that valorizes technical accomplishments at the expense of, or at least against the neutral backdrop of, nature. In *Resurgence of the Real: Body, Nature, and Place in a Hypermodern World,* Charlene Spretnak details how every social transformation toward a more rationalized way of being has been accompanied by opposition movements; these have been dismissed as "romantic," but they weave together politics, philosophy, and aesthetics in salient and poignant critiques of modernity. The value of authenticity is the desire for something real, pure, and true when confronted with modernity: an escape, a rudder, a root, some relief in the face of bewildering change and disconnection. It shows up in how "nature" and the "natural" have been valorized over time. During the industrial revolution, a traditional European perspective on wilderness as something daunting and hostile transformed into the appealingly untamed "virgin" frontier in the American West and elsewhere, offering a counterpoint to urbanization and factories. In America, once Manifest Destiny was accomplished, wilderness changed into the nature of national parks, a sentimental place-set-aside where people could escape the relentless force of progress.[2]

The videographer's work celebrated "natural" birth, pushing against techno-medical aesthetics by substituting sentimentality for rationality. Yet in shying away from a more difficult portrayal, it reveals an uneasiness about bodily experience. Discourses valorizing the natural, embodied, and primal abound in birth worlds, but these are slippery goals, shifting targets. I did not select choice as a value for this book, though it appears throughout the chapters and is certainly an influential concept in the cultural history of reproduction; I also did not select freedom, despite its ubiquity in American propaganda. Particularly for middle-class people, the sheer volume of choices on offer can verge on overwhelming: the flood of content on social media, the taxonomies of consumer goods that signal not only luxury but morality, the proliferation of virtual realities and biological engineering possibilities that call being human into question.[3] Freedom can ring hollow as the "open road" and "wealth-for-the-taking" myths become visible as such, as they become untrustworthy amidst rising inequality and the claims of justice movements. In chapter 3 I wrote that autonomy in childbearing is becoming more about *the process by which one chooses* than choice itself: how is one to navigate? Authenticity is a current answer to this problem, though determining what is authentic is a problem of its own. In a hyperindividualized society the search for authenticity often looks within, as though we could provide our own rudders, our own sense of what's right, an ex nihilo manufacture of truth and desire—a impossibility similar to that of pulling oneself up by the proverbial bootstraps.[4] How, then, to access the real?

When I looked through the videographer doula's website, I didn't recognize the swooning feeling that floods my chest at parturition, a feeling that is equally precipitant to tears and nausea, not categorizable as an emotion. I didn't feel the clammy vice of the birthing person's hand, my fingers' tingly complaints. I remembered a moment when I brushed damp, dark hair from a birthing woman's forehead and was struck by how long ago I had plaited that hair into a French braid; the calm tenderness of that act seemed worlds away from the panting, pungent exhaustion that engulfed us. I recalled the rhythmic drone of one, two, three, four . . . all the way to ten, beet-red face gasping for air. My voice telling her she's doing wonderfully, almost there. The doctor's order to press her knee out and up toward her shoulder at a seemingly impossible angle; students filtering into the room, as if they could understand the hours by watching these few minutes. My aching side muscle as I leaned to peek at the perineum, seeing the black hair matted and waxy and telling her the head is visible, her baby is coming! When I spoke, sometimes my voice would catch; she locked eyes with me, and I felt like I was naked, like I had better not let go.

A rush of fluid, greenish from stool, ruddy from blood, an unharmonious rainbow against the baby's purplish skin. Parturition has a particular smell—

is it the amniotic fluid? Somehow stale and clean at the same time, mingled with sweat, blood, the plastic film on Chux pads and the latex of gloves. A rush of feeling mirrors the rush of fluid, unbidden. It is not what I would call sentimental; it's highly somatic—the nausea—and when I lean down to tell her that her baby is here, she's perfect, she did it, the relief manifests as tears and an oddly impersonal joy. I stay with her, continuity of touch between our hands; I am careful not to move an inch as the rest of the room crowds around the baby in her slimy nudity, the throbbing, rubbery lumps of the umbilical cord still linking her to the womb.

THREE TYPES OF KNOWING:
PRIMORDIAL, MODERN, AND SELF

"There are three types of knowing in labor," explained Kristen, the childbirth educator hired to give private lessons to my doula client, Jasmine. "Primordial, modern, and self." It was a cold and gray summer Saturday in the Mission District of San Francisco, and we were seated in the bedroom of Jasmine's tastefully decorated loft apartment, Parisian prints on the wall and the muf-fled sound of her housemate's tinkering in the kitchen. The two of us were facing the large pad of paper leaning on Kristen's easel, where she was writing down the three kinds of knowledge. "Primordial" she scratched with her marker. "This is like a gut feeling. It's something you know without thinking about it." The scent of green tea wafted in from the kitchen, mixing with the marker's sharp chemical aroma. Jasmine stood up to shut the bedroom's French doors against the ruckus of a delivery truck in the alley below, men hollering as they serviced the Thai restaurant downstairs. She swayed from foot to foot as she walked back to her chair and distractedly stroked her gray tunic where it stretched over her protruding belly, seven months pregnant. Kristen continued to explain "modern knowing" as understanding "logis-tics," combining a biomedical understanding of physiology with information about risks, tools, options, and protocols within medical care. She waved her freckled hand as if to dismiss this as kind of boring but necessary. Finally, "self-knowing" is "knowing who you are and where you come from. It's knowing what you feel comfortable with, and why," explained Kristen. This third kind is the most important, she said, and our session's focus.

Kristen had been trained by the national childbirth education organiza-tion Birthing from Within, which was part certifying body and part franchise; I encountered it multiple times during my fieldwork. Its curriculum, which incorporates spiritual metaphors like labyrinths to guide parents on their "childbearing journey," encompassed many tropes and assumptions about birth that filtered throughout the Bay Area. Jasmine could not fit a standard childbirth preparation class into her schedule of working full-time at a philanthropic investment consultancy; such courses often meet on weekday evenings for six to eight weeks, and many were already full, so she opted for a private crash course over two Saturdays and invited me, her doula, to attend. I had met Jasmine through a mutual friend, and this was her first birth; I eventually attended the birth of her second child as well. Birthing from Within (which I will abbreviate BFW) is not as prescriptively antimedical as some of its contemporaries, such as hypnobirthing, and it is decidedly broader in scope than the classes offered by most hospitals. It shares many similarities with Roxanne's Mindfulness-Based Childbirth Education course. All such courses take up the legacy of the 1970s natural birth movement, but they also incorporate pushback against approaches like Lamaze and La Leche League for being too dogmatic and creating shame and guilt around using medical technology. Although BFW presumes that its audience is wary of medical intervention, it acknowledges that interventions are highly beneficial "if needed." "Like it or not," BFW's website states, "one of the modern tasks of birth preparation for all parents is to learn about the hospital birth culture in their community," including preparing for medically induced labor and cesarean birth.

Natural birth is a fraught term, and alternatives like *physiological birth*, *normal birth*, and the more specific *unmedicated birth* and *vaginal birth* are increasingly used instead. Who wants to be unnatural? On the flip side, how is it possible *not* to be unnatural in a social context so heavily saturated with technology? From genetic testing to plastic birthing balls, from reliable ambulance services to ubiquitous cell phones, technologies shape the embodied experiences of all involved in childbearing. At some point during many of the births I attended, the monitor screen became the central point of attention in the room as partners would report the numerical score of a contraction's intensity or nurses would use its green digital pulses to coach a laboring person when to push. Although people I spoke with frequently differentiated between "natural" and "medicalized" approaches to birth, in practice everyone crafted a bricolage that drew from the epistemological, ontological, moral, and bureaucratic claims attached to each. Being adamant about not having an epidural could be congruent with having several rounds of egg extraction. Scholars have critiqued the overuse of obstetric technology and the ways the term *natural* is deployed, showing how birthing people have navigated a contingent middle ground for decades.[5] The point becomes something other than navigating between nature and technology; rather, it is about *knowing how* to do so.

What I find so interesting about Kristen's epistemology is that it is not binary but tripartite. The self-knowing is the most important aspect. When Kristen describes modern knowing as "understanding logistics," this extends well beyond simply using technology, while primordial knowing indicates an ideological commitment to a specific version of the natural. Connecting with a self that can itself be known and trusted is what allows people to navigate between the primordial and modern; moreover, self-knowledge is produced *through* this negotiation. This self is both innate and designed, something ancient yet endlessly optimizable. Especially for the upper-middle-class professionals I worked with, navigating contemporary childbearing was not so much a question of choosing between technological or natural approaches, nor looking either to expertise or to tradition, nor fulfilling gendered and familial expectations. Instead, it was about enacting a personalized process of self-actualization—a contemporary quest for authenticity through accessing the truest and best self. This is a highly individualized way of understanding and valuing the authentic. As they prepare for birth and caring for an infant, childbearing people in the Bay Area draw from the idea that self-authenticity both stems from an unadulterated, primordial nature and is enabled by a very modern, reflexive strategy of self-design and self-optimization.

This navigation process is an example of the "maternal thinking" Sara Ruddick theorizes as opposed to ubiquitous representations of sentimental maternal *feeling*—yet here the epistemology tries not to reproduce the thinking/feeling divide.[6] Although in conversation with the durable Western legacy of nature/culture dualism, parsing the epistemological conditions of childbearing in terms of primordial, modern, and self-knowing cuts things a different way. Nature/culture dualism resonates with all sorts of other dualisms we have encountered in this book—public and private, regular and contextual, rational and intuitive, control and trust, masculine and feminine, mind and body. If culture is what humans have made, nature stands in for what humans didn't make, what is outside the human realm, or dominated by it. Sherry Ortner's classic piece from 1974, "Is Female to Male as Nature is to Culture?," disputes the claim that it is a cultural universal to value women less than men because women's reproductive capacities associate them with nature instead of culture. By contrast, Ortner shows that women occupy an ambiguous position somewhere between nature and culture.[7]

Two decades later Donna Haraway introduced the simian and cyborg as irreverent figures that trouble the persistent dichotomy between nature and culture. Cyborgs (a term that now rings quaintly of science fiction from before the personal computer) refuse dualism by emblematizing a chimeric fusion of organic and technological components. Simians are primates like us yet located across the human-animal divide. Haraway argues that women are another liminal figure, having been socially marginalized through association with "base" bodily nature and private emotion as opposed to intellect and public leadership, yet persistently claiming membership in economic, political, and intellectual collectives. Haraway calls simians, cyborgs, and women "monsters," which de*monst*rate, which signify: "The power-differentiated and highly contested modes of being of these monsters may be signs of possible worlds—and they are surely signs of worlds for which we are responsible."[8] Although childbearing people would not explain it in these terms, crafting themselves as border creatures between nature and technology was a way many sought to approach contemporary American childbearing and thereby negotiate what it means to be an authentic woman, human, self.

In a context where the cultural, technological, and masculine aspects of dualisms have been dominant, the "natural" can be a category of challenge; advocating for the natural, like advocating for the feminine, is disruptive to the social and political order of things. It is ironic, then, that the term *naturalization* describes how calling something natural obscures the history involved in making that thing—that is, being called natural hides the particularity, the contingency, the story of how something came to be the way it is and how it might be otherwise. Naturalizing something reinforces the existing power relations; it makes the perspective that dominated historical forces seem like the only perspective that exists. What is natural feels timeless, inescapable. We are powerless in the face of the natural. Yet in a way of understanding not shaped by dualism, wherein subjects and objects (people and things) aren't separated from one another but seen as mutually constitutive, enmeshed, and essentially similar, the very category of the natural would not make sense. If nature is what is untouched by technology or meaning making ("culture"), then how could a human take part in it, as all humans use tools and make meaning? Put otherwise, it makes no sense at all to care what is "natural" since absolutely nothing about the way we live is natural.

"Nature" is set apart from what is "human" and both idealized and reviled because of it; concern with the natural reveals a fundamental unease with what humans are understood to be.

. . .

"There's a hormone cocktail in birth that switches moms from left to right brain thinking," Kristen said later in the course, her blunt-cut hair swinging over her shoulder as she leaned forward to explain. "It's about activating that deep brain stem area, the amygdala, not the prefrontal cortex." According to basic neuroscience, the brain stem is responsible for systemic and motor function, the amygdala for emotions and memory, and the prefrontal cortex for cognition. Kristen presumes we are conversant with such neuroscientific facts, a display of expertise that recruits us as educated insiders while lending her claims epistemological weight. She presumed we had heard that analytic/instrumental thought comes from the left brain hemisphere and creative/emotional thought from the right. Both kinds of thinking had a place in the birthing knowledge Kristen was describing.

According to the BFW website, this "hormone cocktail" functions similarly for all birthing people, moving them from controlled, logical thinking to "labor land," where "instinctual, emotional, intuitive, creative, and meditative" thought reigns. The website described primordial knowledge as a state of being: "the innate maternal instinct. Women have this knowing in their bones! And they are in this knowing when they are *not* in their thinking mind!"[9] I was surprised by the extent to which the website's language naturalized the trope of Cartesian dualism, locating primordial knowledge in the (female) body and actively opposing it to the rational (male) mind. Yet Kristen's invocation of neuroscience folded these into one another, locating—and validating—both in the birthing brain. Endocrinology functioned similarly, positing hormones as both a site of innate involuntary response and a medium for self-cultivation. In this way of thinking about how bodies are lived, one's self is always both innate and designed. Biology and culture, nature and technology, the social and the emotional can all be recruited as tools in knowing and making this self. The art of self-making involves knowing which of these tools to use when, and this is precisely what Kristen was coaching Jasmine to do.

To access "labor land," one must put in place conditions conducive to the body's release of oxytocin, for reasons familiar from chapter 2. Kristen explained that this is why birthing in a calm, safe-feeling environment is important, expounding on a contextual physiology theory of hormonal responses I encountered everywhere, from doula training, to birthing people explaining their home birth rationale, to hospital nurses turning the lights down during labor. To some extent, hormones are considered involuntary biological responses, yet one can learn which hormonal responses are beneficial and rationally train oneself, through mindfulness, to be more or less open to their effects. BFW also introduced how and when to use medical technologies. The fifteen-minute animated film "The Elk and the Epidural," which presents the benefits and drawbacks of epidurals, featured in both Jasmine's course and a longer-format BFW course at which I assisted. In this fable, a calving mama elk encounters difficulties in her labor, hesitates at the brink of Epidural Cascading Falls (remember the "cascade of interventions" discussed in chapter 2?), decides to have an epidural, and births contentedly in the hospital. The film presents "animal nature," in the figure of the elk, as not only aspirational (in rosy watercolor aesthetics) but also attainable *with,* not in opposition to, the use of technology. This best-of-both-worlds approach echoes feminist debates over having it all while also showing the supposed distinction between masculine technology and feminine animality to have been a false dichotomy in the first place. (Note, however, that race and class affordances are implicit in the appeal of robust animality as a marker of feminine empowerment, which will be discussed more below.)

Self-knowledge requires cultivating certain kinds of innate awareness alongside rational understanding. The BFW website explained that social conditioning has taught modern women "not to trust or act on our gut knowing," with the result that "one of women's modern tasks of pregnancy is to first learn to feel their gut instinct and to distinguish this feeling from fleeting fear (or the contagious fear of others)." Intention and inevitability merge: one can practice accessing and trusting one's gut instinct using the prefrontal cortex to prepare to bypass the prefrontal cortex. Instinct becomes simultaneously a goal and a compulsion, as one must learn to disentangle trustworthy, desirable, properly innate instincts from emotional responses caused by external factors. This recruits a deeply rooted Western ideology about the interior origins of authentic identity, as opposed to aspects of oneself shaped by relations and context.[10] North American body projects are generally about revealing one's preexistent personal reality (one's "nature") as opposed to approaching bodies as "plastic" fields of potentiality.[11] This is evident in the name "Birthing from Within" itself. In the BFW framework, instincts are desirable not because they are biological but because they are internal, and thus linked with personal authenticity. The cortisol panic response, although equally biological, is not valorized in part because it is seen as resulting from troublesome external factors.

Self-knowledge is needed to override problematic emotional-biological responses. Instructors at both the longer-format BFW class and the mindfulness-based class emphasized the importance of a meditative mental state to enable nonreactive behavior. Such meditative presence is neither instinctual nor analytic but rather is a sort of emotional transcendence entailing self-discipline, self-awareness, and self-confidence. The other BFW instructor, Janice, explained that "reactions" are defenses, and since a properly cultivated birthing space is safe, there is no need for a birthing person to be defensive. However, she explained, "Your body doesn't know that. . . . You can't think clearly when the brain is flooded with adrenaline." Likewise, when Kristen was describing the amygdala, she implied that its functioning would sometimes need to be overridden. Self-knowledge included confidently directing the social situation, which Janice encouraged birthing people to do by "calmly working out problems" from their meditative state, without either creating or avoiding conflict nor speaking from a place of wanting to appease. By deliberately managing one's affect, one could also manage one's hormones and brain, which in turn influence one's rational faculties and enable practical action.

The three kinds of knowing seamlessly merge, not only allowing an optimal birth experience but also producing a more authentic self. Self-knowledge is recruited into a moral imperative that realizes and reinforces a neoliberal version of feminist empowerment wherein self-actualized birthing is the goal. Self-actualization is my shorthand for phrases like "become your best self," "do what's right for you," and "progress on your journey." There is an implicit theory of the self as preexisting yet optimizable, intensely individual yet grounded in universal human biology, requiring the body but not reducible to it. The locus of this self is quite slippery, a moving target that shuttles between being designed and innate. The self is a feedback loop between process and product, subject and object, transcendent and immanent; the personal dexterity needed to navigate contemporary birthing has to account for this complex lived body. As such, Bay Area childbearing can become a management project premised upon a sophisticated understanding of sociotechnical logistics, an attunement to one's biophysical functions, and a quasi-spiritual self-awareness. These capacities are not at odds but interdependent, looping through each other like a Möbius strip. Identity is not figured here as a passive truth waiting to be revealed; rather, the active and ongoing process of seeking to know oneself is understood as equally part of one's identity. This is influenced by the cultural prestige of technology-based "design" and "optimization," and scientific frontiers in which biology is itself a technology.[12] This is not to say that bodies are understood as inherently malleable (as they are, for example, in Brazil among many who tinker with their embodied experiences by taking hormones); here, self-design is not about crafting one's material body within social relations, but rather about creating the proper conditions for internal truth to emerge.[13] Biology is a means to authenticity, digging into evolutionary depths and reconciling them within modern technological contexts.

BIRTHING FROM WITHIN: A DOULA-LED
RITE OF PASSAGE

"We support women—what the mother wants is our priority," asserted my doula training instructor. Being a doula was, in theory, not about furthering our own agendas for a "good birth" or following any prescribed course of action. As service providers, we were to help the birthing person identify her own desires by providing information and opportunities for reflection, and to mediate between her, her partner and family, and hospital staff to help realize those desires. Like most of the women who asked me to be their doula, Jasmine did so because she wanted "support." As a doula, figuring out how to be supportive and not directive involved asking about, listening to, and observing what a person wanted. Navigating childbearing decisions and practices was not so much a question of seeking expert advice or following in the footsteps of friends or family as it was of introspection and choosing "a path that's right for me," in Jasmine's words. In crafting such a path, childbearing people (and their doulas) have to manage not only birth (toward the desired outcome of a healthy baby) but also the meanings of the birth experience (toward a feeling of authenticity, of self-actualization). The achievement of this feeling is aspirational, but in the communities where I spent time, the compulsion to seek it is so normative—that is, understood as the right thing to do—that I consider it a new rite of passage.[14]

Practitioners on the medical periphery, such as doulas, childbirth educators, and some midwives, often decline to be overtly prescriptive while attending closely to the process, and outcome, of others' decision-making. Childbearing people were encouraged, even pressured, by online media and their peers to make their own choices and have opinions, even when they were not particularly interested in doing so. Nondirected decision-making reflects dominant Euro-American ideas of agency and consent (by contrast, for example, Vietnamese childbearing is shaped by practices of collective decision-making).[15] Yet the nonoptional status of this expectation levies judgment of its own. Discourse about making the "right" choices could certainly be moralizing, even in ostensibly supportive reassurances that c-sections or formula feeding are not personal failures, yet for those I worked among, the pervasive sentiment was that childbearing people should be judged not for their choices but rather for the process by which they make them.[16] Not only does this stance presume that various options are accessible at will, which is not the case for most people; it also presumes that people have the time, energy, and money to spend crafting their approach, and themselves. I was particularly struck by this when volunteering at a transitional home for vulnerable childbearing people, where clients needed much more practical assistance than help identifying their desires. Recognizing ways my middle-class doula preparation was largely irrelevant brought into relief how centered it was around shaping such an "appropriate" childbearing subjectivity.

Two rituals associated with this rite of passage stand out to me: making birth plans and "going to" labor land. As rituals, they serve a performative rather than a merely instrumental function, drawing the birthing person's attention to the meaningfulness of the process itself, apart from the outcome. Birth plans, discussed in chapter 3, are a result of research, counseling, and introspection, which are often facilitated by a doula. Crafting a birth plan entails making choices that come attached to ideologies that people use to narrate themselves; childbearing people often explained their practices to me using phrases like, "That's just how I approach life," or "I'm going to do [x] but I'm not ashamed to have [y]," or "I'm doing [z], but I'm not *that* kind of person." Labor land, the intuitive, creative state Kristen referred to above, usually entailed experiencing the intensity of unmedicated labor for a period of time, also often facilitated by a doula. Birth plans and labor land require (and cultivate) modern and primordial knowing, respectively. While birth plans are squarely in the realm of the rational, that is to say the human side of the nature/culture binary, labor land bleeds into the animalistic and the spiritual, at the edges of what usually counts as human. Seeking authenticity through birth involves grappling with the animal/spiritual aspects of embodiment.

Many doulas and midwives I spoke with extolled the beauty and power of "primal," "instinctive," "animal" states during labor, characterizing them in terms of internal awareness, spiritual intensity, and disregard for social and cultural conventions. Alzbeta, an experienced doula, offered this explanation when asked about labor land:

> It's that place where you really need to get out of your head and go within. Just work with it. Go with the flow, and don't go against it. And I dunno if that's the right terminology, calling it labor land, but definitely I've seen it. An animal instinct. You'll ask a lot of women, they'll say, "Oh my gosh," or the partner will say, "She's gone to that place, and it was really surprising but she went there."

Explaining that "we are taught in our culture to stay in our frontal brain," Alzbeta called it a sacred and beautiful thing to trust instead in a knowing body: "Don't try to analyze; just let go and let your body do it." Open-mouthed, guttural animal noises were very much a part of birthing, sounding out everywhere from doula training, to births I attended, to a singing circle for childbearing people and birth workers. Once, in a childbirth class at which I was assisting, I was asked to playact a person in labor, and making grunting or moaning noises was foremost among the trainer's requests. Along with noisemaking, nudity seemed almost inevitable; laboring people would gradually cease to care about tugging their hospital gown into place, and my assisting them while they showered and used the toilet quickly became a commonsense intimacy.

But it is not usually straightforward to embrace one's animal nature. I have a poignant memory of Molly, whom we met in chapter 2, squatting naked on the birth stool after hours of pushing. Her trembling, glowing body exuded both exhaustion and triumph, yet for all her intensity, there was something incongruous and even ridiculous about the scene, which was set against a backdrop of computerized bureaucracy and orderly generic decor. In the way Molly practiced it and we received it, nudity was embraced as a sign and symptom of tapping into primordial power, a far cry from the infantilization of the shaved pubic area that was standard practice of decades past.[17] Yet such power must exist in modern contexts. Reconciling these contrasts is part of seeking authenticity, blending two kinds of reality: raw intensity and practical imperatives. Just as the birth plan's significance is more about design than implementation, labor land is about the personal development needed to "go there" and release into one's innate animality/spirituality while still being connected to high-tech surroundings.

Recall Dani from chapter 3, the mother who mentioned wanting to ram her head against a wall like a goat; for her, animality meant an emphasis on physicality and immediacy. When I asked her how her brain was working during labor, she said:

> I was like an animal. I kinda describe it as like, you know how dogs want to just crawl into the backyard and die under a bush by themselves? That's what it felt like my labor experience was! [Laugh] I didn't want any light, I didn't want any major stimulation, closed curtains, turned off all lights.... I did not want to know what time it was ... so that's what I mean animalistic, just intensely present to what was going on right there.

Midwives and doulas often marked this primal state as essentially female, capable of catalyzing a specifically feminine spiritual experience beyond the social constraints of gender propriety. Spirituality was frequently invoked to frame this foray into the nonrational, as were metaphors of goddesses, quests, or labyrinths. Dani rejected the term *labor land* but nonetheless described an otherworldly experience:

> Labor land sounds like Candy Land, sounds like something really light. I've been describing it as I went to hell. It's birth hell, it's totally birth hell. Going to the moon and back. It's like intergalactic travel. But it really is like going to the underworld and bringing a baby back. You have to go down, you have to meet the devil ... shake his hand and do a little dance, then you have to climb back up from Hades.... Oh yeah, and bleed like hell. It was very Grecian, like otherworldly.

One's personal journey inward marks a radical departure from conventional sociality. In Alzbeta's words, "Ignore everyone around you, think 'I don't care.'" Yet these rituals are not primarily concerned with correctly producing womanhood, much less social identities as "good" wives or mothers; rather, they foreground a person operating at the height of her capacities by skillfully drawing on rationality, animality, and spirituality, all of which are embraced as human.

This politics of the human is situated in a particular context of gender, class, and race. Some can choose to be primitive rather than being dubbed so by others, as some can choose to have a cesarean while others have little say in the matter. Near birth ideas about instinct, intuition, and innate knowing are often infused with biological gender essentialism, as we have seen, and are also often linked with a feminized spiritual power. We discussed this a bit in chapter 3, but I want to return to it here to point out how associations with animality and spirituality might seem divergent but have the same effect: they bring birth out of the realm of the human. Or rather, they push against normative, dualistic ideas of what humans are (and it's worth repeating that this is an easier rhetorical move to make for White women, who haven't been historically dehumanized in the same way as people of color). Claims to animality and spirituality celebrate the corporeal and the nonrational, both reinforcing women's association with these devalued aspects and (re)claiming them as essential and superlative. Mere decades ago feminist insistence on pain medication was at least partially because it was "civilizing"; now, this reactionary push is precisely against the idea that it is civilizing, as a way to embrace different power dynamics.

Reclaiming femininity and animality brings with it an "uncivilized" spirituality that is intimately linked with the body. In Rachel Yoder's fabulous (literally and figuratively) novel *Nightbitch,* the overwhelmed mother of a toddler flickers into a she-wolf, displaying a ferocious animality that emerges in response to her lost sense of self. It makes her mothering easier and ignites her submerged passion for artistic creation but at the cost of her sanity, of belonging in a rational human world. As she surrenders to the transformation, she sees how the violent physicality is also creative potency: "At times she terrified herself, wondering if she was a god, if being a mother was one way of being a god. Of course, she couldn't strike anyone down with a lightning bolt, but she could bring a person into being using little more than a handful of clay. Way less, in fact. How were mothers even a thing? How had they not been outlawed? They were divine, beyond horrifying."[18] She tries to articulate how having a child "allows a woman to see how much infinite potential there is," not sating a deep yearning to create but compounding it.[19]

There is a long history of nature, spirituality, and authenticity being entwined in America, conditioned by how Europeans encountered and made sense of Indigenous societies and their religious practices.[20] Renowned figures in this history who are deeply enmeshed with California's landscapes and cultural mythos include John Muir and Gary Snyder, but also less credited women who were cornerstones of the ecofeminist movement, including Susan Griffin and Carolyn Merchant, as well as Starhawk, a key figure in the pagan revival of the late twentieth century. Very generally, ecofeminism views the oppression of women and nature as linked, while neo-paganism orients around their shared potency. The intensity of childbearing makes one aware of the power of the body and the embodied self, the power of transformation; it is a power linked with surrender more than mastery, and of connection rather than separation.

In her book *Dreaming the Dark: Sex, Magic, and Politics,* Starhawk tackles the problem of dualism head-on. In her own terms, she "attempts to move in the space where that split does not exist, where the stories of duality that our culture tells us no longer bind us to repeat the same old plots," where power comes from elsewhere than the "principle of domination upon which our society is based." She argues for power-from-within—immanence—instead of power-over and aims at "using it to resist the destruction that those who wield power-over are bringing upon the world."[21] She doesn't insist on the terms "witch," "goddess," or "magic," finding similarity of purpose with radical Catholics, Buddhists, Quakers, and atheists, for example, but she uses words that make people uncomfortable precisely because the comfortable words are the language of estrangement.

In this rite of passage, animality and spirituality are framed as deeply personal experiences based on self-knowledge and a kind of timeless embodied truth. Finding and enacting an authentic self is forwarded as a moral and social imperative, part of a ritual framework that allows one to reach toward becoming a more fully developed, self-aware, and empowered person. In taking up this project, childbearing people might fail as often as they succeed. Those I spoke with weighed ideals against the constraints and imperatives of their own lives. Such compromises were made from positions of great privilege, and even then making it all work out was stressful. Similar to how Emily Abel and Carole Browner describe women's "selective compliance" with medical authority, I saw selective compliance with an idealized self-authority.[22] People's resolve wavered, and their opinions could fluctuate under shifting influences, pushing them to seek certainty elsewhere. The pressure to chart one's own path and make decisions from within can be intimidating, particularly when one has little experience of childbearing and is unsure of what is actually possible; doulas are in part a response to this. (Most of the people I worked with were either anticipating their first child or grappling with a negative prior experience.) The injunction to design the proper conditions for natural capacities to emerge led to feelings of failure if one's body did not rise to the occasion. Everyone wanted "what's best for baby"—but it was not obvious what that is, or what the childbearing person's own desires have to do with it.

What is clear to me is that ideas about what people are, and how humanity is possible *with* aspects of animality and divinity and not in opposition to them, are key in this self-making, this birthing from within. It is a many-layered play with decades (centuries!) of adjudicating what human—and womanly—nature is. It mixes neuroscience with nostalgia, blends woman as hyper-self-aware with woman as instinctive animal. Neither "primordial" biology nor "modern" design is an end in itself; rather, people wield both instinct and rationality in service of actualizing an authentic self.

After discussing herself as a cyborg with her breast pump, Eula Biss writes that when her friend asked if her son's birth was a "natural" birth, she "was tempted to say that it was an animal birth. While his head was crowning, I was trying to use my own hands to pull apart my flesh and bring him out of my body. Or so I have been told, but I do not remember any intention to tear myself open—all I remember is the urgency of the moment. I was both human and animal then. Or I was neither, as I am now."[23] Anne Enright rejects the animal metaphor in favor of a technological one, memorably describing her pregnant body as taking on agency of its own: "From week to week I felt my body shift into different cycles, like some slow-motion, flesh-based washing machine. . . . I did not feel like an animal, I felt like a clock, one made of blood and bone, that you could neither hurry nor delay. . . . There was no technology for it: I was the technology."[24]

A "good" birth, then, is one in which a birthing person realizes themselves as agentive in a particular way: as both thoughtfully in control, integrating technology as needed, and able to tap into their inner animality and spiritual power by setting the proper conditions for it to emerge. Crafting authenticity through attention to various aspects of embodiment foregrounds an emancipatory politics of women's self-determination. And yet it falls into a dominant cultural discourse that minimizes thinking about mutual account-ability, allowing the social conditions in which humans actually exist to fall to the wayside.

DESIGNING THE INNATE: GODDESS, ANIMAL, CYBORG, HUMAN

Jasmine experienced the postpartum period after her first child's birth as full of anxieties about returning to work, producing and pumping milk, and the baby's weight; anxious memories of this time overshadowed preparations for the birth of her second child. When I encountered a Silicon Valley start-up founded by three Stanford graduates who were designing a better breast pump and looking for moms to talk to, I connected them with Jasmine. Later, I attended a meeting to brainstorm design goals for their nascent product. The meeting was held at an "incubator" that helps San Francisco tech start-ups by providing them a workspace, funding, and mentorship. I arrived at the refurbished warehouse in the gentrifying South of Market neighborhood, with its banged-up metal door and rusty railings, and checked in on a sleek iPad. Piles of electronics were strewn across tables filling the open space. In a smaller meeting room, pump prototypes of silicone cups and tubing were set out, and refreshments included varieties of Mrs. Patel's "lactation treats" and teas, made with fenugreek seed to stimulate milk production, a gesture toward both the herbal medicine of the White natural birth movement and the prominence of South Asian immigrant cultures in Silicon Valley. The other six attendees were nursing mothers.

Infant feeding is a morally and emotionally charged issue (often reduced to questions of breast milk versus formula, though there are myriad hybrid practices) among White, educated, and/or middle-class communities. There are logistical difficulties in breastfeeding while maintaining a professional life, as Jasmine did, in addition to a swath of anxieties and frustrations about one's ability to produce adequate breastmilk (an ability heavily coded as "natural"). Both concerns were projected onto the fantasy pump we were envisioning. Attendees said it should ideally work under clothing, with people around, and while doing something else (multitasking is essential). It should be easy to clean, with few parts and crevices, simple to use with no instructions, and have mix-and-match components to suit various outfits and contexts. Perhaps it could sense when it was set up incorrectly and alert the user, and it could come with a nightlight. They emphasized that it must be a stress reducer, not a stress enhancer. Particularly interesting was talk of an accompanying mobile app to track data and provide moral support, offering a virtual "high five" and letting the user know how much milk had been pumped—although if the volume were less than usual, attendees worried such information might be "crushing." The app offered a kind of technological intuition, as these nursing people hoped it might not only assuage feelings of failure and guilt, but also help them relax and "connect with the baby's needs" through tracking, praise, reminders, and education—"like a baby health Fitbit." This breast pump was to be a personalized tool that could be tailored to one's own biometrics and emotions.

This fantasy breast pump encapsulates the political aspirations at stake in this version of authenticity. It would seamlessly meld into the childbearing person's physical and emotional contours, enhancing her capabilities and fortifying her wellness, while feeling "like skin on skin" instead of like being hooked to a machine. In this imaginary, the nursing person is a cyborg in Donna Haraway's best sense, empowered by relationship to a machine. Mammalian functioning is valorized via comparison not with the denigrated animality of livestock—nursing people did not want to feel "like a cow" when using the breast pump—but instead with the primordial version represented by the noble wild elk and experienced as naked power. The pump would produce new embodied possibilities—in many ways, new possibilities for being a woman—in a historical context of feminism in which both the mechanical and the fleshly have been romanticized as well as disparaged. Yet there are political stakes not just in this fantastic version of the individual human body and its capacities but in the very focus on it, a focus that eclipses social context.

When paid labor often separates childbearing people from their babies at the same time that the virtues of breastfeeding are extolled by U.S. Surgeon General and there is a rise in what Charlotte Faircloth calls "militant lactivism," breast pumps are a crucial technology, essential for whatever possibility there is for women to "have it all."[25] They contain contradictory politics, blurring domestic work and paid labor in a way that creates "more work for mother,"[26] and providing more mobility and freedom to users while also highlighting the absurd absence of guaranteed maternity leave in the United States. At the meeting with the start-up, we did not discuss parental leave policies or employer accommodations for pumping. Nor were questions of affordability addressed; when I asked what price point the developers anticipated, the range given was out of reach for most American families. The meeting exemplifies how pressure to craft oneself as a nature/culture hybrid results in personal anxieties about failure, and eclipses structural and social issues on which enacting such hybrids depends. The quest for an individualized, exclusive, technical solution for a problem that might otherwise be solved by collectively restructuring working conditions, gender relations, and state responsibility illustrates the neoliberal context in which self-actualization is valorized.

Using ideas about personal authenticity to navigate the options within contemporary childbearing is not simply a new version of the familiar tale wherein a person realizes herself as a proper woman through becoming a (good) mother in a culturally appropriate way.[27] Rather than foregrounding embeddedness in a heterosexual matrix of gender and kinship, these narratives around authenticity share tropes and cultural logics from the Silicon Valley world of innovation, disruption, and entrepreneurship. As childbearing decisions become practices of self-actualization, they become ways of doing feminism, producing a less-gendered womanhood and making reproduction matter—that is to say, they become political. In this sense, they are what Michel Foucault calls "technologies of the self."[28] Yet the way self-actualization circulates as a discourse of authenticity is notably depoliticized, supposedly "just" about oneself. This is a way of not acknowledging the structural and material constraints on making choices, and also a means of disconnecting from relationships, traditions, and responsibilities—connections that might make claims upon one's freedom but might also provide guidance and reassurance.

There are positive things about this cultural emphasis on personal agency. It responds to a history of misogyny in hospital reproductive care. It can neutralize coercive, dogmatic ideas about natural versus medical approaches, and transcend the shaming that childbearing people often encounter tied to accusations of endangering their babies either by not doing things "naturally" enough or by not making adequate use of technology. Focusing on and valorizing the self shifts focus off the fetus/baby, whose interests can eclipse those of the mother in reproductive politics.[29] Yet it also diverts attention from (and therefore perpetuates) the social and structural pressure put on mothers to be the sole fount of security in an insecure world.[30] Seeking authenticity in the ways I witnessed is a response to not knowing how to be in the here and now, to being in a generic, abstracted world, lonely and disconnected—but looking deep into the self for guidance instead of looking outward. This is also alienating, so people reach for other rudders, reach far from their immediate context, from their here and now.

We have already encountered the concepts of "authoritative knowledge" (professional forms of knowing about birth and women's bodies) and intuition (personal, contextual knowledge); a third kind of knowing is experiential knowledge, which draws on cultural tradition and the experiences of friends and family.[31] I rarely heard anyone explain their choices by referring to cultural traditions, and although some people invoked family traditions, like gifting a particular kind of teddy bear or using a heritage cradle, they did not follow received wisdom about *how* to undergo childbearing. Accepting help from parents and in-laws was often coupled with strategies for maintaining personal space and defending one's preferences; Stanford Medicine offered a course for new grandparents teaching them, basically, to back down and respect their children's choices as parents.

While some may feel removed from familial and cultural traditions for reasons of geographic and class mobility or generational length, there is also a cultural pressure to self-invent by crafting personally meaningful rituals and making new traditions. For example, "blessingways" were promoted in my doula training as something we might offer clients, and they were practiced by several people I interviewed. These appropriate a Navajo custom (generally without crediting it) and entail a gathering of friends and family to bless the pregnant person via newly invented rituals like group singing or making bracelets to wear until the baby is born. More recently I encountered White, Euro-American people practicing "closing the bones" ceremonies that emulate a tradition variously attributed to Mexico or Ecuador, in which cotton shawls called *rebozos* are wrapped around the recipient's pelvis to symbolize closure of the childbearing experience. In the Bay Area generally, knowledge accrues influence less from established institutions or heritage than from claims to being innovative, disruptive, and original, yet ironically these self-invented rituals appropriate preexisting practices (or stereotypes of them) that are part of other heritages. They evidence the desire for a root without knowing where to look for one. They demonstrate ambivalence about belonging.

I have even recently seen detachment touted as a virtue in doula work. In 2023 a doula group I am part of in Scotland circulated advertisements about a training (offered by someone based in the Bay Area) to become a "transformational birth coach." This growing approach uses the contemporary entrepreneurial sense of coaching to detach doulas from the outcomes of births, and even from participating in them, in favor of preparing childbearing people's mindsets. This particular advertisement was dense with the jargon of self-actualization. It claimed that, given the unpredictability of childbirth, the "secret" to "a positive experience" is staying "committed to the process." This "new framework" was marketed to doulas presumed to be exhausted, suggesting that one could "avoid over-committing yourself to the point of burnout" and instead increase clients' accountability, ownership, and autonomy. The doula movement itself was presumed to be burned-out: "After five decades of teaching childbirth education classes and providing doula support, it is time to admit that we have not been as impactful, nor successful, in our mission to promote healthy and positive birth experiences. It is time to pivot!" Rather than focusing on birth per se, such coaching could "empower individuals undergoing major life transitions so that they can create a clear vision for the next phase," helping a client "become the expert in her life." Rather than emphasizing nearness and accompaniment, this version of doula support is entirely about coping with the inevitability of being alone.

The breast pump app and its "baby Fitbit" capacities align with a take on nature that looks for truth in both individual bodies and an imagined elsewhere, but not in surrounding context or community. This take on nature is at the root of other popular trends in the Bay Area and elsewhere, such as paleo diets and barefoot running, as well as biometric tracking and biohacking. What links them is a focus on the body itself as opposed to its context, as well as an explicit desire to optimize the body. This is *not* the 1970s version of nature, which evoked anti-consumerism, informal communality, spirituality, harmonizing with the outdoors, and allowing the body to do what it will. Neither is it ecofeminism, foregrounding ecological and intergenerational relations and their concomitant responsibilities (although both of these sensibilities do flicker around the edges of contemporary Bay Area birth worlds). Rather, current ideas about human nature invoke pop neuroscience and the idea that certain traits or aptitudes are hardwired into generic individuals through evolutionary processes, downplaying the role of society, cultural particularity, or material environments. Nature is framed as something both universal and inherent to individuals, rather than cultivated through particular experiences in an interconnected world; it is instinct, not intuition. Self-optimization not only involves managing logistics well and in keeping with one's essential nature (as with the self-actualization discussed above), but it heightens anxiety by suggesting there is a best way of doing so. For many of the people I worked with, such rhetoric both fueled their anxiety by elevating the stakes of their decisions and provided much-desired guidance. Ideas about optimizing the self recruit high-tech biometric practices alongside ideas about a primordial, ancestral embodiment removed from the corruptions of modern life.

The emphasis on individualized desires, self-awareness, and personal responsibility as, in Kristen's words, the "most important kind of knowledge" advances a social politics of non-relationship, of being not-accountable for each other—which, from a position of privilege, can look like autonomy. However, anxieties about an uncertain future beyond any individual's control or influence haunt this sort of autonomy, perhaps in a mutually reinforcing way. In his study of U.S. affect since the Cold War, Joseph Masco argues that technological fallout creates complex problems that exceed existing social forms (such as the nation or the family), take on momentum of their own, and bewilder people's sensory capacity to perceive and negotiate risk; consequently, practices of everyday life are based on insulating oneself from one's environment, not engaging it.[32] Turning inward could be seen as a reasonable response in the face of a future that seems out of one's control; hyperfocus on one's personal decisions could go hand in hand with a sense of disempowerment and social alienation. It is precisely because the material and social conditions that interfere with self-actualization are sidelined from the self-making feedback loop that the whole project is not only untenable, and therefore anxiety provoking at a personal level, but can resonate with feelings of alienation and disempowerment ratcheted up to the species level.

THE SCALE OF THE SPECIES: EVOLUTION AND NOSTALGIA

Evolutionary narratives look to the deep past to locate a form of truth in human origins, a truth that is usually disconnected from the sort of relational issues that might make claims on someone in the present. The science of attachment and attachment parenting fuels a vibrant set of ideas about appropriate human reproduction, including extended breastfeeding well past the toddler years, babywearing, co-sleeping, skin-to-skin bonding, and continuous cooperative childcare wherein the young child is never left alone but is also not the responsibility of one person. This body of research includes some fabulous neologisms, such as "skinship" and "breastsleeping," which tie into ideas about mother-infant co-embodiment. "Allomothering" describes group supervision of children in indulgent, low-punishment, mixed groups doing play-oriented work, using "attachment networks" in which the mother's primacy is not confused with exclusivity. The birthing person's body has been described as the baby's habitat, its micro evolutionary environment of adaptedness (MEEA), and in turn, that babies' cuteness is evolutionarily designed to appeal to adult humans' brains—both longstanding premises in attachment theory, along with the idea that "babies have no wants, only needs."[33]

Sometimes called "paleo parenting," this intellectual heritage recruits evolution to advocate for particular cultural practices. Whether or not these practices have desirable effects is to the side of what interests me about them—although continuous cooperative childcare sounds pretty great. It is odd to evaluate practices via beliefs about earlier evolutionary states, whether cultural or physical. Why would the fact of something having been done in a radically different context automatically recommend the practice? Such recommendations are overwhelmingly applied to individual parenting behaviors, whereas it seems clear that, if anything, they should cause us to reconsider the contexts we have made.

Biocultural research on childbearing, which spans biocultural and evolutionary anthropology, developmental psychology, evolutionary biology, and behavioral ecology, walks a line between producing evidence to support what people are already doing for any number of embodied, contextual, cultural reasons, and adding to the cacophony of pressure on parents to be a certain way.[34] It often looks to primates as bearers of biological truth, and to human cultural arrangements supposedly closer to primate life, such as hunter-gatherer societies. Claims about, for example, the appropriate age to wean (often between three and seven years) or the survival benefits of unmedicated labor source legitimation from ideas about a persistent, underlying nature, as though biology were destiny, which can imply that biology is timeless and static, not itself responsive to context. Bringing biology into interaction with the sociocultural is not easy to do in a society so structured by nature/culture dualism. Biocultural anthropology attempts to do this in a way that integrates the two entities, while feminist science studies is more concerned with how the two were never separate in the first place.

Such work can push, slowly, for broader change instead of adding individualized pressures. For example, the concept of breastsleeping, introduced by James McKenna and Lee Gettler at the Mother-Baby Behavioral Sleep Laboratory at Notre Dame, asserts that infants and their mothers are biologically intended to sleep in close proximity such that breastfeeding and sleeping seamlessly become part of the same activity. Their work offers what the lab's website calls "a major corrective to more traditional infant sleep models promulgated in western societies." They promote the concept in pediatric journals, arguing that babies and nursing people affect each other's "sleep architecture" (the adult's body trains the baby's body in temperature regulation, breathing rhythms, and patterns of deep and shallow sleep), that bed-sharing infants are less susceptible to sudden infant death syndrome (SIDS), that the "sustained tactile interaction" of breastsleeping gives babies more neurological stimulation, leading to better emotional security and problem-solving abilities as toddlers, and that as teens and adults, bed sharers are "more happy, optimistic, confident, and close to their family."[35] They argue that a breastsleeping dyad "comprises such vastly different behavioural and physiological characteristics compared with nonbreastfeeding mothers and infants" that it must be given its own epidemiological category.[36] If the American Pediatrics Association formally recommended bed-sharing on the basis of such research, this would shift the landscape of regulation, expert advice, and consumer products, creating a very different context for individuals to navigate.

In addition to behavioral-physiological research, other contemporary science explores the biology of motherhood through genetics. Abigail Tucker's popular nonfiction book *Mom Genes: Inside the New Science of Our Ancient Maternal Instinct* claims to reveal "the hard science behind our tenderest maternal impulses, exploring the ways a new mom's brain gets permanently rewired."[37] This is different from the "scientific mothering" of the 1940s and '50s, when "better living through chemistry" and all kinds of products and processes now deemed "unnatural," including formula feeding, became aspirational and then mainstream. Not only has the authority of scientific expertise become more diffuse and characterized by multiplicity over the past century, with parents holding more decision-making power and consumers being conceptualized as more scientifically literate—but popular uptake of science has become more about illuminating what's "natural" and therefore true and good, interpreting what is supposedly already deep within us. If it's genetic, it's inarguable; it's hardwired.

Recall Haraway's "simians, cyborgs, and women" analysis. She explains that in observing animals, especially primates, we polish a mirror "to look for ourselves."[38] Feminists have struggled "over the modes of producing knowledge about, and the meanings of, the behavior and the social lives of monkeys and apes."[39] Indeed, paleo parenting ideas are both lauded and decried by feminists. Haraway's feminist critique helped found the discipline of science studies, which keeps returning to questions about the knowing/known subject and the trope that women's knowledge is somatic, primal, and emotional as opposed to rational and scientific. Recruiting the language of supposedly acultural biology to describe the ideal conditions for health and well-being brings scientific frames to bear on ideas about gendered care, asserting that health and well-being stem from proper biological conditions and thereby masking the politics implicit in the recommendations. Both attachment theory and ideas about paleo living have been critiqued by scholars for their naturalizing effects—briefly, attachment theory takes moral ideas from nineteenth-century Anglo-America (which stem from the Romantic response to the woman question) and psychologizes them into human universals, while "paleofantasies" presume that there was a past state of harmony between humans and our environment (when this was, exactly, is unclear), and that evolution only takes place excruciatingly slowly.[40] And yet both ideas persist.

They persist and are so powerful because of the way they resonate with contemporary ideas about nature as something clean and pure, unsullied by human modernity and its malaise. Literally looking to monkeys radically ignores the context in which Americans live today, despite claims about possible modifications. It locates a kind of inexorable truth in primal/primitive/primate states, implying that contemporary culture is a corruption of past purity in a reversal of the techno-futurist progress narrative. In the birth worlds I moved in, rhetoric about humans writ large could take on apocalyptic tones, describing species-level degeneration and echoing anxieties about the Anthropocene, the idea that we have entered an epoch of human-made environmental catastrophe.

Michel Odent's 2014 *Childbirth and the Evolution of Homo Sapiens* is emblematic. In it, the French obstetrician, also a prolific author and much-lauded figure in many Bay Area birth circles, suggests that the rising rate of cesareans is causing the human species to evolve such that it might not be able to birth new generations without intensive medical involvement. He posits a thought experiment: considering how safe and easy cesareans are now, perhaps a cesarean-dependent species is simply appropriate to the times? Odent argues, however, that the "primal period" near birth is crucial in the formation of lifelong (and intergenerational) human wellness, connecting medical interventions into the "oxytocin system" with an increased population-wide incidence of autoimmune, metabolic, and mental-emotional disorders. Odent attempts to cut across conventional chains of cause and effect, positing, for example, that the pertinent difference is not between vaginal and cesarean births, but between births where the "physiological hormone cascade" has been initiated and those where induction bypassed this process, or births where the "trauma hormones" of adrenaline and cortisol are present and those where they aren't. He expresses concern that the proportion of people who bear children "thanks to the activity of their own oxytocin system" is becoming insignificant, arguing that "there are no other examples of physiological systems that have suddenly been made useless. . . . [O]xytocin is involved in all aspects of our reproductive/sexual life, in socialization, and in all facets of the capacity to love, which might include respect for 'Mother

Earth.'"[41] Odent calls for more research into correlations that have not been adequately investigated, including possible near birth origins of noncommunicable diseases from obesity to autism, to which end he started the Primal Health Research Center in London. He extrapolates the possible damage caused by near birth practices not just to maternal-infant outcomes, or even to lifelong health metrics, but to the fate of the species.

The preservation of the species features in other birth media, such as the *Indie Birth* podcast (part of a larger enterprise including doula and midwifery training). One episode states that a natural, midwife-led birth process is "really is what's going to keep us going as humans."[42] It acknowledges that this is a big leap but gestures toward "tons of research," including how undisturbed birth allows for bonding, which is "what holds us together as glue. These are the relationships that we need to grow up into healthy, responsible, caring people." Positing a "worst-case scenario" in which in fifty years no one knows normal birth anymore, they cite the preservation of the species as "the huge picture for many of us that are choosing outside of this system. It's not just to be different." And yet, within an instant, this enormous scope swoops back into the frame of individual risk: "It's not always super politically charged for many women. It's simply that they understand that this is the safest way for them to bring a baby into this world." Personal safety and the fate of the species align around "natural" physiology. This is a different framing than the activism we will visit in chapter 7; by explicitly minimizing the political aspects of birthing practices, nature as an inarguable force comes to the fore—diminishing history and context, which is itself a political move.

Ideas about childbearing on grand temporal scales are entwined with the politics of nostalgia. Nadia Seremetakis argues that the American use of nostalgia involves trivializing romantic sentimentality, "freez[ing] the past in such a manner as to preclude it from any capacity for social transformation in the present, preventing the present from establishing a dynamic perceptual relationship to its history." By contrast, she says, the Greek sense of nostalgia is "the desire or longing with burning pain" to journey home, evoking "the sensory dimension of memory in exile and estrangement," mixing bodily and emotional pain.[43] Bay Area birth worlds' nostalgia for the "natural" past is not based on sensory memory of actual experiences (at least not within individual bodies; transgenerational community memory might be something else), but it does speak to present experiences of loss or lack. It is full of longing for a more sensuous relation with the material world and embodied existence, exalting the perhaps-remembered delights of physical closeness with one's parent and the intensity of labor in an anesthetized world. Practices seeking authenticity in birth worlds suggest that such a longing does transform the present and is not merely "frozen" sentimentality or mere projection.

Feminist thinkers, including Starhawk and Silvia Federici, whom we have met, reference the witch hunts as a historical turning point that "shattered the peasants' connection with the land, drove women out of the work of healing, and imposed the mechanist view of the world as a dead machine," a rupture that "underlies the entwined oppressions of race, sex, class, and ecological destruction."[44] This philosophical, historical insight has had a suppressed but enduring resonance over recent decades, as we saw in chapter 1—and indeed, it holds a place in my heart. But it can evoke a romantic vision of past purity similar to that of evolutionary approaches to paleo parenting. Both versions of valorizing a more authentic humanness in the past reverberate with emotional aspiration and discontent, a malaise permeating "how we do things now." The book about Amazonian tribal childbearing mentioned by the attachment parenting instructor in chapter 4, Liedloff's *The Continuum Concept* (which also surfaced a few other times during my fieldwork), was a crossover between these visions. It bears the subtitle "In Search of Happiness Lost."

Yet expressions of sensuous desire too easily become appropriated into weighty dictates about the "right" way to do things, using the authoritative language of science in a way that ossifies gender politics or forecloses rationales based on spirituality, intuition, or—heaven forbid—pleasure. Most people, of course, would not advocate a return to Paleolithic conditions or pre-Enlightenment feudalism (not least because rates of maternal mortality were quite high!), but there are echoes of a desire for a difference located not in an ever-improving future but in a painfully absent past. Such nostalgia is romanticizing, but it is also potent and transformative.

Time becomes intensified as nature converges with an idealized past and is opposed to a disconcerting future in which technology and its mastery over nature erodes our essential humanity. The twenty-first century's rapid and dramatic development of technologies that reshape life and death have provoked cultural unease, including common processes such as in vitro fertilization, egg freezing, and genetic selection as well as controversial possibilities like human gene editing and ectogenesis. When juxtaposed with the side effects of industrial pollution on fertility and concern that human-induced climate change will make the planet uninhabitable for many of our descendants, technological advances make for a troubling future. Meanwhile, the idea that evolutionary truths represent how humans are supposed to be supports the fantasy that if we look back to primal or paleo states we can find a kind of purity and objective guidance—an authenticity. This echoes the discussion of forward-thinking progress in chapter 1 but inverts it: if paradise is not ahead in the heaven of Elysium, it might lie behind, in the Eden of Arcadia. In Christian mythology, Eden is the original state of humans, prior to sin. In a scientifically oriented mythology, retrospective longing uses the language of evolution.

SIX

Immunity

ECOLOGICAL ANXIETIES ABOUT CHEMICALS, MICROBES, AND STRESS

"HUMAN BEINGS ARE AFFECTED BY THEIR environment as soon as they have an environment, and that means as soon as they are implanted in the womb," Gabor Maté, a doctor and author, says in the trailer to the 2015 documentary film *In Utero*. The trailer continues in an alarming fashion, with statements like "Intra-utero life is not a paradise, as some people try to make us believe. . . . This substance feels every little feeling that the mother feels." The image of a pale hand petting a pregnant belly gives way to footage of people frantically running through a crowded intersection surrounded by skyscrapers and making circuit boards on assembly lines, fast-forwarded clips of traffic and subways, close-ups of women's sad faces, crying babies, dividing cells. "Fetuses of mothers who are anxious are showing differences almost, we want to say, in temperament," a woman's voice continues. "We see reduced brain volume, reduced gray matter density. People are conceiving, carrying, and birthing children under increasingly stressed conditions."

An old, grainy photo of a woman picking cotton transitions to footage of a Black woman with her young boys climbing a tree as she says, "My grandmother had undiagnosed depression, which then contributed to my mother's stress level, and that's gonna get transmitted to me, and I was gonna transmit that to the next generation." The trailer shows images of rioting and violence, with the male voiceover calmly stating, "When we see dysfunction in people, we're actually seeing the imprint of that early experience. . . . An adult trauma is really a fetal trauma." The images shift to home videos of babies, and the viewer is told that this knowledge is "the missing piece, the foundation for our whole life." The trailer juxtaposes exploding skyscrapers and hospital birth scenes, concluding with a fade-in of an image of a pregnant belly.

This film attracted no major attention, either within birth worlds or more general publics. It was alarmist and seemed unaware of its own irony—for how could raising this alarm help but cause further stress? But it illustrates a set of concerns that have surfaced in less extreme ways about how the environment "gets in" at the fetus, disturbing the idea that a newborn is untouched, pure, and innocent, immune from the evils of the world. Such anxieties creep in at the edges of birth worlds, anxieties about too much stress but also about missing microbes and toxic chemicals, about the way our environments may be damaged and damaging.

It is not obvious what a healthy environment is. Some level of challenge is considered beneficial, but too much results in "toxic stress" or "chronic stress." The psychological literature calls the former "eustress" (as in euphoria) as opposed to the latter's "distress." Some microbes are beneficial and indeed necessary, as research into the microbiome is resoundingly showing as it uncovers more and more questions about this "second genome." Efforts to wipe out "germs," which featured in twentieth-century hygiene campaigns, can take things too far, producing what might be called "toxic sterility." And chemicals, both naturally occurring ones like mercury and lead and synthetic ones like BPA and phthalates found in plastics, can disrupt cellular and hormonal processes throughout the life course, revealing toxic chemicals as the shadow side of industrial triumphs. (Despite its reputation for sustainability, the Bay Area is one of the more chemically toxic places in the country, with numerous Superfund hazardous pollution sites, largely from semiconductor waste). A triple toxicity, then—all three of which have ambiguous boundaries and slip disturbingly easily between desirable and terrible.[1]

Concerns about toxicity raise questions about the possibility of protection itself, about whether dangers and harms can be prevented at all. The desire to protect by drawing and defending boundaries seems commonsensical—it is a value and, again, a problem. It's a desire for immunity. Immunity as a cultural concept extends far beyond infectious disease, though it certainly shows up in the politics surrounding vaccinations. Until about a hundred years ago, immunity referred to protection from political and economic damage, to entitlements that exempted people or collectives from political obligations and responsibilities (it is the etymological opposite of "community.")[2] Biological immunity has been emphasized in its place. In both cases, immunity is an attempt to manage the fact that we are constantly in relation to other people and other beings, that we are actually part of our context and not separate from it.[3] In an American sensibility, there is a deep-seated urge to reject what's threatening instead of forming a relationship with it. A relationship implies vulnerability, a recognition that we are affected by something, that we might be reliant on it or harmed by it. It is more appealing to believe that we are invulnerable, exceptional: that we can stand alone and be safe. That we can protect those we love by staving off the world.

Microbes, chemicals, and stress blur the separation between a human and her environment. It becomes difficult to see humans as discrete units moving through an environment external to them, a form-on-field relationship. Rather, humans are part of ecologies, networks of connection and dependency, and our bodies themselves are environments for other beings that are part of these networks. The effects of our interactions with toxicity are not straightforward in time; they may be latent, persistent, partial, symptomatic, ambiguous. They may be carried across generations. Ecological thinking posits organisms as interactions. Ecologies are contingent, evolving, responsive, processual. Changing terms changes concepts: if one is in an environment, then harmful aspects of that environment can be blocked—destroyed, even. Immunity is possible. And likewise, beneficial aspects of that environment can be harnessed, hoarded, commodified ("nature" can only be a resource *for* humans insofar as it is understood as *not* human, as we have just explored). But if one is part of an ecology, the environment is not "out there." Rather, it *is* us. We are inextricable from what surrounds and composes us. We don't exist without it.

CHEMICALS: A RELATIONSHIP WITH INDUSTRY

I was seated on a wooden bench in the beautiful Asilomar conference center just outside of Monterey, attending the 2012 annual meeting of the Midwives Alliance of North America (MANA). A number of the women seated around me were knitting or doing other handwork in the light of big leaded-glass windows, the old floorboards creaking with the collective shifting of our weight. The cathedral-meets-cabin main hall was open to the sea breeze and views of scrubby cypress nestled among sand dunes. I was distractedly admiring the intricate braids of the woman seated in front of me when Sandra Steingraber captured my attention. This was the first time I had heard her speak, and I was enraptured. She was talking about biomagnification, aquatic ecosystems, and the accumulation of industrial runoff in fish flesh. The toxicity under discussion was jarring in this peaceful space—what did toxic ecologies have to do with birth?

Steingraber, an ecologist who has written popular science books about chemical toxicity, childbearing, and cancer that draw from her own experience, explained biomagnification as the phenomenon whereby toxins become more concentrated every link they climb in the food chain; they remain in the flesh of the consumer. Because there are so many more food chain links in aquatic ecosystems than terrestrial ones, carnivorous fish are particularly prone to high concentrations of toxins. Mercury is an industrial byproduct; released into waterways, it bonds with carbon and becomes methyl mercury, a neurotoxin notorious for the epidemic of neurological disease surrounding Japan's Minamata Bay in the 1950s. During fetal development, cells that are being differentiated and knit into organs or into the nervous system are extremely sensitive: one alteration in the unraveling of a zygote into a fetus can have huge consequences. Because of this, there is a well-known advisory that pregnant people should avoid eating tuna, a large carnivorous fish. Disturbingly, Steingraber insisted that not only should tuna be avoided, but there is no fish that is safe for a pregnant person to eat: all of them embody methyl mercury and other toxins in levels that threaten fetal development. *Every fish on the planet.*

I have since learned much about the many ways reproduction and toxicity are related, both through birth worlds and academic networks across the sciences and humanities, but this anecdote stays fresh in my memory because of an exchange that followed. Steingraber, her measured voice ringing across the wooden hall, took a broad view of toxicity, insisting that we are all interconnected and mutually implicated. She described how water *flows*—through irrigation canals and urban river dump sites, into water tables hundreds of miles from the source of contamination, and into the ocean, where it evaporates and travels the sky in clouds. Toxins transcend national borders and their regulatory jurisdictions. Polluted water in warm countries evaporates, condenses over cold countries, and rains down on them. Children living in "pristine" Arctic snow take in seven times more PCBs through breast milk than infants in California.[4] American municipal water is often contaminated with agricultural runoff; most exposure to waterborne toxins comes not from drinking but from inhaling water vapors, so even if one buys bottled water to drink while pregnant, the advantage is undercut while taking a shower.[5] There is no escaping our planet.

Steingraber called out and rejected the ideology of salvation through consumer choice—the common idea that by purchasing nontoxic products and cultivating our domestic environment we can protect ourselves and our family. Nonetheless, a midwife in the audience raised her hand and asked what fish are safe to eat during pregnancy. What can she tell her clients? Does Steingraber have a list of the most dangerous ones? Steingraber patiently explained that that's not the point—everyone's babies are at stake, everyone's babies matter. But the woman repeated herself, becoming frustrated, asking what, then, she should tell her clients?

"Tell them to become abolitionists," answered Steingraber after a small pause. Earlier in her talk she had drawn an explicit parallel between ending global dependence on toxic fossil fuels and abolishing slavery in the United States, stating that slavery was a deeply economically entrenched system upon which rested ways of life cherished by the powerful, a system that adversely affected everyone in society, even if they were not absorbing its worst effects. The same, she said, is true of the petroleum economy. In response to this woman's query, she asserted that "our biggest problem" is "well-informed futility syndrome," or feeling complacent about inaction. "Abolitionists fought and marched and died," she said. "Political action is part of good parenting; it reassures your children that the world will be okay. Mom's on the job."

·   ·   ·

The idea that no fish is safe illustrates the conundrum of immunity within an ecology. On the one hand, toxicities of various kinds impact us all and are cause for universal concern, even though they don't affect us all equally. Rob Nixon uses the term *slow violence* to describe the ways toxic environments unjustly harm poor and marginalized communities, whose livelihoods and neighborhoods are treated as sacrificial zones.[6] Yet wealth can only go so far in staving off harms, and the health of a generation eventually becomes everyone's problem. There is no escaping our planet, though this is precisely what immunity encourages us to think is possible—that we can put up barriers and make ourselves an exemption.

On the other hand, the toxic fish begs the question of what individuals can do to feel a sense of agency in the face of poorly defined threats, to mitigate the damage done by necessities of daily living. Pregnant people need to eat, after all. (And they receive conflicting advice, such as to consume fish for their omega-3 fatty acids.) In a market society oriented around purchasing goods and services, ethical thinking is somewhat inevitably framed by consumption. Much of conducting daily life and performing quotidian practices of care operates via consumer choices. When the impossibility of protecting one's own bubble clashes with a relentless market logic that individualizes responsibility, of course a futility syndrome is likely to result.

There are a number of chemicals other than mercury that cause damage during gestation and breastfeeding. Lead became notorious around the time of its ban in the 1970s, but it is still present in many residential environments via paint and water pipes, and on roadsides via leaded gasoline exhaust dust. PCBs, or polychlorinated biphenyls, are carcinogenic neurotoxins that were widely used in industry prior to the 1980s. BPA, a component of plastics, is still touted by the plastics industry as safe. At a birth activism conference I attended, a speaker shared that there is an average of two hundred chemicals known to be toxic in the umbilical cord blood of a given American baby. She explained that fertilizer use in California's Central Valley was causing a campaign of concerned citizens to warn people not to drink the water or eat food cooked in it. "Babies are dying from it," proclaimed handmade signs that proliferated in the area. In an issue of the alternative birth magazine *SQUAT,* a spread featuring "TED Talks we love" included "Toxic Baby" (alongside "Peace Begins at Birth" and "What We Learn Before We're Born"), which passionately expounded on the pesticide atrazine.

The way synthetic chemicals are woven into everyday life is what cultural historian Michelle Murphy calls "chemical regimes of living."[7] Synthetic chemistry flourished during World War II as industry engineers sought to replace commodities blockaded by the war. Afterward, during American capitalism's "golden age," the stockpile of unneeded chemicals was re-marketed and developed for domestic use, including PFAS, substances that make surfaces impenetrable. Their utility is inextricable from their toxicity, as Timothy Neale explains: "Just as they can easily slip between absorbent fibers and staining oils, these substances can also penetrate deep into strata, aquifers, and mammalian bodies," where they interrupt endocrine (hormonal) systems.[8] Glyphosate, which began as Agent Orange, a defoliant used during the Vietnam War, was re-marketed as Roundup, a commonly available herbicide that is touted as harmless to humans; it was later linked to horrific rates of cancer, birth defects, skin diseases, and other serious health issues, yet it is impossible to extricate from the fabric of our lives.[9] Many synthetic chemicals—notably plastics—are byproducts of the petroleum industry. Endocrine-disrupting chemicals, or EDCs, are present even in household dust, and all of us have traces of them in our urine.

Chemical engineering itself is not necessarily a problem, as recent explorations of "green chemistry" demonstrate. Rather, the problem is the myopic priority placed on industrial profit in how products are developed and regulated. Currently, the vast majority of the eighty-five thousand chemicals registered for use in the United States have not been deemed safe. The American regulatory approach has generally been to require proof of guilt from those who believe themselves harmed, not proof of innocence from the manufacturers. But proving guilt—that is, cause—is not easy because there are too many variables in chemical ecosystems, in a given individual's exposome. In Neale's words, epidemiological studies of environmental pollutants over the past two decades have "struggled to delineate the signal of one chemical cause amid the noisy reactive miasma in which we live. . . . We are bodies without baselines."[10] There is no original purity to be recovered; there is no way to effectively draw boundaries.[11]

When asked in an interview why we're not having public conversations about chemical toxicity, Steingraber answered, "We have a kind of cultural blindness. People don't think of themselves as vulnerable or permeable somehow. Sometimes the most obvious biological facts bear repeating. . . . [O]ther than the forty-six chromosomes bequeathed to us by our parents, we are simply rearranged molecules of air, food, and water."[12] Her articulation of the way our bodies and environments are inseparable is poignant, but the cultural blindness she describes is utterly unsurprising. Of course people don't think of themselves as vulnerable or permeable. A value on immunity—on protection via separation—is ubiquitous. This extends into how we view *intentional* endocrine disruptors, meaning hormonal drugs, from birth control pills to antidepressants. Taking such drugs is framed as an individual choice, at best a socially influenced one, but the hormonally active chemicals in pharmaceuticals exit bodies via urine and get into waterways, affecting wildlife and, in oblique ways, other humans' bodies. Antidepressants are so common in some waterways that fish exposed to them begin behaving weirdly, bobbing vertically instead of horizontally.[13] Synthetic chemicals have lots of effects, but we frame some as "primary" and relegate the others to "side effects," like collateral damage in war. From the fish's perspective, which effect is primary?

Unintended effects of drugs span generations as well as species. Many toxins are transferred via the placenta, despite the fact that physicians used to think it acted as a barrier (another interesting manifestation of the immunity bubble).[14] The placenta actually facilitates the transfer of chemicals, including harmful ones, which can become even more concentrated in umbilical cord blood than in the pregnant person's blood. The barrier myth was shattered in the 1960s with the thalidomide scandal, in which mothers given that drug for morning sickness gave birth to babies with severe deformations, like missing limbs. The diethylstilbestrol (DES) scandal followed swiftly in the 1970s, in which teens and young adults suffering from unusual cancers and deformities of the reproductive system were discovered all to have been born to women who took the drug DES during pregnancy in the 1930s, when it was commonly prescribed to prevent miscarriage. And yet this permeability is still headline news: the *New York Times* featured an article in 2017 proclaiming "The Womb Is No Protection from Toxic Chemicals."

Many other toxins are shared through breast milk, which has higher concentrations of toxins than the nursing person's body. In her MANA talk, Steingraber used this fact to claim that it is not the adult human at the top of the food chain but the human infant. When I looked her up after the conference, I found an interview in which she says that one of the most daring things she's ever done was passing a cup of her breast milk around the United Nations while speaking about embodied toxins.[15] Breastfeeding people actually lose toxins from their fat stores in decreasing proportion to the number of children they've nursed; the first child to suckle serves as a kind of detox. If the childbearing body is taken seriously as requiring a reconceptualization of (individual) persons, and consequently a different politics, it offers an important window on the broader fact that bodies and environments are woven together across generations, a fact also highlighted by chemical toxicity.

Where childbearing and chemical toxicity overlap, the limits of consumer politics are evident. Norah MacKendrick shows how putting the onus of protection on consumers through a "better safe than sorry" model of green shopping, which she calls "precautionary consumption," barely scratches the surface of the toxicity problem.[16] In addition to being socioeconomically exclusive, it puts a huge share of the burden on women, especially mothers, who do most of the quotidian shopping and household management. During fieldwork I thought of this as the "politics of Whole Foods," referring to shopping at the elite grocery chain as a way of purchasing peace of mind. It was a widespread ideology even among those who could not afford to put it into practice. Choosing safer food and household products requires vast amounts of label reading, mental tabulation of brands and ingredients, less efficient routines, and efforts to become informed. It also requires that accurate information be accessible to consumers, which is often not the case, due partially to inadequate labeling and selective branding but moreover to the egregious dearth of research about chemicals. Consumer access to information is the focus of San Francisco–based consumer advocacy group MOMS, which stands for Making Our Milk Safe. Relevant information is unevenly distributed; many cosmetic products used by Black women are not represented on environmental consumption sites and lack printed ingredient lists. Like consent, discussed in chapter 3, the purchase relation is a contract not usually entered into on equal terms, as consumers never have complete information about a product's production and effects, its before-lives and afterlives.

In science and policy, women's bodies are treated as womb environments that can pollute a fetus. This (unsurprisingly) subordinates potentially pregnant people's needs and desires, but it also disconnects the maternal body from the environment in which it is itself immersed, looking past shared responsibility for that environment and targeting interventions at women's decisions and lifestyles.[17] Some scientists attribute the drastic reduction in male sperm count and the rise in infertility to the ubiquity of EDCs, yet female reproduction continues to receive disproportionate attention in the United States.[18] This missing science of men's reproduction not only under-investigates male health but directs undue responsibility and regulatory control toward women.[19] Steingraber's call to activism—"Mom's on the job"—draws on and perpetuates ideas of maternal responsibility.

Feminist scholars have elaborated on the gendered politics of EDCs, and there is a robust activist-scholar movement highlighting environmental justice, which for many overlaps with the concerns and platform of reproductive justice. The environmental reproductive justice (ERJ) framework, proposed by Mohawk midwife Katsi Cook, is concerned with how environmental degradation, pollution, and climate change shape the conditions of possibility for biological, social, and cultural reproduction.[20] Along with the effects of extractive industries and arguments about human population growth, the experience of toxicity and pollution is a key area of concern.

Toxic exposure is often greater for those working and living in proximity to industries like agriculture, oil refining, manufacturing, or mining, and in places with less geopolitical power and ability to resist corporate exploitation—a geographical violence entwined with race. Exposure is also gendered, as women are more likely to suffer poorly understood diseases correlated with toxicity: multiple chemical sensitivity, fibromyalgia, endometriosis. Margaret Lock distinguishes between "situated biologies" that show how everybody is affected by human-induced environmental changes and "local biologies" that are stratified within this universal exposure.[21] Yet emphasizing class and racial inequalities in the distribution of harm can stigmatize groups of people as "damaged"; rather, we should direct attention to our shared need to find better ways of living.[22]

This is precisely what consumer politics is unable to do, at least not in any fundamental way. Consumer politics is an individualized, market-mediated response to the increasingly pressing need to think ecologically. It rechannels the problem back into the original mold. Consumer choice and the "informed consumer" are, in many ways, a distraction, like the mommy wars over parenting choices discussed in chapter 4. But the question of what to do instead isn't straightforward. Steingraber's solution relies heavily on governmental agencies: "I'm not interested in trying to put my family inside a bubble.... It's the government's job to protect us from danger, whether it be enemies abroad or chemicals within."[23] Scholars like Lochlann Jain, writing on toxicity and cancer, likewise argue that change needs to happen "upstream" via regulation, and that consumer-citizens need to exert pressure to make that happen.[24]

Yet this is ever more challenging in a context of increasing deregulation. In 2018 the Environmental Protection Agency placed the director of its own Office of Children's Health Protection on administrative leave, which raised concerns about the potential closure of the office that has promoted regulating industrial pollutants. And too often "protective" government intervention gets things horribly wrong. For example, in 2016 the FDA recommended that fertile women not using birth control refrain from drinking alcohol even if they don't intend to get pregnant, recruiting fetal alcohol syndrome to police female sexuality, but it doesn't ensure municipal water supplies are safe (as the 2015 lead scandal in Flint, Michigan, showed). Many communities historically persecuted by governmental agencies understandably feel ambivalence about such a strategy. The tension between taking individual action and strategizing based on relational interconnection is what I have called the double bind of environmental toxicity.[25] Neither option is adequate, and both are necessary, but the two sit awkwardly together. Both Steingraber's call to abolition and the pragmatism of the midwife in the audience have a place.

MICROBES: A RELATIONSHIP WITH THE NONHUMAN

I was walking down a Santa Cruz sidewalk on a warm September Friday toward the Ugly Mug coffeeshop. Its window was lined with clay mugs sprouting grotesque faces in the tradition of gargoyles, with a hippie-craft twist. In the coffeeshop I met Juno, the doula whose childbirth class I had been helping at, her pale hair spilling out from her messy bun, soft face smiling warmly, tired creases at the corners of her eyes. I remembered that I owed her money— she paid my dues at the Meet the Doulas night a few weeks before, where doulas and potential clients "speed date," so I bought her a chai latte.

Other familiar faces began to circulate, including Emily, elfin and dark, a young San Francisco transplant I met when we sat next to each other on a log around a mountain bonfire at a doula retreat in June. My first impression was that she seemed too cool for me, with her flowing black clothes and tattoos, but I soon warmed up to her goofy earnestness. I knew Barbara, her face fabulously creased with age and sun above her brightly colored polar fleece, from volunteering at the home for childbearing women in difficult circumstances, where she was well loved and respected. Methadone baby? Struggle with Child Protective Services? She "just loves on them," she said in an interview with a dismissive wave of her hand. It was clear from the stories, though, that she won her clients' trust through a fierce loyalty, refusing to leave their side, even during forty-eight-hour hospital debacles. There was the doe-eyed, intimidatingly witty Alzbeta, with her Eastern European accent, and Meg, who used to be my boss at a foreign language teaching gig; she dropped me an email at the end of the program saying that actually, she loves babies and was going home to the United Kingdom to train as a midwife, and could we chat birth sometime?

We were gathering for a film screening of *Microbirth*. The title is a play on the term *microbiome* (a concept that had not long been in public awareness at the time of the screening in 2014), which describes the microscopic life-worlds making up human bodies. The film's poster is Earth seen from space, a faintly luminous horizon beneath dark sky and stars. There is a magnifying glass over the "O" in the title, within which floats a shadowy fetus. The play on scale is not coincidental—here are minuscule ecologies with enormous consequences. Communities of microbes live in the gut, on the skin, in the eyes and mouth and nose, and in the vagina, yet the womb was thought to be microbe free, the fetus sterile in its amniotic sac. Where does our microbial universe come from, it provocatively wondered.

A year earlier, celebrated American food journalist Michael Pollan published a *New York Times Magazine* cover story, "Some of My Best Friends Are Germs." This was back when the American Gut Project was relying heavily on stool samples from its scientists' own families, before "microbiome" was, if not quite a household term, at least one that doesn't raise many eyebrows in an educated crowd.[26] The piece lays out much of the science that inspired the filmmakers: there are ten microbes per every human cell (making us "10 percent human"), and American guts are considered microbially impoverished due to an industrial diet of processed foods, high antibiotic use in medicine and agriculture, living in increasingly sterile environments, and low rates of vaginal birth and breastfeeding. Pollan describes how, during birth, the baby is "colonized" by the vaginal microbiome through which it passes, followed by contact with the birthing person's skin and breast milk, each of which has its own microbiotic ecology. Babies born by cesarean miss out on this colonial event and have different microbial gut communities than vaginally born babies, he reports, a difference that might affect their immune development and account for higher rates of allergy, asthma, and autoimmune problems in babies born by cesarean.

Pollan recounts how the "mystery of milk" was one of scientists' earliest clues to the microbiome: breast milk should be food "perfectly engineered by evolution," so why does it contain sugars that are indigestible by infants? Scientists puzzled over these sugars, called oligosaccharides, for decades, and formula companies didn't include them. Oligosaccharides are actually prebiotic—that is, food for bacteria. These sugars are eaten by *Bifidobacterium infantis,* healthy levels of which "crowd out less savory microbial characters" and nurture the intestinal lining, preventing infection and inflammation. Breast milk transfers the nursing person's immune system to the baby in real time, priming them for the actual pathogens they encounter, and it contains antibodies that kill harmful bacteria and viruses on contact, yielding old wives' tale remedies like using breast milk to relieve infant eye infections. (More recent research suggests the placenta might have its own microbiome and that it can transfer microbes as well as chemicals, meaning neither the womb nor the fetus is sterile, which troubles the "colonizations" metaphor of the newborn's body as *terra nulla*, empty land.)[27]

Back at the Ugly Mug, *Microbirth* picked up where Pollan's article left off. It emphasized the importance of vaginal births, breastfeeding, and immediate skin-to-skin contact between an infant and birthing person. Then it introduced "vaginal inoculation," a practice of swabbing a surgically born baby with vaginal fluid, under formal clinical trial by Maria Gloria Dominguez-Bello, who is interviewed in the film. Dominguez-Bello does not vilify C-sections themselves but rather their overuse, saying they are misdistributed globally. The film takes microbiome science in an apocalyptic direction, describing the "initial colonization" in the first few moments of nonsterile life as the "one chance" babies' guts have to learn which microbes are good and which are bad. It describes bodies as ecosystems, which, like other ecosystems on the planet, are shrinking in biodiversity; people are not sick, "the system" is. The film gestures towards an "antibiotic winter" when antibiotic-resistant bacteria will be unstoppable, and it expresses concern that an interconnected world will soon make pandemics inevitable (this was, of course, before the COVID-19 pandemic). It warns that noncommunicable diseases like diabetes and asthma, which already account for 60 percent of deaths globally, will bankrupt our healthcare system, bankrupt our world.

Most striking was the idea that compromised microbial ecosystems are not just related to the diseases of a generation, but that the consequences are heritable. Microbial genes outnumber human genes in a human adult by a factor of at least one hundred to one; it appears increasingly likely that this "second genome," as it is sometimes called, exerts an influence on our health as great as and possibly even greater than the genes we inherit from our parents. But while inherited genes are more or less fixed (with some environmental exposures changing gene expression, known as epigenetics), it may be possible to reshape, even cultivate, the second genome—a process that spans generations: "You are what your grandma ate." The film describes a "maternal microbial heritage" compromised by C-sections, synthetic hormones, and formula feeding, among other things. There are important ways that gut bacteria affect the nervous system and brain; the film asserts that the stress of unmedicated labor hormonally primes the baby's immune system, and that this process has long-term effects on metabolism. Asking whether Pitocin has transgenerational consequences, the film claims, "We don't have a clue!" In a grand statement, it asserts that "emotions [in birth] set the template for future life." The film ends with a call for big research into the question "How do we know we're not altering the course of humanity?"

After the credits ran and the lights were turned on, the atmosphere in the Ugly Mug was heavy. The thirty- to forty-person audience, mostly doulas and some midwives and nurses, all stayed for the discussion. We talked about the prevalence of antibiotics: if a birthing person runs a fever during labor, the baby gets antibiotics, and antibiotics are prescribed for many infant and childhood illnesses. There was a lively discussion about the virtues of clorhexidine, an inexpensive antiseptic that has been shown to be as effective as antibiotics at preventing the transfer of group B streptococcus (GBS) from birthing person to infant when used as a vaginal wash during delivery

(30 percent of women are positive for GBS and almost all receive antibiotics). Regarding the need to reduce cesarean rates, Juno said, "Everybody's jumping on the bandwagon now, and that's fabulous." Tara, a midwife whom I knew only by name, observed that the film mounts further evidence from within the scientific community against casual cesareans, widening the gap between evidence-based medicine and common hospital protocol. "Obviously we're not using evidence-based practices," she asserted. Someone else complained, "We interfere instead of defaulting to nature." Since there is no medical protocol for vaginal swabbing, a third person enthusiastically suggested, "So let's make one! We'll *force* evidence-based medicine!" Remember from chapter 2 how evidence-based medicine becomes used among reformers in birth communities to push against protocol by calling for better science on its own terms?

The audience largely agreed that this film is for birth practitioners, not mothers. What we have just witnessed is depressing, heavy, and huge. Some suggested that moms could watch a shorter version, perhaps to sway those on the fence about home birth, but above all it should not be shown to women who have had C-sections—"they have enough guilt!" (That this is taken as a truism speaks to the birth worlds I circulated in.) Surely, I thought, it's true that washing another layer of anxieties and responsibilities over childbearing people is not helpful, but these statements struck me as promoting their own form of paternalism. Shielding people from what might harm them can be a form of care, but it can also promote the idea that they are vulnerable and helpless, incapable of capable of navigating the complex terrain of motherhood. The overwhelming sentiment was that this film screening was preaching to the choir. To conclude our discussion, Clara, wearing a colorful peasant skirt, laughingly but seriously suggested, "We should swab our grandmothers' vaginas, before it's too late!"

. . .

Since Louis Pasteur catalyzed the development of germ theory in the late nineteenth century, microbes have popularly been painted with the same bad-guys brush. Germs cause disease, and therefore eliminating them is healthful, the conventional wisdom goes. While the germ theory of disease is more nuanced than that, there has not been a lot of room for nuance and ambivalence in cultural practice. The complex web of concerns spanning outward from the microbiome and its reproduction should be thought of in conjunction with concerns about chemical toxicity in daily life. Antimicrobial cleaning and hygiene products are ubiquitous in American households and workplaces, and our food systems (notably antibiotics given to livestock) have largely unknown effects on our resident bacteria. The "hygiene hypothesis" describes how too much cleanliness is linked with health problems like asthma and allergies, while children exposed to soil, plants, and animals and their feces don't have such problems. Germ theory had immensely positive consequences for medical practice and public health, but where is the boundary with "too much of a good thing"?

In chapter 3 I mentioned Ivan Illich's argument about "technological watersheds," points beyond which beneficial developments outgrow their utility and become burdens. Penicillin, the first biomedical antibiotic, and germ theory's implications for hygiene are among his examples of fantastically useful discoveries that have now crossed the threshold into negative effects.[28] Antimicrobial resistance and the microbiome were not being discussed in the 1970s, but how much more is his point illustrated now! Synthetic chemicals could also be said to have crossed the threshold, taking on a life of their own and affecting humans in ways we don't fully recognize, which are neither determined by us nor for our benefit—not to mention their effects on the complex ecologies of which we are a part. The technologies now being vilified for microbial degeneration, including hospital birth, industrial food, and antiseptic products, were hailed as wonderful during the period in which they became common. Heidegger discusses short-sightedness about new technologies, stating that technology's power and danger come from "enframing," where humans seek to manipulate a set of possibilities but without being able to see all the contingent possibilities and their consequences.[29] Technology acts on the occult level, where it cannot be directly experienced—its effects are unknown, and they outlive its creators. This makes technology insidious. A given technology itself is the tip of the iceberg, as it were; its implications are far greater than meet the eye.

Eva-Maria Simms, who develops a "placental ethics" based on material interconnection, argues that to redeem technology, we must recognize that it operates beyond human control or even perception and interact with it accordingly.[30] She references Goethe's poem "The Sorcerer's Apprentice," which in my mind is inextricable from Disney's animated *Fantasia* sequence. Mickey, the young apprentice, cleverly puts a spell on a broom to make it carry water, relieving him of his chores. However, he soon realizes he doesn't know the spell to make the broom *stop* carrying water. Desperate as the house floods around him, he breaks the broom in half, but now he finds that there are two brooms carrying water. He chops them into splinters with an axe, and the shards rise up into an army of enchanted brooms that drown the house. Modern technologies—from television to plastics, from pesticides to epidurals and C-sections—have introduced a host of unintended social practices and biological/ecological consequences that were not foreseen by their creators or promoters.

The impossibility of foreseeing consequences is another reason consumer choice is a poor paradigm for addressing problems. Vaginal swabbing, for example, is an appealing "fix" that someone can (theoretically, from a position of consumer power) choose to have performed, but it is poorly understood too. *Slate* ran a story in February 2016 titled "Forget What You've Read: Swabbing Your Baby with Vaginal Juices Is Pointless and Weird." The obstetrician who wrote the article has a sense of humor and considers birth "natural and humbling," but she is not convinced by the evidence that vaginal swabbing is helpful and sees a few reasons it could be harmful. Or consider the anti-vax or vaccine choice movements, which could be interpreted as a backlash stemming from anxieties about unforeseen consequences.

The microbiome raises questions of how humans are interconnected temporally between generations, both via transfers of actual microbes during gestation, vaginal births, and breastfeeding, and via inherited epigenetic markers influenced by the presence of microbes and their genomes. Microbiomes also raise questions of how humans are interconnected with surrounding ecologies. People who live with a dog have more diverse gut microbiota. Keeping infants secluded in single-family homes is not necessarily good practice, leading to Pollan's somewhat tongue-in-cheek observation that "the nuclear family may not be conducive to the health of the microbiome." (This is fitting as the nuclear family offers its own sort of social immunity, a norm of separation and boundedness.) The human body is increasingly being seen as teeming with nonhuman life on which its survival and health depends. Biomedical epidemiological concerns attend to ecologies in new ways, from antibiotic-resistant "superbugs" to zoonotic (animal-transmitted) diseases causing pandemics. Cultural theorists have turned their attention to such interspecies relationships, to a "microbiopolitics" that calls for a different valuation of nonhuman life.[31] What does it mean to think of an individual's health not only as having consequences for human communities—the labor of caretaking, the cost of long-term diseases, the potential for pandemics—but of health as a collective property amongst many kinds of beings?

The formerly ubiquitous metaphor of immunity as a bodily war against microbial invaders is fading away to one of competing colonizations: Which populations are entrenched first? Which get more environmental support? Which grow and decline at which rates? Chikako Takeshita, who uses the term *motherfetus,* reframes pregnancy not as a bidirectional exchange of substances but rather as a symbiotic process involving complex networks of microbial activity.[32] This allows her to think of the childbearing body as a holobiont, an assemblage of different species forming an ecological unit. Microbiome scientists have proposed a project of "restoration ecology" in the human gut, but this requires not only understanding each person as host to a teeming ecology, but also understanding the health of our species as a *collective* property of our microbiomes.

STRESS: A RELATIONSHIP WITH MODERNITY

A year after my fieldwork I went to meet Harmony at a strip of shops near the beach in Santa Cruz. The coffeeshop was packed and thick with coastal hipness. I ordered a "bowl of soul"—chamomile tea steeped in steamed milk—and staked out a table. We were meeting to discuss Roxanne's Mindfulness-Based Childbirth Education class, with which I had assisted early on. Harmony, a hospital midwife who had trained at UC San Francisco, one of the best American medical research hospitals, had taken the class as a pregnant person. Roxanne had passed away the month before our meeting, and Harmony was preparing to take over teaching her immensely popular class at the hospital where she worked.

She arrived wearing a ponytail, soft gray blouse, and jeans. Shrugging her bag full of books onto the chair, she apologized for being late; she had had trouble putting her son down for his nap. Over hazelnut cookies and tea, we shared anecdotes and compared notes. Toward the end of the meeting I recalled that the first time I met Roxanne, I asked her if she thought birth has effects that shape a personality, that stay with you throughout your life, and Roxanne had replied, "Oh, goodness yes!" with a huge smile. Harmony enthusiastically agreed, adding, "That's why I do the work I do!" Fifteen years ago, Harmony told me, local birth activists had started a now-national group focused on fetal/infant psychological experience. Though parts of the story were familiar to me, Harmony connected them in new ways.

The organization was APPPAH, the Association for Prenatal and Perinatal Psychology and Health. I first encountered it in the corridor of an Arts and Crafts–style office building in North Berkeley, on a community shelf scattered with a variety of postcards and advertisements. APPPAH's card caught my attention: it featured a spherical belly, hands forming a heart shape around the navel. It advertised a retreat for those who would like to become pre- and perinatal educators. I slipped it into my bag along with one on baby sign language classes and stepped outside into the warm eucalyptus-scented air. As I walked down Shattuck Avenue, with its clusters of gourmet eateries, I remembered that I had actually first encountered APPPAH a year earlier at the midwifery conference where I met Steingraber, at a table manned by one of the very few men present. I now wonder how poorly I concealed my skepticism when I chatted with him, as I did not quite believe that people would attempt to relive and heal traumas suffered during their own births through techniques like group hypnosis.

Remembering my initial reaction is instructive to me, since APPPAH's premise has come to seem pretty normal. Perinatal psychology, a field of study and practice that originated in California in the 1980s, is concerned with psychological experience in the womb and during birth and infancy. Its premise is that humans carry these psychological effects with us throughout our lives, whether we know it or not. My initial impressions notwithstanding, APPPAH is less concerned with the healing of adults and more with shaping the emotional fabric of future humans through educating birth practitioners and parents. APPPAH's cofounder, Thomas Verny, was featured in the documentary film *In Utero,* which opened this chapter. Attachment parenting takes up this line of thinking by framing infant experience as setting an affective template for life.

This logic can be found throughout birth worlds; the very popular trend of postpartum skin-to-skin contact emphasizes that the moments after birth form infants' first impression of the world and will be less traumatizing if they sense a familiar warmth, smell, and voice. Beliefs about formative trauma motivates more marginal groups like "intactivists," who oppose infant circumcision. Over the years I encountered craniosacral therapy, a mode of healing that uses light touch to "listen" to the body, a process that is predicated on the idea that babies remember and are processing the challenges of their birth experience in nonlinguistic ways. I heard the maxim that for the baby in the womb to feel safe, she needs at least three empathetic interactions between the adults in the room for every conflict interaction.

A *New York Times* article written by an unhoused woman who left a destructive relationship and experienced a long custody battle describes the toll it took on her infant, and her own guilt as a mother: "I'd failed her even in my womb, dragging her through my stress and heartache. When she was born, she had two scabs on her hands called sucking blisters from trying to self-soothe."[33] In different guises, it's easy to find the idea that near birth qualities shape emotional qualities.

In our conversation in that cafe, Harmony took things a step further back, to the materials of conception. She recounted that the founders of APPAH believed that "the mom's stress level determines what kind of egg she releases. If she's stressed, she produces a being with more emphasis on the midbrain, where the fight or flight instinct comes from, instead of the front brain, where thought and empathy happen. So [a child's temperament] can start in the mom's health, even before conception." This take is rather unconventional, although some medical research does suggest links between egg quality and maternal stress. Harmony continued, "And it makes sense that a lot of cortisol production during pregnancy would make for a highly tuned nervous system in the baby. Cortisol, you know, the stress hormone." She went on to say that her one-year-old son is jumpier than his peers, probably because she was overworked and stressed out while pregnant. "And that's not like a war zone or anything," she said with wry humor. It went without saying that the mindfulness classes were related to these claims: mindfulness practice reduces stress, and stress is a toxic affect. The womb is not a safe shelter, she implied, but a vulnerable ecology where the psychological capacities of future generations are formed.

. . .

Sarah and Roger, two of the parents introduced in chapter 3, believed similarly. They were strongly opinionated about the well-being of their calm, chubby eight-month-old son, Gabriel, and deeply skeptical of institutionalized medicine. We were seated in their backyard after a pancake breakfast shared in their small mountain studio, talking quietly while Gabriel amused himself with a stone mortar and pestle and listened for birds. They told me they considered beginnings and origins to be crucially important. Sarah explained, "Not that you can't ... transform and heal traumas later on, but as a parent, I want to do my best to give Gabriel really positive healthy experiences to build his life on rather than traumatic ones that he later has to overcome and heal." They considered infancy to be a time of exceptional openness, receptivity, and wisdom in realms with which adults have lost touch. They don't have a TV or use screens of any sort in front of Gabriel, neither Sarah nor Gabriel left their home for the first six weeks after birth, and they waited for two months before putting him in a car. They protected him from loud things, mechanical things, and chaotic spaces like the grocery store. Sarah explained:

> He felt so, so *open*. The newborn is in a state of what as adults we would call enlightenment ... they're not separate ... they're absorbing [what surrounds them], so I was extremely protective of that space he was in.... We let him say when he's ready to do something else, give him all the time to do whatever he's doing rather than interrupting with "How about this, let's do this." He's in a place of completely in the present moment, in a way that most adults *long* to be.

Sarah shared how Gabriel and "any little person" could immediately read adults' emotions. She valued and "celebrated" this interpersonal attunement and receptivity alongside his ability to be in the present moment, believing that it is something he will be able to access as an adult if he is encouraged to cultivate it in infancy. She and Roger link this belief to Waldorf philosophy and Indigenous cultures, which they learn about through reading. Their approach to parenting is incredibly demanding, as discussed in chapter 3, yet meeting what they perceived to be their young child's needs was their unquestioned priority because of the lifelong implications they understood such efforts to have. Sarah shared her belief that when parents "take the easy way out" and "make the choice to not be fully available for the baby, for the rest of the child's life, every person it's around is going to pay the price." Though she reported, "It has been incredibly hard for me this year, super intense!" she thought her efforts would enable Gabriel to go "into the world as a secure, healthy person who reaches out to interact out of joy of connecting, rather than need of attention. That is worth whatever challenge and struggle I have been through." Roger talked about the love that he knows Gabriel can feel when he's in his parents' presence. He explained "limbic resonance" as "what mammals have that makes them mammals": an emotional-somatic attunement to other mammals in their presence. It's what enables empathy.[34] He said that Gabriel's birth was healing for himself, Roger, who had been born not breathing during a C-section; he remembered his mom fighting with the doctor during this time and knows that he became jaundiced soon afterward. "With [Gabriel] it was so natural."

Roger's main work was "doing nature connection" with kids and sometimes adults, which involved leading survival skills courses at UC Santa Cruz, summer camps, and different groups during the school year. He held up Indigenous lifeways as a model, seeking to connect with "parts of our being that have been covered over by [the] modern industrial lifestyle." Sarah chimed in, saying that "that's another theme question" of their lives, in addition to understanding children and babies: "How do we bring what is really healthy about past times when people were connected with each other and themselves and the Earth, how do we bring it forward in a way that is truly in our current time?" Toward the end of the interview, after the recorder was off, Sarah earnestly posed a question I found very strange. She asked how can we get people to value their children's health. She was concerned about all the "skinny, crying babies" she saw and was genuinely perplexed why people didn't want to fix this apparent problem. I considered this for a moment, a bit taken aback, then said I didn't think it was a problem of desire. The people I knew cared about their babies' health very much, perhaps even too much, and as a result they became anxious and sometimes depressed about how daunting, demanding, and confusing it could seem. Perhaps because she had so determinedly avoided more conventional parenting spaces, this wasn't part of Sarah's awareness.

Sarah and Roger's approach was unconventional, but their views resonated throughout different spaces and people I encountered. Roger and Sarah really tried to exempt themselves from modern life, going to lengths others did not consider possible, and indeed, given different access to social and material resources, would not have been possible for many. Yet material and social resources were not in short supply for many of the people I worked with. It was instead, and understandably, difficult for them to integrate the idea that doing something very different from what is conventionally accepted would be important for their babies' health. Even if they were inclined to think so, putting this into practice was far from straightforward. In differing ways, people near birth grappled with the paradox of stress, which is a problem of immunity.

Stress is a capacious and naturalized/naturalizing concept that blurs distinctions between material and psychological experience. In popular discourse, stress can both result from and produce experiences of anxiety, pressure, insecurity, and negativity. These affects can accumulate in the body and manifest as tense shoulders, stomach ulcers, headaches, nausea, cortisol production, or a sense of unease. The term *stress* did come up for those I engaged with, but references to stress were usually implicit. They emerged in childbirth classes and doula training as ways of speaking that were meant to assuage anxiety and promote emotional security, or among parents as initiatives to "go easy on themselves" and be nonjudgmental of others. Stress is a recursive and paradoxical idea, especially when projected onto childbearing: not only is living in a toxic, aggressive, and fast-paced world stressful, but it is stressful to contemplate that one's baby will grow into this world, and that one's parenting (and one's own stress) might be able to mitigate—or exacerbate!—these impacts. Meanwhile, the demands of parenting itself are really stressful in a context that is so unaccommodating. Causes of stress are contradictory and unavoidable: stress about losing one's individuality to constant caretaking coexists with stress about damaging one's baby by being selfish and attending to one's personal needs.

Stress is the condition of our social lives. Protecting ourselves against stress would require exempting ourselves from that which sustains us all, a very stressful thing to contemplate doing (even as it might be enlivening to imagine other possibilities), and something impossible to fully achieve. Exposure to chaotic and overstimulating environments, uneven access to emotional-somatic expressions of love, and precariousness that threatens our ability to meet material needs are ubiquitous problems across American society. In *Cruel Optimism,* Lauren Berlant details how increasing precariousness provides the dominant structure and experience of the present moment, as the "neoliberal feedback loop" efficiently distributes and shapes the experience of insecurity throughout the class structure and across the globe. The pressure to pursue happiness regardless of circumstance, as though it were possible but just out of reach, generates a cruel optimism. The phenomenon is also described in books like Ruth Whippman's *America the Anxious,* a British travelogue through a strangely optimistic culture, and Barbara Ehrenreich's *Bright-Sided,* a takedown of positive psychology. The jarring, impossible juxtaposition of positivity and insecurity further increases stress.

Popular, medical, and critical uses of the term *stress* are blurred, and the nature of stress itself is lost in this tangle. In 1980, the same year that PTSD (post-traumatic stress disorder) was recognized and named, Allan Young wrote critically about the term, arguing that this relatively new concept (prior to 1965, "stress" was not used to describe human experience but rather things, as in structural engineering) was being used in a decontextualized way that reproduced "conventional knowledge."[35] Scientific and medical researchers of stress "produce evidence that certain historically particular beliefs about the social order actually describe a universal reality."[36] In other words, what seemed stressful to a given group of researchers was being assumed to be stressful to humans in any context, a type of universalization that usually recruits biology (and often evolutionary biology) to support it. If biological markers of a given stress could be found, then that stress could be interpreted to affect bodies in "real" (universal) ways. But also the converse: given the assumption that stress affects bodies in "real" (universal) ways, it makes sense to look for biological markers of it. Young critiques the professional medicalization of everyday tension and friction, which turns tension and friction ("stress") into both a syndrome and a cause. Young's basic claim is that research into stress serves to confirm middle-class Americans' beliefs about themselves and their social structure—in particular, tacit knowledge of the "abstract individual." Stress is decontextualized even as it purports to bring in context (by drawing attention to the social life of the individual in question), replacing conflicting class and group interests with a "desocialized and amorphous *environment* ... a pathogenic environment-out-of-control."[37] For example, a "stressful work environment" could be recognized in this frame, but not the sexism, racism, and economic precarity that cause the workplace to be stressful to a particular person in the first place.

With stress, as with chemicals and microbes, anxieties about the state of our world are projected onto the near birth period as a problem of origins, which is another way of looking for causes. Concern with fetal and infant experience as formative of personhood is not confined to marginal activist organizations. Researchers at Harvard's Center on the Developing Child claim that "toxic stress" in early childhood detrimentally impacts "the architecture of the brain, the body's stress response systems, and a host of health outcomes later in life."[38] International and interdisciplinary research on the developmental origins of health and disease (DOHaD)—an endeavor also concerned with early exposure to toxic chemicals and, increasingly, the microbiome—attracts much money and effort from prestigious organizations. Tools like the index for measuring adverse childhood experiences (ACEs) attempt to quantify and research psychological trauma in early life.

We produce scientific evidence that stress makes, and remakes, our nervous system, immune and inflammatory system, and metabolic system. Cortisol, which Harmony mentioned as "the stress hormone," has been described as public enemy number one because of a population-wide chronic stress epidemic that correlates with a plethora of noncommunicable diseases.

While some activation of the stress response is considered good, called "eustress" (like euphoria), too much causes "distress" and becomes pathological. A 2015 *Nautilus* article, "When Stress Comes with Your Mother's Milk," delves into cortisol in breast milk, concluding that "a mother's stress . . . may nudge her baby one way or another, but cortisol alone doesn't dictate destiny."[39] Some studies claim that chronic high cortisol is toxic to unborn and infant children; placentas transfer cortisol as well as mercury (along with *all* chemicals essential for healthy development). Research reporting on childhood stress and class disparities "suggests that the roots of physical impairment and underachievement are biologically embedded, but preventable" if acted on during the crucial window near birth.[40] Yet to reframe it somewhat glibly, it's not the stress that's causing the problems; it's income inequality and capitalism.

When detrimental social power dynamics become articulated in terms of stress, they are sought in the biological (which in turn makes them seem more "real"). Arline Geronimus's "weathering hypothesis" contends that the stress of discrimination essentially results in early aging. She proposed it in the 1990s after researching high rates of preterm birth among Black Americans, later linking it with the concept of allostatic load or "cumulative wear and tear on the body's systems" due to repeated exposure to stressors, and recently explained it all in a best-selling book.[41] Weathering is the best explanation for why horrifying racial disparities in maternal health outcomes persist after socioeconomic status is controlled for; it is not simply about access to resources like prenatal care, education, nutrition, or financial means. To some extent, the decontextualization of stress has begun to shift toward broader social articulations.

Stress is used in contexts ranging from police brutality to standardized testing, from threatened loss of life to threatened loss of status, which neuropsychological theories explain as basically the same thing—as stress. Stress-related illnesses are often attributed to an interaction between genes and environment, in which genes are turned "on" or "off" in response to a stressor. What counts as stressful is not self-evident, universal, or timeless, but research about stress makes it seem like it is. Around the turn of the twentieth century, the commonly diagnosed disease of "neurasthenia" was a nervous condition understood to result from a pathogenic modern environment with rapidly changing technologies, work relations, and gender relations.[42] Moving into the twenty-first century, "trauma" is beginning to take over from stress as the master medical trope of experience, including in diagnoses of PTSD. These are ways of individualizing and pathologizing experience, making it one's own instead of embedded in specific relations.

When I spoke on the phone with an eminent Bay Area researcher on reproductive health and the environment, she defined stress as "a generic term: relationship stress, family, poverty, race, *all things affecting balance and well-being.*" But despite the ubiquity of the idea that we as individuals need to find balance, that's not something a person can manage on her own. The fact that stress is conceptualized as both a cause and an effect of imbalance is one reason it's so compelling—and vexing. How might we move from thinking of an environment (what surrounds an individual) to an ecology (the relations in which an individual is enmeshed)? The difference between saying that stress caused a given person's preterm birth and that embodied racism causes preterm birth for those who live in a society that continually undermines and disrespects people who look like them moves in this direction. Dumont phrases it this way: "The truth is that our culture is permeated by nominalism, which grants real existence only to individuals and not to relations, to elements and not to sets of elements."[43] Consider a set of weighing scales or a playground seesaw, a classic metaphor for balance: the "balanced" entity is not the element on one side or the other but the bar and fulcrum in between them.

CAN IMMUNOLOGY REFRAME THE ENLIGHTENMENT?

I asked Dani and Jonah, the new parents with a two-month-old daughter whom we met in chapter 3, whether they thought drugs during birth mattered. Jonah quickly quipped that he wasn't particularly concerned about that; microbes were far more important.

JONAH: I think it matters that [the baby] got a really, really large dose of Dani's vaginal juices on the way out; that's what I think is the most important.

ME: The microbe—

DANI: Inoculation—

JONAH: Yeah, and I was really surprised that no one has talked about how to reinoculate if you come out C-section . . . you need to do something to inoculate. Breastfeeding of course, but you need the vaginal fauna.

ME: There's a study that's being done about vaginal swabbing—

JONAH: Yeah, I would've stuck that kid up in Dani's crotch, for sure, for sure [laughter], absolutely. It's so obvious that wherever our microbial activity is taking place on our body, that culture is our immune system, is our intelligence.

While crickets chirped in the background, Dani breastfed the baby and a friend made dinner for them. In retrospect, it's interesting that they described microbes as an "inoculation," but rather than bolstering a defense system against "bad guys," a microbial inoculation seems more like building a protective network of "good guys"—an intelligent cultural system that enables a healthy relationship with the world.

Jonah continued to elaborate with good-natured intensity on how the physical and emotional, the environmental and interpersonal, are interwoven as part of his child's developing consciousness: abundant milk and touch create a positive emotional state, and a stress-free infant psyche enables the physiological processing of the material world. Food nourishes the mind, hugs comfort the gut. Furthermore, it's the microbes, the "symbiont" in Jonah's words, that enable these feedback loops between mental and physical effects, between parent and infant embodied subjects. Microbes support "the material digestion of the nurturance." Jonah grappled with the category-blending implications of his philosophy, saying that one could try to separate out the physiological from the emotional or the microbial from the interpersonal "and basically sterilize everything and just have a lot of contact, or flip it around and have all of the probiotics without as much psychological-emotional contact stuff"—that these improvised categories are separate but intertwined. He went on to speak about chemicals and their place in the interlocking processes he has been describing. He noted how "we are awash in so many" synthetic chemical compounds in consumer products and how various people in his life made different choices, calling those choices "distracting" and "confusing, because our kid does not smell like our kid" to describe how chemicals interrupt growth and connection.

Jonah was among the few people I encountered who discussed ecological concerns so explicitly. In the nearly ten years since I interviewed him, such concerns have exploded in scientific literature and have become a topic frequently discussed among childbearing Californians. Research into the microbiome's effects on metabolism and mood are affecting medical treatments, from antidepressants to stool transplants. Endocrine disruption is being taken seriously as a public health issue by some groups, such as UCSF's Program on Reproductive Health and the Environment. Books on embodied trauma, like Bessel van der Kolk's *The Body Keeps the Score*, have topped bestseller lists. Social science and humanistic research on ecologies, toxicity, and their implications has blossomed in the past decade, including within the environmental reproductive justice framework.

Chemicals, microbes, and stress reference problems in our collective conditions of existence that, while worse for some than others, cannot be solved by protecting oneself from the conditions. Yet this persists in being the dominant way solutions are framed. Immunity is about protecting *by exempting*, by taking someone out of a bad situation, rather than protecting someone by building desirable connections, or thinking of protecting *the entirety* of the thing, or changing the nature of the situation. Immunity relies on clear good and bad actors: self and nonself, us and them. But ambivalence is brought to the fore by the problems discussed in this chapter: dosage and timing of chemical exposure, harmful and beneficial bacteria, eustress and distress. A focus on protection itself puts other possibilities off the radar, such as sacrifices that might be required from within the collective to enable mutual flourishing.

In this chapter I emphasize the similarities between stress, microbes, and chemicals because I noticed birth activists talking about them in the same interesting way, in a way that disrupts the idea of health as a property of an individual human, as a condition of either behavioral choices or genetic makeup. Instead, I was made aware of a growing scientific and lay understanding of health as dependent on environmental factors, dispersed in time and space, interpersonal and partially predetermined generations in advance. The origins of well-being are being traced earlier and earlier, not just to childhood and infancy but sometimes back to fetal existence and epigenetic inheritance, and very occasionally through the generational chain of childbearing people's bodies, through links of milk and blood that carry past experience into the future. In this view, health is an ongoing outcome of chemical, microbial, and affective ecologies outside any individual's purview.

Eula Biss, in her aptly titled *On Immunity*, explores the idea of immunity as a broad American cultural phenomenon that spans medical science and parenting practice, how we think of laws and bodies, and the ways we govern countries and households. A central theme in the book is fear. Emotions, and especially fear, are highly influential in directing our attention. Culturally speaking, it is neither the statistical facts about danger (for example, cars and even beds kill a lot of babies) nor the scientific explanations about harm that matter most, but rather whether people are frightened. Tracing fear, as Biss does, shows us how the desire to protect came to elide with creating a state of exemption. It also reveals something interesting about how the object of fear—what we feel the need to protect ourselves *from*—both shifts and stays the same. Chemicals, microbes, and stress get recruited into old and familiar storylines that are just as likely to reinforce individualism as to encourage ecological ways of thinking and acting. The idea of toxicity, for example, takes up much of the class-inflected cultural legacy around cleanliness and purity while also overturning old fears of dirt itself. Contemporary movements to get kids playing outside, immersed in dirt and microbes, embrace exposure to the messiness of nature while reinforcing a class hierarchy in which other kinds of exposure are associated with marginalized, impoverished ways of living. Biss writes that "the idea that toxins, rather than filth or germs, are the root cause of most maladies is a popular theory of disease among people like me," alluding to her White, well-educated, and middle-class social position.[44] She details how such a theory of disease, far from reinforcing the vulnerable idea that we are all in this together, perpetuates the romance of the untainted body and the illusion of a pure system from which the "undesirables," whether agents of disease or classes of people, can be excluded. An illusion of control. This same cultural impulse toward purity has been responsible for some of the most sinister social events of our age—eugenic policies and laws against miscegenation and sodomy—while leaping over the many ways we are all already polluted, even at birth.

Immunity was first a legal term. The legal status of conscientious objector was first used in the context of vaccination and coincided with an ambiguity between conscience as a social property and an individual one, an ambiguity at work in law as well. Morality can't be fully private, as one's actions affect others. The Enlightenment brought the idea of the body as a bounded and whole individual property; prior, it was bodies within bodies, the political body, national body, cosmic body. Of course such bounded and whole bodies that could be self-owned were only for an elite group that did not include women, amongst others. (Interestingly, the 1912 definition of biological individuality was that which is "rendered non-functional if cut in half"—but being split is precisely pregnancy and birth, in one way of looking at it.)[45] There are a host of political metaphors that echo across law, governance, individuals, and biology, merging contexts. The body politic has immunity too, and the national body can be described as "polluted" and "invaded" by immigration, for example. Biss writes, "If our sense of bodily vulnerability can pollute our politics, then our sense of political powerlessness must inform how we treat our bodies."[46] The problem of immunity could also describe the emotional state of citizenship within an American democracy, as a "problem of ecology, of interrelationships, of interdependence."

Such issues are echoed in medicine, from the anti-vax movement to immunological science. Biss describes how a large part of the appeal of "natural" medicine is in providing an alternative language that uses metaphors that address our base anxieties: "cleanse," "supplement," "detox"—get out the bad guys. Ecological thinking asks us to deal with ambiguity, but habits of immunity require clear good guys and bad guys. And so "intuitive toxicology" by people who aren't toxicologists ends up emphasizing all-or-nothing exposure rather than a nuanced calculation of dosage and timing, admonishing people to avoid man-made chemicals—including vaccines—at all costs. In Biss's words, when we feel bad we want something unambiguously good: "The idea that our medicine is as flawed as we are is not comforting."[47]

In the realm of immunological science, we can readily see how scientific concepts are always changing in dialogue with cultural concepts. Emily Martin's classic ethnographic work from the 1990s, *Flexible Bodies,* chronicles how biological immunity moved from a simple defense metaphor, in which the immune system fends off harmful invaders, to one of flexibility in the age of HIV/AIDS. She elaborates how this transition mirrored changes in the labor market, which required newly flexible workers. The immune system is itself a metaphor, as Martin points out: thinking of bodies (and environments) in terms of systems instead of machines developed in the 1970s with the rise of cybernetics and became entrenched in the following decades. Martin explains how one of the consequences of understanding bodies as complex systems is "the paradox of feeling responsible for everything and powerless at the same time."[48] This paradox is where individualist values and ecological realities clash and implode. During the COVID-19 pandemic metaphors of immunity came to the cultural fore again. Efforts to communicate more effectively about vaccines popularized the idea that they are *teachers* instead of defenders, that they help the immune system become skillful (even if ultimately in the service of defense). The idea of herd immunity was used by scientists to describe collective immunity, the point when enough people have been vaccinated that the virus cannot really spread, but when taken up in public dialogue the term evoked ideas of sacrificing vulnerable individual members of the group for the good of the whole, a Darwinist logic that inverts the original sense. It was challenging in so many ways for Americans to integrate their selfhood within a larger systemic whole; in Biss's words, "What gets reported back to us most often from the land of science is that which supports our existing fears."[49]

It is not just the public uptake of science where cultural ideas about immunity have influence. I credit David Napier with the title of this section.[50] He discusses how cultural concepts of immunity have impeded scientists from interpreting their data more accurately and creatively: "What is so often overlooked throughout these debates over models of immunity is the degree to which immunological identity hinges on culture-bound notions of a wholly autonomous 'self'" predicated on "a singular assumption: that a 'self' must preserve its integrity through a protective mechanism." He draws a paradox: as an eminent immunologist reminded him, "Were a 'self' not salient, persistent, and protectionist, that 'self' would soon become ... a toxic dumpsite." Yet if, as we now know, the self is constantly being redefined through defensive antibody production and related acquired immunity, isn't that another way of saying "that it doesn't really exist at all"?[51] Immunological science makes more sense if the self is not a "prior and persistent" Cartesian entity but an ongoing negotiation. Napier speculates that the tendency to characterize viruses as active agents when they are at least equally passive "arises partly from the cultural belief that harboring otherness within us is principally dangerous," a belief that yields the need to protect against things "foreign," and which made studying the maternal–fetal so unsatisfying for immunologists prior to the arrival of stem cell research.[52] New questions have now arisen about why autoimmune symptoms often subside in pregnancy and why women have rates of autoimmune infection that are seven or eight times higher than those of men, and whether childbirth itself might be understood in terms of immunological rejection. Napier concludes by elaborating another possible view of identity, one widely evidenced in the anthropological literature: we know who we are by the risky, dynamic, and sometimes painful process of discovering what we can and cannot accommodate. Antibodies can be understood as creative attempts to engage difference and risk at the borders of self, where immunity is more about exploring otherness than battling to eliminate it. What is foreign is not necessarily dangerous, but assessing danger is more complicated; indeed, the danger may often be ourselves, and recognizing that "the enemy is us" is "faintly un-American," says Biss.[53]

In childbearing, the self/other boundary is unclear. In the remarkably unremarkable co-embodiment of pregnancy and nursing, the childbearing body gives lie to the autonomous individual. In her meditation on the placenta and the relationality of care and nourishment, Emily Yates-Doerr shares that placentas "taught me that even as we are unevenly individualized, *we have never been individuals.*"[54] She elaborates on how the placenta's dual nature, belonging both (or neither) to the pregnant person and the baby, is uncanny for those raised in environments that celebrate individuality because of how it turns what is self and what is other inside out, makes apparent how conduits can be barriers while barriers can be porous and adaptive, and pushes us to develop languages that can account for the dynamism of barriers, differences, and unities.[55] The placenta does what Heather Paxson calls "thresholding," marking both the establishment of a boundary and its transgression.[56] In Yates-Doerr's words, "It mediates between insides and outsides, selves and others, sameness and differences—crossing lines, setting limits."[57] Childbearing embodiment causes us to rethink not only the distinction between human individuals, but also the distinction between being merged and separate. There are ways of being both; we need new terms for the conversation.

In Euro-American intellectual history, one's body not being one's own is monstrous—and, indeed, popular culture is full of references to terrifying pregnancies and the fetus as alien, as a parasite. "Monsters" are what demonstrate, or warn, etymologically speaking—that is, they show us what we are afraid of, what is difficult or uncomfortable to acknowledge. They reveal danger, often within the shadows of our own consciousness.[58] The pregnant body, the microbially colonized body, the chemically saturated body, the overstimulated nervous system—these monstrous figures demonstrate that we have never been individual. A different ontology is visible via childbearing: bodies teeming with overlapping, mutually dependent life and nonlife. This ontology exemplifies not just the inadequacy of choice but its impossibility. Control is illusory, ecosystems are fluid, places are all, inevitably, interconnected. This verges on dystopian. But it also has the utopian potential of rupture, of disjuncture with what has come before because it is no longer tolerable. And childbearing populations are in a unique position to respond to threat, risk, and damage because childbearing is, in overlapping senses, a critical period where our shared vulnerability is visible alongside a newly powerful impulse to make a better world for the next generation.[59]

Childbearing brings our collective past and present into the creation of a future being, yet children are often romanticized as a clean slate. It is because of the way these sit together—the new beginning and the fact that there is nothing new under the sun—that childbearing is a poignant site for activism, for unsettling the individual. This is scary—terrifying even. But staying the same is scary too. To return to Biss, who claims having a kid is the most dangerous thing a person can do: "We have been made fearful. What we do with our fear is central question of both citizenship and motherhood." The fact that discourses about toxicity of various sorts were rather marginal in the birth worlds I worked in speaks to this fear, and to the daunting task of change: you have to change the entire world in order to truly birth a new one.

SEVEN

Redemption

ACTIVISM AND IMAGINED FUTURES

"WHITE WOMEN, UNDERSTAND THAT your having babies is part of a settler colonialism project!" Loretta Ross spoke with conviction and humor on the warm May Saturday. The largely but far from exclusively White audience of the first annual BirthKeeper Summit in 2015 was gathered in the Berkeley City College auditorium. "Not that you shouldn't," Ross added in a lighter tone. "But examine that."

Ross is a key figure in the reproductive justice movement. Recipient of honorary doctorates and a 2022 MacArthur Fellowship and leader of the March for Women's Lives, she is frequently in the media. She began her talk by saying that since she only had one baby and then was sterilized against her will, she thought she "mightn't be a good fit to talk at BirthKeepers" but was eventually convinced otherwise. Ross mentioned the irony of talking about "choice in birthing when you didn't even have a choice about the sex," yet her attitude was resolutely practical and purposeful: "I don't care who fucked up, I'm here now." She talked about how she was born at home unassisted, and she was unaware for a long time of how rare that was. When she feels she is being treated unfairly, she thinks of her mother raising eight kids while cleaning houses on her hands and knees. Someone at the conference had offered her a wider chair to sit in onstage, as she's a large woman. She didn't have to ask for it. "*That's* what paying attention to women's lives looks like," she said. She asked the audience to consider whose motherhood is valued, and whose is disciplined, and she proposed that it's impossible to talk about birth without talking about genocide. A Black woman herself, she stated, "If we weren't living in a context of genocide, 'Black Lives Matter' wouldn't need to be uttered." Later, she led a session called "Appropriate Whiteness" about alliance building.

Ross was emphatic that the reproductive justice movement was not a response to the framework of reproductive rights, familiar from the pro-choice movement that grew in the late twentieth century. "That would mean Black women couldn't get White women off their minds; no, we did it for ourselves." Ross was instrumental in founding SisterSong, the preeminent reproductive justice organization, created by and for women of color in 1997 and based in the American South.[1] SisterSong defines reproductive justice as "the human right to have children, not have children, and parent the children we have in safe and healthy environments . . . the human right to bodily autonomy from any form of reproductive oppression."[2] Reproductive justice is expansive in scope because to truly parent in a safe and supported environment encompasses the prison pipeline, environmental toxins, climate change, deportation, militarized police, gentrification, hunger, and any number of social-systemic problems. "Reproductive justice applies to *everybody*. Everyone has reproductive potential," Ross claimed. "It's more universal than anything I've ever heard feminism talk about." Ross was more expansive than anyone else I had yet heard speaking publicly about what was really wrong with American childbearing. *How* babies are born is inextricably tied up with *whose* babies are born and seen as worthy of being born and cared for. When people I encountered tried to get to the root of the problems with birth, the problems became . . . everything.

This final chapter has been the most difficult to write (and subsequently trim!) and the one that seemed most important to bring up to date; it will inevitably feel inadequate. It is about largely White birth activists and activist organizations working to build coalitions and, in the process, grappling with race, settler colonialism, capitalist rapacity, and how personal intentions are inadequate means of righting wrongs. Redemption, a religious concept that encompasses seeking and receiving relief from sin, is not something that I considered when starting this research. Yet the intriguing activist sensibility that a birth's significance extends beyond the event itself—the idea that births are the root of the problems and the source of the solutions—is imbued with a desire for salvation that exceeds the conventional ways religion, social movements, and politics are entwined. There are other ways religiosity creeps into secular birth worlds. A kind of evangelism clings to the ways natural practices are advocated, and the way American reproductive atrocities are brought into popular awareness evokes an exorcism. Yet the pull toward individuality makes it challenging to grapple with the sins of a community as opposed to the sins of an individual soul. What can one do when the nation itself, or even the world, needs to be redeemed?

Religious sensibilities are woven into the American project, from Puritan colonists fleeing religious persecution in Europe to the way new religious sects, from Mormons to Seventh Day Adventists to Scientologists, continued to seek new frontiers. The desire to reinvent the experience of divinity can be seen in the transcendentalists' worship of the sublime in nature, New Age spiritualism that easily slides into self-optimization, and the Evangelical drive for rebirth and direct communion with God. In California, the Peoples Temple Agricultural Project, a cult known for the mass death of its members in Jonestown, Guyana, in 1978, shared many qualities with the socialist and religious communes being established in that era; before its disgrace, it became thoroughly entwined with California politics in its search for a revolutionary utopian future. In her essay "How America Talks about Itself," Marilynne Robinson suggests that "Puritanical" might simply mean "reformist," the idea that tradition can be questioned. She claims that the American Revolution's most revolutionary idea is "that society as a whole can and should be reformed. This Puritan energy does indeed continue to animate American life."[3]

A key aspect of frontier mythology is the drive to find a clean slate so one can do things differently and better, a desire that slips between abandoning the past and trying to redeem the past through seeking a better future. Insofar as America and the frontier are progress-seeking projects that have left destruction in their wake, progress is what needs to be redeemed—but it is also the vehicle for redemption. As we've seen, questioning progress involves destabilizing science as a quasi-religious social authority. And yet technological innovation, which braids into the cultural narrative about science, persists in seeming inevitable. We see a caricature of this in the manic way Silicon Valley has marshaled technology to shape the future, in the idea that what's to come is worth any damage done, so "move fast and break things."[4] Progress is, in some ways, a form of temporal immunity: immune from the past, protected, cut off. We can *move on*. That's the fantasy of progress. But the past haunts us. Progress presumes origins, genesis. But what if everything moves in cyclical recombinations? What if there are neither origins nor clean slates, as many scholars of Indigeneity and environmental justice remind us?[5] Birth justice activism in its various manifestations encompasses both the desire to reform the origin of persons, at their birth, and the desire to reform the ongoing cycle of reproduction.

Progress and redemption, the values that bookend these seven chapters, are intrinsically linked. Redemption attends to the past, yet like progress is in service of the future. Where progress is hubristic, redemption is humble. The dominant framework for understanding progress is the techno-scientific quest, historically framed as fundamentally different from that of the pilgrim traveling toward redemption or the humanist maturing into a stoic able to face death; it is an infinite search for knowledge whose telos is mastery, not reconciliation. The rise of science as a social force distinct from religion helped separate the species subject (humans writ large) from the contingent subject of individual happiness or salvation—thus salvation became personal, not social. Yet religious sensibilities underlie the scientific project, too—a secular salvation story not only motivates the drive toward innovation but the implicit goals of the social sciences.[6] Saviorism is a key trope of our time: "Everything seems to need saving," writes Risa Cromer, who analyzes the well-worn tactics of fomenting moral panic around a particular figure framed as vulnerable and worthy of protection (fetus, child, gun owner . . .) and cautions us to be wary of saviorism in all its forms.[7]

Progress and redemption both imply optimism, but redemption's optimism is more complicated, with sadness and anger and regret mixed in. Optimism is stereotypically American, manifest in bluff and bluster that is often associated with a kind of innocent, earnest confidence: the belief that things can be put right, evident from Mark Twain's *Innocents Abroad* to a 2023 *Atlantic* article arguing that the current "cultural pessimism" is actually rooted in "our tradition of idealistic cultural narratives that things ought to be better than they are."[8] Yet innocence is a short slide away from defensive outrage, or head-in-the-sand beliefs in convenient stories like meritocracy.[9] For redemption, one needs a relationship with what came before; redemption centers the idea that we have sinned. Redemption is not so much remarkable for its religious language (all values have religious valences) as for how well it speaks to the complexity of the present cultural moment. Identifying wrongdoing underpins both conservative and liberal narratives in contemporary American culture wars, albeit with incommensurate ideas about which wrongs matter and who is guilty. It is easier to look to social extremes for scapegoats, be they refugees or billionaires, than to examine our own multifaceted complicity and the messy logistics of reparation. Redemption confronts the American impulse to reject complexity, sadness, and the wrongness within us, to be the hero and the savior instead of the object of salvation.[10] It requires receptivity and humility—which not coincidentally are qualities encouraged in doulas.

Molly Arthur arrived in neat business casual, a White woman with close-cropped gray curls. Over tea lattes on the leafy open-air patio of a Berkeley cafe, she explained her expansive vision for a BirthKeepers' movement that would unify all social justice causes, from environmentalist groups to anti-racist and anti-military groups to the people who had been active in the Occupy movement a year or two prior. I had first heard about the BirthKeeper Summit via a postcard laid out on the entrance table of the Bay Area Doula Project, which met that month in someone's loft-commune space on a cramped side street in San Francisco, across from a tangled community garden enclosed by chain-link fencing. The postcard offered the provocative motto "Save birth, Save the world." I signed up for the email list and contacted the organizer, offering to volunteer and asking if we could talk.

At our meeting Molly shared that she was not a birth worker of any sort herself but instead a mother seized by a sense of culpability for perpetuating environmental harm to her now-grown children's bodies, and for bringing them into an unsafe and toxic world. Arthur explained how she understood the oppression of women to be inextricably linked to the oppression of the Earth, invoking the witch hunts, colonialism, and male desire to control the reproduction of the workforce. She shared with me her awe at the knowledge that her body, and therefore her children's bodies, were made of (and therefore compromised by) the material that had surrounded her grandmother in her youth. She told me about epigenetics and perinatal psychology, evolutionary biology, ecofeminism, and the thalidomide scandal. She described how the "motherbaby" must be thought of as "a being irreducibly in relationship" and named numerous like-minded people she had learned from and been in contact with, citing their ideas as evidence that this was a matter of widespread interest. Molly told me how her personal background was laced with privilege that she sought to recognize. She had just retired from working in corporate sales when she had a kind of awakening in which she was appalled to realize her own complicity in structures that destroy the environment and oppress people. In a later interview she said, "I did not consent for this to happen in my body. It turns me into a perpetrator. and I do not want to perpetrate harm to my children and my grandchildren. . . . This is an intimate story, this is an intimate endeavor for us." That the feeling of intimate violation was a shock to her speaks to the privilege she mentioned.

But Molly didn't want the BirthKeeper Summit to represent privilege, she told me at that initial meeting, and over the next ten months of organizing she and the other members of the team worked to not have well-off White voices dominate the planning or the ultimate conversation. An early organizing email stated that "the goal of the BirthKeeper Summit is a deep transformation in the paradigm of birth, and life, on this earth. Voices from diverse demographics and disciplines are needed to make this happen." In order to "model the society we want to create" while recognizing that "we don't necessarily have the skills to do that," Molly talked about using NVC (nonviolent communication) trainers to facilitate consensus-based methods among the organizers. They offered scholarships for attending the conference, as Molly noted that it can be "farther" for poor women in East Oakland than an eminent speaker on Black rights from Mississippi. She recognized that "the women on the front lines, suffering the most from the things this movement is opposing, are poor women of color, so they need to be included." But this is easier said than done, not least because inclusion presumes that excluded groups *want* to take part in something they didn't design. Some speakers had to be persuaded and cajoled into attending, as was the case for Ross. Linda Jones, a well-known Black feminist doula, said onstage that she fought Molly for a long time over being part of BirthKeepers, but that, in the end, she was glad she consented.

I don't intend to hold up the Birthkeeper Summit as particularly unique or successful. Indeed, despite a somewhat lackluster follow-up event in Washington, D.C., in 2017, it seems to have lost its momentum. But it was an attempt at "staying with the trouble," as Donna Haraway enjoins: that when we run up against the difficulty of co-creating a respectful vision for a better society, we must keep engaging that difficulty and not let it turn us away.[11] Many of the birth events I attended included allyship and anti-racism training. Indeed, it was more through engagement with birth worlds than academic critiques that I underwent my own (ongoing) reckoning with racial injustice. Figuring out what was done wrong, and how it can be healed, is uncomfortable work that requires grappling with some ugly realities. It required Molly Arthur to step back significantly from her own environmental agenda and recruit organizers who centered different concerns, or who approached environmental concerns in a different way.

The four-day-long Birthkeeper Summit took place during the final stretch of my fieldwork. It was focused on (but not limited to) the United States, and the 350 attendees included parents, midwives, doulas, doctors, nurses, activists, artists, policymakers, and alternative-care providers; most fit within more than one of these categories. Panels and workshops dealt with a wide range of topics, including racial disparities in care and outcomes, embodied historical traumas, Indigenous birthways, postpartum depression in fathers and mothers, perinatal psychology, the social impact of new reproductive technologies, environmental effects on fertility, and LGBTQ experiences with reproduction. Speakers included Dr. Shelley Sella, a third trimester abortion provider who does so "in the style of midwifery" and who worked with Dr. George Tiller before his notorious murder, and Suzette Johnson from the Perinatal Substance Abuse Task Force, who spoke about institutional racism and how doctors are no "higher" than doulas, quoting Alice Walker that "anything you love enough can be healed." Others spoke about how to educate one's elected officials and run for office, about toxic chemicals in consumer products, and about how capitalism perpetuates fear through language.

The emotional tenor of the event vacillated between fascination with the depth and miracle of the birthing process and impassioned anger at the indignities and abuses birthing people suffer. Tensions over feminism, race, and privilege surfaced regularly. In the many panels that grappled with sensitive topics, touching and enlightening dialogues ensued: the patient who felt wronged and the nurse who asked what could have been done better; those with a deep mistrust of hospitals confronting those who experienced poorly managed home births; and midwives who fought for professional legitimation honoring Indigenous midwives who gathered knowledge and skill in unofficial ways. The conference presentations repeatedly stressed that even though differently situated mothers and children suffer unequally, the well-being of all mothers and children is linked. A healthy new generation is imperative to everyone. Yet some of the tangled threads in the event speak to broader, durable concerns about the roots of problems.

Let's look at the motto that first attracted my attention: "Save birth, Save the world." Who and what is included in those capacious placeholders, "birth" and "world"? Furthermore, save them *from what*? Partially, the phrase fetishizes human origins—that people (or better said, individuals) begin at birth, and therefore this is where problems may originate. Much of the BirthKeeper materials discussed the "primal continuum" as a critical period that starts before conception and continues through infancy, in which the dispositions and aptitudes of the next generation are cultivated in the "MotherBaby" as "one biological system," often merged with "MotherEarth" into an all-encompassing whole: "MotherBaby MotherEarth." And so, paradoxically, linking birth and world also recognizes birth as a site of interconnectivity and transmission between bodies, generations, materialities, communities. Speakers in the introductory panel introduced themselves by remarking on the oppressions and violences that darkened the generational chains leading to their own births: born into legacies of slavery, rape and incest, genocide, famine, abuse, and scopolamine and cesarean trauma. Lastly, the phrase is an explicit call to salvation. The summit was suffused with the recognition and interpolation of childbearing as the site of passionate concern, care, anxiety, and love, predicated on the idea that things are *not* alright.

An early organizing email conveys these aspirations. Addressed to "Friends, Supporters, and Activists for a better world," it defines a BirthKeeper as "one who guards our most precious birthright—being born healthy and loved into a flourishing and just world." It recruits both ancestors and possible futures into the vision of prioritizing "the immutable relationship we have all been born into—that of "MotherBaby MotherEarth"—projecting that this would yield "healthy, caring humans and a healed earth home" where we "act in solidarity with all who are endeavoring to change the systems of destruction in our culture ... withdrawing our consent from a culture that commodifies and privatizes our Mother Earth and intervenes with MotherBaby." The email asks for help collaborating with "frontline communities enduring the largest impact" and says that "we will hear from Black activists, Indigenous elders, youth leaders and birth workers" about steps toward "a world of care and compassion ... inspired by the confluence of grassroots movements from diverse segments of our society." There is, of course, no single, simple answer about how to bring such a vision into being.

One of the more literal interpretations of "Save birth, Save the world" was a memorable session focused on redeeming individual birth experiences. The speaker was describing craniosacral therapy, which, like other touch therapies, aims to address fear and trauma by building in "love." She described newborns in terms of their social and sympathetic nervous systems, explaining how their bodies express distress and overwhelm, that they cry not only when they need something but when they are working through troubling memories about their births, and that bodily movements (like the "breast crawl") can reenact and heal early embodied experiences even years later. Yet how is this focus on individual trauma relevant to world building? When an audience member questioned the speaker's assertion that "we're here because this is to help humanity, [to] address a bigger picture," she elaborated that "secure attachment is the goal. If we develop it in our babies and children, and get them in their bodies, they'll have empathy for themselves and others, and then they'll care about society, culture, environment, the Earth. That's one of the best ways we can heal the world." This is a beautiful illustration of fetishized origins—that one good beginning will have infinite ripple effects. Shaping feelings in this highly embodied way is affective instead of emotional. In William Mazzarella's description of affect, "society is inscribed on our nervous system and in our flesh before it appears in our consciousness. The affective body is by no means a tabula rasa; it preserves the traces of past actions and encounters and brings them into the present as potentials."[12] The craniosacral therapist—and many others we've encountered in this book who hold similar beliefs—posits affect as redemptive. That is, past harms can be atoned for on an embodied feeling level so they don't persist as potentials for perpetuating harm in the future.

Other BirthKeeper events took a more social angle. In addition to Ross, reproductive justice activists who spoke at the conference included Samsarah Morgan and Linda Jones, East Bay–based doulas of color who explained their work supporting vulnerable mothers. Morgan advocates for young pregnant women in foster care, defending their need for resources: "They are wards of the state, which makes us all their parents, and they are receiving abuse and neglect. Yes, *any* woman who makes the choice to bring children into the world needs lots of help, that's normal, that's human." She connects them with doulas and explains that "mothering is learned, so there's no shame in not knowing what you're doing." She focuses on primary skills like cooking meals to feed themselves: "You need to have three square meals in your body to fight for social justice, or even to care about it." Morgan explained that these women often fire their doulas, and that that's okay because it's the first time in "the poor young lady's life she gets to fire someone—you can't fire a social worker." They usually make up. It's the process, the right to complain and be listened to and acknowledged and have power, that is transformative.

Jones used to own a baby shop in upscale North Berkeley called Waddle and Swaddle, which I remember from my days as an undergraduate student. She said she started it because she saw women "wandering the street pushing $600 strollers" (which now retail for twice as much), crying because they had no one to listen to them or help them care for their babies. So the store began as a kind of community space, where she hired moms who walked in looking for something more than a purchase. They worked there together with their babies wrapped on their backs, she recounted. Jones cofounded Black Women Birthing Justice (BWBJ), which published an anthology of over a hundred birth stories from women who don't often get to tell them. Jones said emphatically, "I want people who are not afraid to be around Black people to help Black people have their babies. And I want them to get paid for it." She acknowledged that her present doula clientele is primarily wealthy White women from the Berkeley Hills, but "they need help too, and I'm okay with that."

In all sorts of activist movements in the Bay Area and more broadly, people claim their particular issue is *the* one that everyone can mobilize around, whether it is climate change or mass incarceration. For Molly Arthur, as for many well-off White people, environmental issues can slip into the foreground; Molly would not have disagreed that gender, sexuality, race, capitalism, colonialism, and the environment are inextricably linked.[13] Yet people have different starting points in coming to this realization that can make building alliances tricky. In our interview Molly insisted that mothers are in denial about their responsibility for the burden of cellular-level intergenerational transfer; she wanted to make them understand that they "are culpable as a mother for this toxicity." Her own culpability had been the catalyst for the whole event, after all. Yet she recognized that "the last thing mothers need is more guilt and responsibility." Her solution was that moms need to be in a community where everyone supports and nurtures mothers; if they don't have to carry the whole burden, they won't have to deny the whole burden. Yet getting to such a new society requires managing the present phase where individuals, and especially individual mothers, carry the burden. Trying to change the system also presents a problem of purity: there's no escape from present toxicity, yet an idealized pure space is often the inspiration for change. Arthur praised the film *Birth Day* for showing "what natural birth looks like," yet followed this by bemoaning "you can't go somewhere where there's an untouched culture" and, moreover, "there is so much pollution [that] there's *no* place you can see a natural birth anymore." This short film was eventually screened at the BirthKeeper Summit. Trying to redeem birth is trying to redeem the world, which spools out of control and *is everything;* that's the point, and the problem.

The Birthkeeper Summit captured the visionary spirit that I found so intriguing since starting this project. It encapsulated the idea that changing how birth happens will ripple outward into some form of utopia, that the problems of the world start near birth and therefore need to be remedied there. Many of the birth workers I spoke with insisted that childbearing practices have broader consequences than the health and well-being of mother and baby—as Roxanne did in chapter 1. A memorable, but typical, APPPAH graphic features an image of a White pregnant person, head cropped, with a satellite view of Earth superimposed on her belly next to the words "Ultimately, womb ecology reveals itself as world ecology as the seeds of peace or violence are sown ... during birth." The premise of the BirthKeeper Summit was that if the well-being of *all* mothers and babies were prioritized, the planet's problems would start to be cured and a whole different reality would emerge. This ideal introduces chicken-and-egg-style questions about which needs to come first. Only if White supremacy and imperialism were replaced with structures enabling all to flourish would elite, influential American parents begin to feel safe enough to stop frantically reinforcing their privileges so their children don't slide backward in a competitive, precarious society; only if influential Americans acted against their immediate self-interest would social structures change. That there is no linear map of how social change should happen, that things spiral along together in their heterotopian way, leads me to not read too much into the present dissolution of the BirthKeeper Summit. The term *birthkeeper* circulated long before the event and continues to do so, as does the visionary spirit.

HAS THERE BEEN SIN? HISTORY AND INNOCENCE

The day after the BirthKeeper Summit, a small crowd of us gathered outside the annual conference of ACOG, the American College of Obstetricians and Gynecologists, held at San Francisco's Moscone Center. Hand-drawn prayer flags waved above us; I had drawn one myself the day before at a table in the exhibition hall featuring squares of brightly colored fabric and markers with which attendees were urged to create messages about birth. This was the summit's final event, and the crowd who showed up for the demonstration numbered about thirty, a small number in contrast to the 350 or so who populated Berkeley City College during the prior three days. But they had a lot of energy! A blond woman was speaking at a podium, a sparkling turquoise cape thrown behind her shoulders (I learned from a conference vendor that "turquoise is the color of the birth revolution"). She proclaimed, "We demand evidence-based care! Don't induce for large babies, low amniotic fluid, or anything before forty-two weeks—acknowledge forty to forty-four weeks as the norm! Ask before you do something, episiotomies, putting your hands inside. This is my body. I get to decide!" Her words merged evidence and politics, as discussed in chapter 2, in righteous indignation at paternalism. She proudly proclaimed that she is "just a mom," founder of the Just a Mom League, which advocates for changes in maternity care from outside the medical profession. She later told me the organization is for "everyone who's willing to support moms as the primary decision-maker regarding their body."

Other speakers included Laura Perez, a *partera* (midwife) I knew from the community, who emphasized her gratitude for surgeons in appropriate contexts, which in her opinion did not include the majority of births. An older man in a plaid button-down shared a written speech about the impact of living conditions and social and economic inequality on health. A brusque and businesslike woman advocated evidence-based medical care that would alter many of ACOG's policies and tacitly upheld practices, which, she explained to me after her talk, are done for liability reasons. She said obstetricians are "asking women to . . . bear the weight of their liability issues," which is not okay for either party. The only person from the ACOG conference that engaged with the group was a doctor from Brazil, who stepped outside to casually investigate and chatted with Molly Arthur; she told me he agreed with lowering cesarean rates, which in Brazil are some of the highest in the world.

This demonstration illustrates how complicated it could be to engage with guilt in the BirthKeepers' explicit goal of redemption. Through positioning themselves outside the ACOG meeting, the demonstrators identified obstetric practice, and to some degree obstetricians themselves, as not innocent. "We're all in this together," the event seemed to say as individuals tried to draw attention to ways the groups' purposes overlapped, "but *you* have done wrong." In many ways it is fair to call out the faction holding the majority of the power and resources as culpable for the manifest problems in their sphere of influence. Yet pointing fingers at obstetricians is also a kind of simplified scapegoating. When I asked Molly Arthur why she was present at the demonstration, she rhetorically posed the question, "What would happen if the first consideration was MotherBaby, MotherEarth? There would be no more violence against women, no more violence against children, no more violence against the environment. There would be care and compassion as the new definition of human beings." But obstetricians aren't violent as a matter of principle (though they often are in practice); indeed, they usually understand themselves as working for the benefit of mothers and babies.[14] And yet it is worth noting that very, very few of them came to the BirthKeeper Summit or other events on improving birth that I attended.

On my way to the demonstration, a man handed me a leaflet denouncing infant male circumcision, and I noticed a group across the road, the "intactivists" whose white pants had a red circle sewn across the groin. American doctors (usually pediatricians) regularly perform circumcisions, a procedure that can be described as both elective and nonconsensual. Some activists consider this genital mutilation and link it with adult sexual violence. Are doctors culpable if they don't see it this way? Are parents who request the procedure? How can one even have such a conversation? I asked a woman at the BirthKeeper demonstration about the intactivists, and she said she had worked with them before but didn't care for their shock tactics. Building alliances is not a straightforward proposition.

Obstetricians stand in for—and in real ways carry forward the social legacies of—the racist and classist agendas, misogynistic professionalism (since the witch-hunt era, professionalized medicine has taken birth care forcibly out of the hands of women), and eugenics that were inimical to the BirthKeepers' mission. And yet the BirthKeeper Summit emerged from a context alive with similar cultural forces and ambiguities. Trying to improve things is not neutral; it presumes a certain idea of "the good" and a plan for attaining it, which vibrates with utopia and all its problems. There is a creepy undertone to betterment, as evident in the eugenics platforms discussed in chapter 1. The BirthKeepers did not have some covert eugenicist agenda, but a legacy of ideas about progress is integral to the sensibility from which it emerged. Social movements haunt each other in ways that are not immediately obvious.

Quintessentially progressive, at the forefront, the frontier, California is good at whitewashing its history. The generative seat of a particular kind of neoliberalism, it easily mutes context by focusing on individuals and mutes history by focusing on what comes next. But California has been the site of genocide, internment camps, forced labor, and racial cleansing on a scale unmatched elsewhere in the United States (the fact that plantation slavery didn't happen in California seems to overshadow this fact). Despite explicitly studying birth culture in California, the sense of the regional kept escaping me as I worked on this project. In a workshop, a colleague pointed out how unsurprising this is: California claims to be everyone's future, and nowhere. It is unmarked as a frontier place. It is pure potentiality. Relatively few people know California was an epicenter of eugenics. I didn't, not from growing up there, nor from my elite California education in the humanities. I didn't realize it until I was well into my research for this book. No one I interviewed or hung out with during my fieldwork spoke about California this way. I grew up in an almost exclusively White community alongside the tacit understanding that "racism doesn't happen in California." Racism doesn't happen in progressive Oregonian cities, either, their White residents having forgotten that the state prohibited Black people from settling there during the prior century. As Loretta Ross exclaimed in an animated Q&A session, "There's so many White people allergic to history, I can't even fathom that!"

Another reason Californian eugenics doesn't have a more negative reputation is that it was intimately tied up in euphoric ideas about the place itself, in what California was imagined to be and enable for those entitled to it. It was not only the manifest destiny of American settlers to expand all the way to the West Coast, but once they were there, the "perfect" environment would enable racial perfection to be attained. Joseph P. Widney, founder of the Los Angeles County Medical Association and dean and president of the University of Southern California Medical School, believed California was going to be the center of health *for White people;* he talked about an "Aryan climate" and Southern California as a "Garden of Eden," and he was a virulent racist. For Widney and others, a misguided love of place was entwined with explicit ideas about intellect and morals. A superior "race of Californians" was said to "seek vigor in the open whenever possible," a version of the Protestant work ethic that implied physical robustness and adventurous courage. It was a utopian project, building both paradise and those suited to live in it.

Place and race are entwined in many versions of blood and soil nationalism, but California's version had an unusual edge, a blood and soil bohemianism that brought creativity to the forefront. In the early 1900s cultural institutions like the Bohemian Club in San Francisco and writers' retreats in coastal beauty spots like Marin and Carmel helped creatives make biological claims to intellectual legitimacy. These writers emphasized the health and virility of a rural bohemian lifestyle featuring the outdoors, positioning it against the neurasthenic anxieties of the time. The concept of creativity emerged from this crowd and became part of California's brand, with clear ties to the present-day Bay Area's embrace of fitness, nature, and innovation, manifest in cultural phenomena as diverse as biohacking, mindfulness, and disruptive enterprise. The isolation of various places—Carmel-by-the-Sea, the Berkeley Hills, California itself—was embraced as a buffer against racial mixing in this earlier era; currently, ideas about creativity and the creative class are entwined with gentrification practices.[15]

Ronald Reagan, in his successful 1967 campaign for the California governorship, introduced the Creative Society, a program to reduce federal dependence in favor of personal freedom (in contrast to Lyndon Johnson's Great Society), championing that "there is no major problem that cannot be resolved by a *vigorous and imaginative* state administration willing to utilize the tremendous potential of our people."[16] What is now known as neoliberalism took off when Reagan moved into national leadership in the late 1970s. Although creativity may be liberated by government policies favoring individual entrepreneurial freedoms or protected by exclusive spatial arrangements, in this intellectual legacy it is resolutely imagined as an individual property. Nikolas Rose elaborates how neoliberalism "responsibilizes" individuals in ever-deepening ways.[17] This is entwined with the Californian emphasis on pursuing individual improvement: the practices of mindfulness and life coaching emerged from California in the early 1990s, and New Age spirituality, self-optimization, and market enterprise have deeply entangled roots. This has deepened into the current creative class regimen of personal branding, wherein everyone needs to turn an entrepreneurial lens on their employment, leisure, opinions, and myriad side hustles, cuttingly embraced as both a route to self-actualization and a way to hedge against economic precariousness.

Political expression in contemporary American society is closely related to normative ideals of private life that revolve around consumption and the family, what Lauren Berlant calls the intimate public sphere. Unpacking the cultural history of the early 2000s, Berlant describes how American politics became centered on the intimate space of the family during the "rise of the Reaganite right."[18] This conservative cultural politics diluted the far more oppositional politics of the 1960s and '70s that exposed the oppressions of stereotyped groups, highlighting differences and inequities instead of patriotic assimilation. The privatization of citizenship changes legitimate claims for redress from a frame of historical wrongdoing to one of present loss. This is key to why redemption is both now being called for and so challenging to engage. Within a frame of historical wrongdoing, the claims of women, Black people, gay people, and others are justified. A frame of present loss legitimates the nostalgia of those who "lost" the American Dream and the freedom to feel unmarked. This nostalgia enables "a scandal of ex-privilege ... a desperate desire to return to an order of things deemed normal, an order of what was felt to be a general everyday intimacy that was sometimes called 'the American way of life.'"[19]

Berlant claims that in this conservative norm, to be American is to be unconflicted. Introducing identity politics of any sort, or indeed calling out wrongdoing, is itself felt as a transgression. Citizenship is more a feeling than a political relationship. When private life is posed as the core of politics, the unborn child becomes the ideal citizen because of its quintessential innocence; it has made no public claims, and it has no controversial history. Private cultivation of the domestic realm, including by buying products and services (even those that should be public goods, like healthcare and education), seems more relevant and pressing than political struggle. And indeed, vanishingly little activism near birth involves lobbying, protesting, petitioning, or running for public office; the majority looks to empower, inform, and support individual moms and babies in their private contexts. If it no longer makes cultural sense to take to the streets with grievances and aspirations, and if childbearing is the core of heteronormative domestic family life, then there is significant gravity tugging those who believe we need to transform society toward individual infants and the context in which they come into being. Ironically, this also undermines the intention to transform and "save" society because it so easily reinforces the alienating anti-politics of middle-class private life. The landmark Supreme Court decision protecting abortion, *Roe v. Wade,* protected private, individual relationships between a woman and her doctor—not civil rights or gender equality; its recent overthrow is linked with a fierce nostalgia for the child-centered, "innocent" America that Berlant describes.

California, and specifically the Bay Area, has been on the forefront of civil rights movements that have in turn been hampered by the hyperindividuality of the creativity legacy that pushes against public collective action and naturalizes the success of those who are already seen as worthy. Some have called third-wave feminism "libertarian feminism," exemplified by tech executive Sheryl Sandberg's "lean in" messaging. Due to the intense gentrification happening all over the Bay Area, resulting in the highest-rent areas in the nation and much of the world, the remnants of civil rights movements are pushed to the economic and geographical fringes. Social movements flare up in California but break down quickly because individualism rules the day. On one hand, championing government interventions like free provision of reproductive healthcare, accessible quality childcare, and expansive parental leave is a way out of the neoliberal politics of privatized individuals, but, on the other hand, it advocates giving a concerning amount of power to a state that is fundamentally and perhaps irredeemably colonial. People have excellent reasons not to trust the state or the professional organizations involved in civic governance (including medical bodies), and this is especially true regarding reproduction. Eugenics is still very much with us.

The number of Americans in prisons has increased more than 450 percent since 1980 despite a steadily falling crime rate, and California has led the way with what government analysts have called "the biggest prison building project in the history of the world."[20] In *Golden Gulag*, Ruth Wilson Gilmore describes how the defeats of radical struggles, along with a weakening of labor and shifting patterns of capital investment, have been key in this prison explosion. Mass incarceration is reproductively devastating and disproportionately affects poor and non-White people. Yet, as Carolyn Sufrin details, the San Francisco jail system is one of the very few ways people who are not valued by society can access basic life-sustaining care.[21] Police violence against entire communities is reproductive violence that implicates victims' parents and future children. All three pillars of reproductive justice—abortion, procreation, and parenting—have been violated under recent U.S. immigration policy, including the refusal to grant teen migrants abortions even in contexts of rape, the forcible separation of parents from their children, and forcible sterilizations at a for-profit Immigration and Customs Enforcement (ICE) detention center.

CHOICE, RIGHTS, JUSTICE: SCOPE OF A NEW WORLD ORDER

"We need to bring birth to the forefront of the feminist agenda!" cried Kathi Valeii, speaking at the opening panel of the BirthKeeper Summit. She had started a website called BirthAnarchy.com—it is now defunct, but I vividly remember its graphic of a genderqueer pregnant lion breaking through its shackles. Valeii's talk was full of righteous anger about how mothers with infants are excluded even from feminist spaces, how young women should learn about birth as well as abortion, how only in birth do we accept a woman being held down, shushed, told to be good. In the following Q&A Karen Ehrlich, a much older woman whom I knew as one of the founding midwives in the Santa Cruz natural birth movement, stood to respond: "You forget," she said, "that all the birth activism of the past decades was done by feminists." Another woman said she was "deeply saddened" by their forget-fulness, reminding them that childbirth "came up even in the suffragists, with the desire for pain relief." Valeii and the other panelists acknowledged this but pushed back, claiming that today "childbirth is *not* mainstream as a feminist agenda. People think 'reproductive justice' means contraception or abortion." Yet the people of color who originated the reproductive justice framework—who don't necessarily identify as feminists—were referring to something quite different. The idea of feminism was revealed to be a fascinat-ing multigenerational, cross-racial stew of tension. Throughout the summit, cascades of interruptions insisted on specificity: someone's protest of "excuse me, you mean *White* feminism" was followed up by another's addition of "you mean *conservative* White feminism." An audience member passionately reminded people that "Black women have been fighting for the rights of our births for four hundred fucking years! Indigenous women have been fighting colonial oppression!" Over and over, heated questions were raised about whose feminism counts and whose perspective and history are recognized.

On the panel with Valeii was Khatera Aslami, an Afghani immigrant who lost her baby daughter in a wrongful death in a Bay Area hospital midwifery practice; she hadn't been believed during the three days she had been saying something was wrong. The audience discussion splintered with tensions related to how to interpret this. Finally, someone hopefully suggested that "we can come together on the idea of autonomy—that women can choose where and how and are treated respectfully in that." We have seen how autonomy is complex for a given person to put into practice; it's no more straightforward on a social level. Choice, rights, and justice are the lexicon of autonomy—but like diversity, inclusion, and equity, these concepts try to draw more people in while struggling to account for difference. While there is a neat story about how reproductive justice is broader in scope than repro-ductive choice and that they respectively align with the interests of people of color whose reproduction has been curtailed and White feminists whose reproduction has been encouraged, I witnessed a lot of blurriness, appropria-tion, enfolding, and rejection in how politics near birth were framed. In particular, the term *rights* was used across contexts, sometimes quite casually and inconsistently. The right to choice could bleed into the right to autonomy, scaling up into rights to access, rights to possibilities, rights to states of being.

Consumer rights discourse has been a staple of White feminist birth advocacy championing the right to choose a midwife or home birth.[22] As recently as 2014 Californian midwives were still being persecuted for practicing at homes; in 2013 I attended a large demonstration outside the Sacramento capitol building protesting the patronizing rule that required midwives to have physician supervision (it was lifted for LMs that year, and for CNMs in 2020). Valeii's rights-based position focused on absence of constraint rather than proliferation of choices; she argued that "vaginas aren't for regulating" no matter how well the person (politician, physician, woman) understands female anatomy, because autonomy "is not science based. It's rights based." An international movement for human rights in childbirth usually draws on the UN's Universal Declaration of Human Rights, which invokes both the obligations of governments to support human rights to life, health, privacy, and equal treatment through providing accessible and affordable maternity care, and "specific medical rights" to refuse treatment and give informed consent that are grounded in rights to autonomy and authority over one's body. The movement both pushes against an obstetric model of care and promotes the accessibility of obstetric interventions. Sometimes rights are invoked more nebulously than either civic entitlements or self-ownership. At a midwifery training Tamara Taitt differentiated between the right to access healthcare and a right to health *itself*—a clean environment, a nurturing social group, nutritious food—which would be truly revolutionary. Expansive views of rights can infringe on each other. Black Women Birthing Justice published an article on a child's right to breast milk, which might seem similar to a right to healthy food, but breast milk must be provided at a significant personal expense of time and energy, skirting into the ways children's rights have been pitted against childbearing people's rights.

Expansive as a reproductive justice framework might be, it often circles back to individuals' human rights. Ross was emphatic about this in her talks, as in her and Rickie Solinger's authoritative 2017 book on the topic. She argued that the human rights framework has been deradicalized but that fighting for one's rights is the pathway to justice, that human rights are unifying, not individualizing, a way of bridging differences between racial groups, generations, and pro- and anti-abortion camps: "We need a movement where we all come together. That's the movement of the twenty-first century." Certainly, rallying around equal rights has fueled massively important civil changes around voting and desegregation. But the idea of rights originated in Enlightenment-era views that foregrounded property ownership and implied subservient lesser persons like slaves and wives. Is rights-based organizing a fight for inclusion in a fundamentally problematic system, inviting people to play a rigged game from which they were formerly excluded instead of changing the game's rules? Some justice advocates talk about the rights of communities, or the "rights of nature" in Indigenous South America. Rights have a lot of discursive power (and questioning them as a White person is presumptuous, dismissing what people of color have never fully had). But rights are complex to reconcile with interdependence. All life is not equal, nor are all persons the same; yet all life is valuable and interconnected; all well-being is contingent on other well-being. What would it look like to shift the frame? Instead of rights, some Indigenous and Black scholar-activists talk about "right relations" as a goal and guiding principle.

It is an understatement to say that right relations are complicated to put into practice. Over the ten years this book has been in the making, I witnessed the imperative to promote diversity become more and more emphasized within traditionally White organizations. At one Bay Area Doula Project meeting in San Francisco that was overflowing with people—I was perched on the kitchen steps—a Black midwifery student declared that "affirmative action for midwives of color is the answer!" UCSF offered such scholarship programs, as did DONA and MANA, and the majority of trainings and conferences I attended included sessions on White privilege, allyship, and structural bias. *SQUAT: An Anarchist Birth Journal* aimed to be "a radical celebration of midwifery and birth" and featured gorgeous, colorful images highlighting racial, ethnic, and body-shape diversity. It was a self-published quarterly from 2010 until the volunteer editors retired in 2016; I met one of them at a workshop on abortion care in Oakland, though I never had a chance to attend the annual SquatFest. The magazine was an explicitly political, younger generation's version of *Midwifery Today,* an iconic natural birth publication going since the 1970s, yet it had limits. The author of the blog/zine *Outlaw Midwife,* an "out of system, out of compliance" midwife of color who wanted more leeway to express anger, critiqued *SQUAT* for merely being a hipster version of the older publication. A typical *SQUAT* article profiled Claudia, an African American woman training to be a midwife and inspired by her time at Ina May Gaskin's Farm Midwifery Center, where, in her words, "no one births in fear"; she "understood that a community that cannot birth itself will not survive" and shared her vision for a more representative midwifery community.

This has been a bumpy transition. Nasima Pfaffl, who worked with the Midwifery Education Accreditation Council (MEAC), shared that MANA was having a "big controversy over midwives of color," calling it a timely, delicate issue. At the 2012 conference where we spoke, there was a planned fireside vigil about racial health disparities, which became a singing circle featuring songs largely from the White natural birth movement of the 1970s; the next morning some of the organizers issued an awkward public apology for a "slip-up in focus." Such attempts reflect conversations happening more broadly in America, wherein White communities realize that good intentions are important but inadequate, and they struggle to accept that abstinence and ignorance are not innocent. Indeed, MANA was dissolved in early 2024 over such controversies. The statement issued by the National Association of Certified Professional Midwives explains that "for some, MANA was primarily a gathering place that felt like coming home, and for others, it highlighted their lack of inclusion, power, and access within midwifery leadership."[23]

My notes from that 2012 event are full of what seemed an unofficial motto, "We need to get our eyes off the perineum!" The perineum, the tissue between the vagina and anus that stretches (and often tears) to accommodate the passage of a tiny human, is here a metonym for birth proper. It is problematically limited to think only about how babies are literally born, yet it can be overwhelming to consider the entire context of possibilities and affordances that shape this pivotal moment for different people. Despite the widespread belief that "midwifery is the answer," sometimes people wondered if the world was becoming too broken even for midwifery to fix. To quote a speaker at that gathering, "Midwives may be experts in low-risk 'normal' birth, but the world is becoming a high-risk world," especially in low-income communities of color. "The population who can enjoy low-risk, normal pregnancy is shrinking." Although it was not directly in response to this sentiment, it is not a coincidence that in 2024 UCSF announced plans to eliminate the midwifery master's degree and require all future nurse-midwifery students to graduate with a clinical doctorate, dismantling one of only two such programs in the state in a move that will majorly disrupt the workforce (no existing faculty can teach in the new program as they do not have doctorates), with no clinical or safety benefits to patients. The California Nurse-Midwives Association unanimously opposed this, highlighting how it will worsen the reproductive health and maternity care provider shortage in California and asking UCSF to recognize the significant importance of midwifery as a strategy to improve the U.S. maternal health crisis. White birth worlds have been stretching—and confronting the inevitability of tearing—though it is not clear what new paradigm might be being birthed.

Outside of birth work, White, middle-class feminist politics is also shifting, though it often repeats old patterns. Eugenic mass incarceration for the poor is twinned with an opt-out revolution of women leaving prestigious and powerful careers to embrace domesticity and intensive mothering. Natalie Fixmer-Oraiz links American security culture after 9/11 with the Victorian idea of reproducing the Nation as a White settler state through what she calls "homeland maternity."[24] Rather than subservience to men (regressive), this new domesticity is about subservience to children, adopting "postfeminist vocabularies of 'choice' and 'empowerment' in service of an agenda that individualizes women's struggles, strips feminism of its radical import, and reduces the political to the personal once more."[25] This White, idealized motherhood is increasingly turned into curated social media businesses, muddling traditional public-private distinctions even as opting out reinforces them. Jong Bum Kwon writes about White mothers' roles in the reproduction of racial inequity and structural violence through "transforming home spaces and suburban landscapes into white fantasies of childhood," showing how racialized suffering is not necessarily perpetuated through animus, neglect, or ignorance.[26] "In the US, motherhood is inextricably linked to whiteness in almost every way" claims Sara Petersen, yet she notes, "The construction and upholding of maternal ideals has always been in service of white men in power. It's never had much to do with mothers"—a fact that echoes backward across decades of abortion debates and eugenicist propaganda.[27]

Other middle-class women have rejected the third-wave feminism mantra that they can have it all by pushing for the social acceptance of voluntary childlessness. Shadowing both voluntary childlessness and opting out is the increasingly untenable social situation in which "successful" women simply cannot manage the demands of careers and mothering given the near-total absence of state support, pressure to relocate far from family for work, the necessity of two-income households, and the dearth of equally educated male partners.[28] Women who are highly educated, used to being taken seriously and paying money to do "all the right things," can experience a particular disillusionment as part of birth trauma, resulting not just from difficult events and the experience of not being listened to or respected, but also from *surprise* at not having been able to advocate for themselves. Of course it's a privilege to not have been aware of how contingent women's autonomy is, to take for granted the value placed on one's existence even while being angry at false narratives; the more difficult question is whether this indignation can motivate empathy and coalition building.

The environmental politics of reproduction are also morphing, complicating the idea of global overpopulation that emerged from the 1970s White community (and which demonized the "excessive" childbearing of Black and Brown people without considering colonial histories or outrageous disparities in resource use).[29] Young people worried about climate change are negotiating what it means to bring children into a catastrophe-ridden planet, sometimes refusing to do so.[30] Donna Haraway recently urged people to "make kin, not babies" and faced significant pushback, eventually working with scholars of color to elaborate the problem in multiple ways.[31] Michelle Murphy incisively critiques the politics of population; building on her book *Seizing the Means of Reproduction,* which elaborates the colonial power dynamics of the 1970s women's health movement, *The Economization of Life* exposes the colonial resonance of the view that poor women can be "invested in" through education and contraception and that having fewer babies makes women and their children "more valuable" to society.[32] Murphy asserts that life cannot be separated from its conditions. A cosmology positing human individuals as isolatable from "conditions of becoming with the many" is what enables elite, consumptive, low-fertility lifestyles that are supported by others' exposure to violence. Instead, reproduction could be thought of as a politics of redistribution, as a struggle over different futurities, not differential fertility.[33] She proposes "alterlife" as an alternative to population, a concept recognizing how we are all already altered by the economic logics of value and waste, which means we hold the capacities to alter and be altered again. In this, there is a possibility not for return, but for something like redemption.

There is an inherent tension between universal goals and valuing difference; in other words, it's complex to allow for multiple views of "the good." This problem is not unique to birth activism. Building an all-encompassing movement requires making bridges between worldviews that seem incommensurate. In the talk that opened this chapter, Ross described herself as a bridge maker, referencing Cherríe Moraga and Gloria Anzaldúa's classic women-of-color anthology, *This Bridge Called My Back.* She emphasized how bridge building is taxing work, not something everyone is suited for or willing to do. It requires that the bridge maker become invisible. She jokingly said, "Guess I'm not a radical because I have a bad habit of seeing my enemies as people to talk to." In Ross's view, one of White supremacy's ripple effects is to make us feel there's only one way to be something—a feminist, a doula, an activist—such that we're damaged by trying to fit into that ideal while also damaging others for not fitting into it. She also disagreed with the "women's movement myth" that "we can create safe spaces where people don't have to feel pain." Birthing something new is painful; grappling with history is painful. Bridge making is becoming ever more essential to feminist politics as political visions are increasingly composed of heterogenous possibilities and priorities. Something other than feminism is happening here, when the hope and goal is to redeem the world.

SAVIORS AND SCAPEGOATS:
DOULAS RIGHTING WRONGS

It happened relatively inconspicuously, at a regular meeting of the Bay Area Doula Project, held in a downtown Oakland business center—but it etched itself in my memory. During a discussion a doula stood up with a child wrapped on her back, a long, bright skirt and tall bun enhancing her regal bearing. Clear voiced and unapologetic, she said, "I refuse to make choices based on fear." This simple statement was the basis for an approach to life, babies, and everything as the doula went on to explain with an appreciatively received economy of words. An orientation toward fear—and, by extension, courage—underlaid much of the anxiety, dissatisfaction, and aspiration I saw near birth. Not being afraid is not the same as being reckless, of course, and so embracing courage doesn't necessarily simplify things, but it puts them in a different light. By rejecting outright an imperative to be afraid and anxious, this woman implicitly raised the question of what alternative values and affects might be. Perhaps it is not a coincidence that she was Black, as this positioning opens up possibilities for not only idiosyncratic choices and community solidarity but also powerful anti-colonial politics.[34]

The Bay Area Doula Project (BADP) met monthly in the East Bay or San Francisco. It hosted evenings with reproductive justice activists, "resistance art parties" and game nights, and biannual full-spectrum doula trainings that prepared doulas to support people through abortions. Essentially, it was a platform for doula work as political activism. Some of the topics we met around included sex during labor and childbirth, Chinese medicine for menstrual health, home abortion care, processing pregnancy loss of desired babies, mental health training for doulas, and racism and disparities in reproductive care. We met with organizations supporting young parents and gathering "untold stories." BADP maintained distance from the word *doula* on their website, recognizing it as "a racially charged, class stratified, and gendered word ... typically said to come from the Ancient Greek word δούλη meaning 'female slave' or 'woman who serves.' That makes us feel complicated feelings."[35] Indeed.

Miriam Zoila Pérez, a doula who describes herself as a queer and genderqueer Latina of Cuban descent, self-published *The Radical Doula Guide* in 2012 and maintains a blog of the same name. In the guide they define reproductive justice as "building a world where everyone has what they need to create the family that they want to create." Pérez was a key figure in these early days of doula activism, when doula work was becoming not just about reproductive experience or feminist autonomy but about building a just world. Upon encountering the community spearheaded by *SQUAT,* the anarchist birth journal mentioned above, Pérez was delighted: "Needless to say, I no longer feel alone. Instead I'm in awe of the incredible growth in the doula movement, and particularly in the movement of doulas who see their work as part of a broader social justice vision. . . . [I]t's about changing the systems altogether."[36] Pérez's Radical Doula blog features numerous profiles of self-identified radical doulas from around the country. The profiles, mostly gathered around 2015, critique racism, capitalism, institutionalized medicine, institutionalized violence, systems of privilege, and fear. They advocate things like autonomy (including for infants), nonjudgment, strong communities, evidence, sex positivity, beauty, and reimagining language, explicitly framing doulas as agents of change and childbearing as an activity wherein the qualities of humans and their world are shaped.

Since then, doula communities building on this activist sensibility have not only grown but are on the cusp of profound change. In the past few years doulas have been hailed as the answer to the U.S. maternal mortality crisis. In 2017, the American College of Obstetrics and Gynecology acknowledged that "continuous one-to-one emotional support provided by support personnel, such as a doula, is associated with improved outcomes for women in labor."[37] In 2020, twenty-two birth justice organizations and prominent scholar-activists took out a full-page advertisement in the *New York Times* to call for national "birth justice and accountability," asking "How many Black, brown, and indigenous people have to die giving birth?" and invoking a reality where "midwives, doulas, and perinatal support services are fully integrated into maternity care." Jennifer Nash, who wrote the book *Birthing Black Mothers* about doulas in Chicago, published a 2021 op-ed in the *San Francisco Chronicle* titled "Black Maternal Mortality Rates Are a National Embarrassment. Doulas Can Help," one among many similar pieces.[38] An influential 2019 position piece on community-based doula models as a standard of care for advancing birth justice was collaboratively published.[39] The federal Black Maternal Health Momnibus Act of 2021, which is moving through Congress, includes funding for community-based organizations, diversification of the perinatal workforce, and innovative payment models to incentivize nonclinical support.[40]

Jennifer Nash describes how women of color (WOC) doulas have become "foot soldiers in a birth-justice movement rooted in black feminist praxis," whose efforts have been incorporated by the state "as a crisis-mediation tactic rather than as an oppositional stance."[41] The work of this birth justice movement, with all its internal tensions, complicates efforts to resolve the crisis, not least because it reinforces Black maternal bodies as adjacent to danger and death. The state embrace of doulas "effectively recasts the maternal black body not as a medical or embodied category, but as a political one . . . both underscoring the utter necessity of doulas' life-affirming labor and placing doulas' rhetoric surprisingly close to the state's rhetoric: for both, black maternal bodies are the paradigmatic site of crisis." Nash describes a WOC methodology of "togetherness" as an imagined form of crisis mitigation and way of mediating against obstetric violence. While she honors the work WOC doulas are doing, she concludes by pointing out that "the struggle for black children and mothers to quite literally live is still exclusively and entirely in our own (underpaid or unpaid, largely untrained) hands."[42]

No matter how much doulas collectively improve outcomes or how amazing an individual doula is, they cannot be the answer to a set of much bigger problems. They cannot solve broken maternity systems and save those who are vulnerable. Absolving American maternity care of its crisis is an enormous burden that requires grappling with centuries of history. I see this view of doulas as saviors as something less glamorous—as a form of scapegoating, but inverted. If a scapegoat is something onto which you put the sins of the community and kick it out, an inverse scapegoat bears all the sins and is brought in. It seems government institutions and policymakers are beginning to realize what a bargain it would be to loop doulas into systems of insurance and Medicaid, to encourage marginalized people to take on a challenge that they already care so deeply about that they work toward it with little or no pay. Because the thing about a scapegoat, of course, is that it absolves those who use it of responsibility for changing themselves. That's the point.

And yet doulas resist such scapegoating even as they are incorporated into always-already capitalist-colonial systems. For all that calling doulas "saviors" puts too much weight on their shoulders, the politics of a savior is a little different than that of a scapegoat: a savior invites the question of whether something is required in return. Branches, sects, and denominations of Christianity, the implicit American religion, disagree on this matter: Is salvation freely given? Does it need to be deserved or earned or asked for? Are there chosen people entitled to it? Doulas resist becoming scapegoats through all the ways they induce, request, and require changes from the systems within which they work.

· · ·

When the Alameda County public health department solicited proposals for assisting adults reentering society after incarceration in 2013, the Birth Justice Project, which provides doulas for women in the San Francisco County Jail, partnered with Black Women Birthing Justice, which Linda Jones discussed in her address to the BirthKeepers. They received a $191,000 grant to train formerly incarcerated women and other low-income women and women of color (grouped together to avoid stigma) as doulas to serve in their communities and make a living doing so.[43] The initiative received crowdsourced community financial support to continue with another cohort in 2016. In 2017, a similar initiative training Latin/Hispanic people as doulas to support migrant birth began in San Francisco; it was soon consolidated into Doulas Telar (meaning loom, or place of weaving). In 2020 Doulas Telar opened a doulas' house in San Francisco's Bayview neighborhood to continue supporting the Latinx community. They are part of a broader San Francisco organization of community doulas called SisterWeb, founded in 2019, which facilitates Latinas, African Americans, and women from the Pacific Islands serving their communities.[44] SisterWeb not only trains doulas but is a powerhouse of organizational change; it organizes its doulas into teams that support each to prevent burnout, pays them a starting salary of $25 an hour with health insurance and other benefits, and partners with UC Berkeley's School of Public Health to evaluate the program (which it does glowingly) and provide evidence and models for other such initiatives.[45] The care they deliver is free to those receiving it, which is possible because they have received over $200,000 in donations from organizations as diverse as the San Francisco

Mayor's Office of Housing and Community Development, the CA Public Utilities Commission, Anthem health insurance, Merck pharmaceuticals, charities like Every Mother Counts, and the Zuckerberg San Francisco General Hospital Foundation, as well as individual donors.[46]

There are at least ten similar California doula pilot programs with a primary focus on addressing racial health disparities, and in particular on providing free doula services to childbearing people of color or enrollees in Medicaid (government-provided health insurance for low-income people), reported to be the largest number of such programs in any state. In the 2018 survey "Listening to Mothers in California," a majority of people who gave birth in California affirmatively expressed interest in having doula support for future births.[47] An array of governmental and nongovernmental organizations across five Bay Area counties launched the #DeliverBirthJustice campaign around this time, stating that "the fight for racial justice begins with birth justice."[48] California's Department of Health Care Services began rolling out sponsored coverage for doulas as part of the Momnibus Act of 2021; after a multiyear process that included monthly meetings with stakeholders to design the benefit, it went live in 2023, though will take time to come into practical use.[49] Other states have included doulas in their Medicaid programs, starting with Oregon in 2012, followed by a raft of others in 2019. Some integrations didn't work very well, which is why effort has been made to design the California rollout in consultation with over three hundred doulas and four focus groups across the state, including longstanding community organizations like Black Women Birthing Justice and recent innovators like SisterWeb.[50] The National Health Law Program, which led the consultation, maintains a large repository of articles advocating access to doulas as "an evidence-based intervention" that can reduce risk of cesareans, preterm birth, and postpartum depression and improve breastfeeding rates. External recognition of doulas' power to advance social justice has exploded since I concluded my fieldwork, alongside the Black Lives Matter protests and the COVID-19 pandemic that highlighted deep-seated inequities and made many people hesitant to birth in hospitals.

Jennifer Nash identifies three tensions in women of color doula work: professionalization (which implies standardization), differing reasons for opposing medicalization (critiques of medical racism and capitalism versus an aesthetic and spiritual preference, which respectively support ideals of autonomy and authenticity), and birthing as a personalized yet universal experience. These tensions, versions of which play key roles in White birth work as well, emerge from trying to carve out space for connection with something larger than oneself alongside self-recognition and self-respect within broader norms that discourage both. On another level, all three tensions are manifestations of a broader tension between WOC and White doula traditions and commitments, wherein WOC doulas make use of the momentum and visibility established by White birth activism (or, in Nash's terms, the "feminist birthing industry") while reinterpreting it with their own communities' ends in mind.

The California pilot project reports are interesting because they are an instance of those with social power listening to community doulas, which shifts the doula from an inverse scapegoat into a savior. Implementation is another thing, but reports of the consultations indicate humility and receptivity. An Alameda county representative said that engaging with community doulas "was initially a challenge; government systems and institutions have done so much harm to community care providers," requiring ongoing and active work "toward accountability with our birthworkers and doulas who have been filling the deficits of government programming long before there was funding." One report emphasized "letting doulas take the lead," stating that programs "should not claim they are trying to integrate doulas, when what they are actually doing is asking doulas to assimilate and subordinate themselves to medical systems of care," insisting that community doulas must be involved from the beginning in all decision-making.[51] The term *cultural congruence* is used throughout reports to indicate racial, ethnic, and socioeconomic alignment between doula and birthing person, a shift away from "cultural competence" or its successor, "cultural humility," both of which imply the provider is not from the same community.

The challenges of integrating doulas within health systems are a microcosm of political paradoxes. They reveal how access is both dependent on existing systems and facilitated by the flexibility to act outside those (broken) systems. They proliferate ways of recognizing expertise while acquiescing to oversight. They encompass the constitutive paradoxes of wage labor, which require doulas to balance their politics of solidarity with their need to survive by obtaining a wage, to balance birth work within one's community as a spiritual calling against recognizing the value of this work with money that might introduce other motives. As a participant in the California pilot reports said, "It can't turn into something else where it's not heart driven.... [People should] do it for the outcome, not the income."[52] Meanwhile, an evaluation of SisterWeb's compensation approach advocated "simultaneously advancing birth equity and equitable labor conditions."[53] This is more than a tension between care work and professional ideology, but rather a central tension of capitalism.[54] Parallels can be drawn with midwifery's professionalization, which in many ways is a cautionary tale. While midwives I spoke with emphasized that professionalization was undertaken to increase access, it severely limited access to midwives for people of color.[55] Speaking in Edinburgh recently, Dána-Ain Davis answered the "tricky" question of doula payment by saying, simply, give Black women money to spend as they wish. If they want to hire a doula, they will—or do any number of the other things that are required to reproduce, parent, and thrive.

Home birth, as well as the tiny but growing movement toward free birth, attempts to stand outside existing options, to refuse to participate. Indigenous theorist Audra Simpson's theory of refusal (related to Damien Sojoyner's theory of Black fugitivity), does not mean refusal to consent, which is simply resistance, but refusal to play a rigged and hostile game.[56] Both consent and resistance are "easy answers," Simpson says, while refusal is profoundly difficult because it opens the door to the unthinkable, to options not currently on the table. Erica Weiss describes refusal as "an affirmative investment in another possibility."[57] Opening toward other modes of politics begins with recognizing that established channels of dissent themselves bolster the fundamental conditions in which possibilities are registered. For some I spoke with in the White midwifery community, professionalization took refusal and transformed it into mere resistance. Doula politics illustrate how refusal/resistance is not a simple binary. Doulas are a bridge between worlds of political possibility, illustrating the paradoxical difficulties of trying to refuse from within existing conditions while nonetheless doing what needs to be done.

Doula work absorbs these contradictions, mediating between different registers of possibility and risk, enabling care, attunement, and togetherness in a space that is not built to encourage them. There are so many levels on which refusal or resistance or change making might take place, from personal choice to settler-colonialism to the species to the Earth. While people have different gravities in this respect, and the scalar incoherence can make coalition building complicated, the search for redemption is unifying—as a problem, as an aspiration. Political imaginations flourish near birth. Activism here, as elsewhere, simultaneously enacts difference and reinscribes sameness, a dance between unification and heterogeneity. If progress is about the future, redemption is about *futures*. Rebecca Solnit writes that both optimism and pessimism are passive, while hope requires action. Action is implicit in progress and redemption—but redemption highlights that a relationship with what came before is necessary to take appropriate action. What came before was not the same for everyone, nor should be what comes next. Redemption is neither nostalgic nor aiming for mastery. It opens a window onto sideways utopias, onto proliferating heterotopias where things are, and continue to be, different.

Conclusion

FEARS AND FANTASIES

IN ONE WAY OF STATING THINGS, this book has been about fantasies. Birth might be seen as a moment to simply endure and move on from, but that is not what I encountered. In California, where fantasies of all sorts are magnified, birth and everything near it is an increasingly ambitious space where people seek to influence biology, ecology, medicine, history, spirituality, and social systems of race, class, and gender; it's a space of world building that grapples with contradictions in foundational values. If values are emotionally laden notions of what is desirable, and myths weave those notions into stories that are invisible because they are understood as truth, then fantasies connect such stories with desire. Fantasies take the stories and personalize them; they bring our emotions to life and keep us attached to our desires. Fantasies are not always pleasant or positive; our desires are often muddled by fears, and fears can take on fantastic proportions. Fantasies grip us in ways we are not often able to articulate, even while the situations that give rise to them are ever so real.

Near birth, fantasies give emotional purchase to the problem of valuing individuality. Individuality, so foundational to American culture and society, just doesn't work very well during childbearing. Conflicts around individuality may be latent in many social spaces and practices, but they are highlighted near birth. Childbearing is a liminal state, and because of this becomes a site of projection. A host of political projects and anxieties are becoming understood as something that can be organized through childbearing—through that portal where understandings and experiences of bodies and social systems are shaken up, destabilized. This loosening indicates possibility, which is frightening as well as enticing; it can attract a reactive doubling down on what came before. As biological knowledge about childbearing becomes more refined, the fetus-infant, that stand-in for the future, is understood as vulnerable to affect, toxicity, microbial influence, overuse of technology, the *longue durée* of structural violence, and so birth becomes central across different scales of imagining and producing what is to come. This is reinforced by people's growing realization that the entire environment we are in is changing, an expansive notion of threat that bounces from endocrine-disrupting chemicals to racism to climate change to neoliberal class precarity with barely a blink.

The chapters in this book have examined the cultural problem of valuing individuality from seven different angles, showing how individualism is both challenged and reinforced as people grapple with bringing a new person into being. We began with fantasies about what California is and might be: the final frontier, simultaneously the cutting edge of technological progress and a return to nature, a regenerative utopia and degenerate dystopia, counterculture and cyberculture, where conventions hold less sway but the grip of neoliberal consumerism is ironfisted. Innovation of personal and entrepreneurial sorts is fused. It is an ideal place to examine the fantasy of progress: that we can move on instead of being haunted, cyclical, knitted into relationships with histories, complicit. Different fantasies of the past circulate throughout American birth worlds: claims to connections with early modern European peasants called witches, with communally oriented female sociality among settlers, with Indigenous and traditional practices from all over the world, with communities that survived in the face of violence—counterpoised against the fantasy of neutral, beneficial, scientific progress, presumed to inform professional medicine.

By delving into ideas about physiology, we explored fantasies of where and how experience counts, of intuition and embodied knowing that might release us from dependence on institutional expertise, that might correct our alienation. There were fantasies of how the tool of evidence might be repurposed to dismantle the house from which it came. Fantasies of trust and control in the birth room speak to a simultaneous desire for autonomy and meaningful connection. A fearful fantasy saw autonomy slipping into abandonment, buffeted with judgment, isolation, and too much responsibility—a war on women, within which mommies lash out at each other to stave off dread. Equality itself was revealed to be a fantasy in a society where the full participation of some is designed to rest upon the partial participation (and manifest exploitation) of others. It is closely related to the fantasy of inclusion, that we can *all* win the game without changing its rules and without the current winners stepping down.

Nostalgic searches for an elusive authenticity are, as we saw, fantasies of nonmediation, of raw truth. They indicate a longing to feel connected to something outside oneself in a context of rapid change yet are taken up as a way to express, optimize, and recognize oneself as an individual. They are closely related to utopian ideas of primacy and a fantasy of human origins. They are foils for the fantasy of techno-medical triumph over pain, death, and uncertainty—and yet get swept up into the drive for technologically mediated mastery. The desire for mastery is related to the desire for immunity, the fantasy that barriers can protect us and that we don't need to be in conversation with what we find threatening. It springs up when faced with transgressive, ubiquitous toxicity and the startling intimacy of other life forms, challenging the fantasy that our health is an individual property we can own and defend, that our health indexes our moral worth—counterpoised with the fantastic hope that an ecological view will provide an easy route to reconceptualizing what it means to be human. The fantasy of a "root" movement, a search for a cause that would link all injustices into a redemptive solution, is in its way also a fetish of origins, seeking a problem from which all others stem and around which diverse coalitions can align. We encountered eugenics, a fantasy of improvement gone awry, and its more palatable cousin meritocracy, a fantasy of individual worth that makes distributions of power and resources seem just such that there isn't any need to come clean or fix things. Meritocracy undergirds the fantasy of inclusion, that we can address the problems without actually changing.

These fantasies act out social, political, and ethical questions that are latent in other U.S. contexts. American birth is becoming the site of different levels of investment, raising questions about what life is, and what it could and should become. Anxieties and aspirations about the past and the future are projected onto this beginning. Bodies are seen as endangered and transformed at the same time as their resilience is trusted to get us out of this mess. Inequalities are understood to be perpetuated through the physical and affective qualities of early experience, linked with the very survival of communities and the drive to engineer a type of human who will be able to thrive. Though such projections are all too easily reincorporated into dominant narratives, they are also real openings onto other possibilities.

The American fantasy of the autonomous individual, exaggerated from its European Enlightenment roots by "rugged individualism" and the historical importance of the settler frontier, has been a foil throughout all these agitations to understand and be otherwise. Childbearing exposes and undermines the truism that being an individual is what it means to be human. Near birth, I keep encountering thematic questions that transcend the individual subject, that transcend a given social moment, social situation, or society itself. The questions don't fit these conventional scales for inquiry: small as a molecule, big as the human species' degeneration. They are the wrong size to be managed through such American frames as rights, self-reliance, choice, or fresh starts—which doesn't mean that those individual-scale tools aren't doggedly employed for the job! Ironically, individualism is entwined with the reasons many people are still committed to (biological) childbearing. Having a child is the most socially obvious way to not be alone, to have belonging, security, care relationships, and a family when a sense of community has become threadbare. Yet having a baby dramatically reduces one's ability to be an individual in the free-floating autonomous sense, and more so the thinner one's community is, a phenomenon linked with the increasingly common desire *not* to have children. And so bearing children becomes framed as a way to self-actualize, to find personal meaning (or not), in a deepening catch-22 that doesn't recognize the ways bearing children is a social good and social responsibility. Questions about continuity are implied in decisions about having children—which invites questions about death, and endings.

Death is the shadow to fantasies about birth. Both have been medicalized and taken out of the home; both death and birth doulas try to mediate this experience differently. Hospices and birth centers are both quasi-institutional spaces that seek to humanize these transitions. It seems self-evident to prefer births to deaths, but this is exaggerated by valuing progress and productivity, always looking toward expansion with no room for cyclicality, rest, and finitude. There is very little room for the ambivalence that can accompany both—that deaths can be good is medical sacrilege; that births can be unwanted is a political minefield. The totalizing ideology of scientific progress is a way of transcending individual mortality. As a result, the contextual view of physiology that aims to step outside a framework of technoscientific medical control skirts uncomfortably close to having to embrace death and injury as normal and unpredictable aspects of living.[1] Biopolitics, the governance of life, is always shadowed by necropolitics, arbitrating who is allowed, or encouraged, to die; this difference overlays how White and Black reproduction has been treated. In the cultural formations surrounding both birth and death, we can see attempts to bring context to a supposedly neutral value on life that obscures its qualities and affordances.

The past five decades or so have entailed significant cultural shifts in the United States. A new race politics has evolved with civil rights, Black Lives Matter, and the "browning" of the U.S. population. The queering of social life has posed questions and possibilities about family and intimacy. Class narratives of an attainable American dream or egalitarian middle have been exposed as illusory and exclusionist. Political apathy and reactionary political horror are two sides of the same distrust and disaffection, signaling the dominance of the neoliberal private consumer mode. Heteronormative, White, middle-class people are reacting and adapting to this swirl that decenters our collective perspective and privileges, in many ways reflected in this group's childbearing practices. The older style of anthropology I have indulged in here, one that encompasses a breadth of interests to return to culture and how it works, has allowed me to explore how American values are problems, and the ways those problems have become more visible and present in people's practices and discourses.

In moments during my fieldwork I believed I saw transformative social potential near birth. These were moments that transcended the personal transformation so often hailed in birth story narratives of trauma and empowerment. I found these glimmers of radically different knowing and being remarkable, and deeply alluring. The fantasies we have explored are almost never engaged as such, wholesale, explicitly. The way they flicker between seeming utopian or dystopian depending on perspective makes them slippery; they disintegrate if you look at them too closely. When it comes to practicalities, people constantly make hybrids and make bricolage and make do. Yet these fantasies are the terrain through which they navigate, the visions around which they orient. Sometimes childbearing practices are creatively anti-hegemonic and other times they re-entrench heterosexist, racist, exploitative, neoliberal capitalism. Often they do both simultaneously. The questions raised near birth are nothing less than what is the future of society and what kind of human is being built for it? The world appears to need reinventing, and in quotidian ways people are doing so, near birth.

NOTES

INTRODUCTION

1. My formal fieldwork took place between September 2013 and September 2015. I lived in or near the Bay Area until 2017 (and before that from 2004 to 2009) and worked as a doula both before and after my fieldwork.

2. See Morton, *Birth Ambassadors.*

3. A note about practitioners in the United States: *Doctors* involved in childbearing are usually obstetricians, who are trained in birth pathology and surgery, but can also include gynecologists, pediatricians, neonatologists, general practitioners, and naturopaths or osteopaths. *Nurses* work in labor and delivery units and well-woman clinics under the auspices of any of these doctors. *Nurse practitioners* take on more of the duties of a doctor. *Certified nurse midwives* (CNMs) are nurses with a master's degree in midwifery who usually work in hospitals and can oversee "uncomplicated" births; they are legal in all fifty states. *Certified professional midwives* (CPMs) and *licensed midwives* (LMs) are trained in nonpathological birth and well-woman care and sometimes called *direct entry* midwives; they oversee out-of-hospital births. Their legal/licensure status is variable across the United States. (In California, the physician supervision rule was lifted in 2013 for LMs and in 2020 for CNMs.) *Doulas* are childbirth attendants who provide nonmedical support. *Lactation consultants* and *childbirth educators* specialize in breastfeeding and prenatal preparation; they involve a variety of training and certification routes and are often also nurses, doulas, or midwives.

4. See Franklin, *Embodied Progress;* Dow, *Good Life.*

5. Joas and Wiegandt, "Cultural Values," 3.

6. Ortner, "Dark Anthropology."

7. Barthes wrote about contemporary mythologies in 1957 and Mills coined the term "sociological imagination" in 1959. A critical anthropological interest in culture swelled in the 1990s after the "writing culture" turn, which became politicized in various ways. Clifford and Marcus, *Writing Culture;* Wright, "Politicization."

8. See Marcus, "Experimental Forms"; Jobson, "Letting Anthropology Burn."

9. Strathern, "Nice Thing," 161.

10. Sloterdijk, *Stress and Freedom,* 7.

11. Latour, *Never Been Modern,* 3.

12. See Lauren Berlant's "national sentimentality trilogy," *The Queen of America Goes to Washington City, The Female Complaint,* and *Cruel Optimism.*

13. Dumont, *Essays on Individualism,* 260.

14. See Sahlins, *Western Illusion;* Rees, *After Ethnos;* and Cohen, *Body Worth Defending,* for different approaches to this insight.

15. See Starr, *Americans and the California Dream,* and his entire "California Dream" series.

16. Irigaray, "This Sex," 24.

17. Haraway's concept of "situated knowledges" in her eponymous article is emblematic.

18. Intersectionality was conceptualized by Crenshaw in "Mapping the Margins." Nash's recent critique, "Re-Thinking Intersectionality," encourages tightening the concept.

19. Haraway, *Simians, Cyborgs, and Women,* 3.

20. Notably, I am excluding conception and its shadow side, infertility, from childbearing. Issues surrounding fertility and conception have received disproportionate attention in recent anthropological literature, largely around novel and controversial reproductive technologies such as in vitro fertilization, egg and sperm donation, and surrogate gestation. As this excellent body of work shows, such issues also illuminate "big picture" cultural problems and reproduction more generally.

21. Appiah, "The Case for Capitalizing the B in Black."

22. For example, Addams, "Why I Don't Use the Word 'Doula.'"

I. PROGRESS

1. Grusauskas, "Labor of Love."

2. A full-spectrum doula supports a person through all reproductive outcomes or decisions. Full-spectrum practice often overlaps culturally with support of queer and trans family making, and awareness of poverty and racial justice. That friend was the only full-spectrum practitioner I knew of among the many doulas in Santa Cruz. Abortion is a divisive issue in the birth worlds I encountered.

3. Cattelino, "Anthropologies," 275.

4. Miller, "Mapping Our Disconnect," 64.

5. Missions have been described as carceral (Teran, "Violent Legacies"; Madley, "California's First") and as heterotopias (Sánchez, *Telling Identities,* 50). Orfalea links California's unique history to its present exceptionalism in "Exceptional State."

6. Reyes, *Private Women,* examines how these hierarchies were maintained and challenged.

7. Sánchez, *Telling Identities,* 142.

8. Madley, *American Genocide.*

9. Warren, "California Dream," 260.

10. Barbrook and Cameron, "Californian Ideology," 44.

11. Olmsted, *Right Out.*

12. The occupation of Alcatraz was largely responsible for catalyzing a sense of pan-indigeneity among native peoples. In California, tribal structure was destroyed in the genocide and eventually reorganized into "hubs," and as such California has an interesting place in Native politics. Indigeneity doesn't exist anywhere else in the United States in the same way, although this uniqueness is often erased. Ramirez, *Native Hubs.*

13. Didion, *Slouching,* 171–72.

14. Franklin, *Biological Relatives,* 263.

15. Pastor, *State of Resistance.*

16. Pellow and Park, *Silicon Valley of Dreams.*

17. Maharidge, *Coming White Minority.*

18. Weston, *Families We Choose.*

19. Badger, "Immigrant Shock."

20. Kline, *Building Better.*

21. Lira, *Laboratory of Deficiency.*

22. Kline, *Building Better,* 33.

23. Le Guin's wonderful essay "Non-Euclidian View" is a particularly Californian example of feminist critiques of utopia.

24. Singh, "California Wildfires."

25. Foucault, "Of Other Spaces, Heterotopias."

26. Sánchez, *Telling Identities,* 50. For fun, see Simeon, *Foucault in California.*

27. See, for example, Johnson, "Situated Self."

28. Cooper, *Everyday Utopias;* Gordon, *Hawthorn Archive,* viii.

29. Gordon, *Hawthorn Archive,* viii, quoting Raymond Williams. "Sideways" references Le Guin, *Non-Euclidian View.*

30. Basso, *Wisdom Sits,* xv.

31. Boal et al., *West of Eden.*

32. Shapiro, "Mommy Wars."

33. Wilson, "Immaculate Deception."

34. Kline, "Little Manual," 174.

35. Turner, *From Counterculture to Cyberculture.* See also Farber and Bailey, "Afterword."

36. Kline, "Little Manual," 111.

37. Kline, "Little Manual," 200.

38. Currid-Halkett, *Small Things.*

39. Osnos, "Doomsday Prep."

40. English-Lueck, *Cultures@SiliconValley,* cover copy.

41. Dowling, "Love's Labour's Cost."

42. As my presence at births took place exclusively in hospitals, this work answers Morton's call, "Where Are the Ethnographies of US Hospital Birth?"

43. Martin et al., "Lost Mothers"; Villarosa, "America's Black Mothers."

44. Petersen et al., "Vital Signs."

45. American Medical Association, "Birthing While Black."

46. Womersley, "Why Giving Birth."

47. Oparah et al., *Battling Over Birth.*

48. Sakala et al., "Listening to Mothers."

49. Scott and Davis, "Obstetric Racism"; Reyes-Foster, "No Justice."

50. Chen, Robles-Fradet, and Arega, "Building a Successful Program."

51. Sakala et al., "Listening to Mothers."

52. Ross and Solinger, *Reproductive Justice.*

53. Cook, "Women Are the First Environment."

54. Goodman, "Midwives at Dakota Access."

55. See Wagner, *Born in the USA.* The medical industrial complex was discussed in medical journals as early as 1991; Relman, "Health Care Industry."

56. Fisher, *Capitalist Realism,* 1.

57. Starr, *California,* 247.

58. Kapsalis, *Public Privates,* 31.

59. The More Up Campus website, www.anarchalucybetsey.org.

60. UC San Francisco's Motivating Interdisciplinary Lactation Knowledge (MILK) Research Lab website, https://milklab.ucsf.edu.

2. EXPERIENCE

1. The movement she did perform is called the McRoberts maneuver. Shoulder dystocia is rare, unpredictable, and has no widely accepted protocol for prevention or treatment.

2. For a beautiful anthology, see Lock and Farquhar, *Body Proper.*

3. Nelson, *Argonauts,* 13.

4. Kirmayer, "Mind and Body," 82.

5. Martin, *Woman in the Body,* 59.

6. Gaskin, *Ina May's Guide,* 172–74.

7. Enright, *Making Babies.*

8. Gaskin, *Ina May's Guide,* 182.

9. Rothman, *In Labor.*

10. Davis-Floyd, *American Rite,* 6.

11. Martin, *Woman in the Body,* 59.

12. Rothman and Simonds, "Birthplace."

13. See Ford et al., *Hormonal Theory,* building on critical classics like Roberts, *Messengers of Sex,* and Oudshoorn, *Beyond the Natural Body.*

14. For example, the author of the oxytocin book, physician Kerstin Uvnäs-Moberg, also publishes in prestigious medical journals (Olza et al., "Neuro-Psycho-Social Event"). See also physician Sarah Buckley, who self-published "Ecstatic Birth" and coauthored Sakala, Romano, and Buckley, "Hormonal Physiology of Child-bearing," which appeared in a major obstetrics journal.

15. See Bell, Erickson, and Carter, "Beyond Labor."

16. Martin, *Woman in the Body*, 61.

17. Owens, "Too Much," 848.

18. It is very common for monitor readouts to be visible at the nurse's station outside the patient's room, where every staff member can see them. Presumably, if there were any alarming variations, other staff members would have intervened.

19. Sanabria, *Plastic Bodies*, 203.

20. Quoted in Jay, *Songs of Experience*, 216.

21. See, e.g., Rountree, "New Witch"; Sempruch, "Feminist Constructions." Rina Nissim, a key figure in the women's health self-help movement in continental Europe, entitled her book on the subject *A Contemporary Witch (Une sorcière des temps modernes)*.

22. Patterson, "Inactive Spectators."

23. Morris et al., "'Screaming.'"

24. Harjo, "Three Generations," 130.

25. The concept of experience has been called "one of the most obscure that we have." Jay, "Experience Without a Subject," 47.

26. Quoted in Jay, *Songs of Experience*, 49.

27. Haraway, *Primate Visions*, 355.

28. Fraser, "Modern Bodies," 46.

29. Fraser, "Modern Bodies," 48.

30. Apple, *Mothers and Medicine*.

31. Apple, *Mothers and Medicine*, 140 (italics mine).

32. See also Swanson, "Milk as Technology."

33. Armstrong and Kenyon, "Choice Becomes Limited."

34. De Certeau, *Everyday Life*, 91.

35. Daston and Galison, *Objectivity*.

36. Ford, "Attuned Consent."

37. Jay, *Songs of Experience*, 41.

38. Pérez, *Radical Doula Guide*, 31.

39. Davis-Floyd and Davis, "Intuition," 315.

40. Csordas, "Somatic Modes," 147.

41. Mazzarella, "Affect," 291.

42. Mazzarella, "Affect," 293.

43. Mazzarella, "Affect," 293.

44. Federici, *Caliban*.

45. Heidegger, "World Picture."

46. Wendland, "Vanishing Mother"; Ford, "Advocating for Evidence."

47. Star, "Boundary Object," 602.

48. Stengers, "Doctor and the Charlatan."

49. For detailed citations and elaboration, see Ford, "Advocating for Evidence."

50. Stengers, "Doctor and the Charlatan," 30.

3. AUTONOMY

1. This was considered extremely rare when I started fieldwork around 2012, but by 2023 it has become noticeably more common. Interesting trend toward the tactile!
2. Sandelowski, *Devices and Desires.*
3. See Löwy, "Prenatal Diagnosis"; Taylor, *Public Life.*
4. Apple, *Perfect Motherhood,* 135.
5. Martin, *Woman in the Body,* 62
6. Illich, *Tools for Conviviality.*
7. Illich, *Medical Nemesis.*
8. Rapp, *Testing Women.*
9. Owens, *Medical Bondage.*
10. Owens, "Too Much."
11. Lyerly, "Shame, Gender, Birth."
12. Furedi, *How Fear Works,* and Masco, *Theater of Operations,* for example, describe a "culture of fear" in different ways.
13. Ford, "Attuned Consent."
14. Buckley, "Ecstatic Birth."
15. Gonzalez and Lusztig, "Birth of Motherhood."
16. Roberts, *Killing the Black Body;* Washington, *Medical Apartheid;* Owens, *Medical Bondage.*
17. Rothman, quoted in the header of her own website, www.barbarakatzrothman.com/2021/12/offline-how-others-see-us.html.
18. Craven, "A Consumer's Right."
19. See Bordo, "Are Mothers Persons?"
20. Solnit, *Paradise,* 29.

4. EQUALITY

1. See Williamson, *Maternal Ambivalence.*
2. Heti, *Motherhood,* 21.
3. Belkin, "Opt-Out Revolution." See also Jones, *Women Who Opt Out.*
4. Petersen, *Momfluenced.*
5. See Kline, *Building Better,* and Roberts, *Killing the Black Body.*
6. Collins, "Shifting the Center."
7. TallBear, "Making Love and Relations."
8. Sasser, *On Infertile Ground.*
9. Roberts, "Genetic Technologies."
10. Liedloff, *Continuum Concept;* Small, *Our Babies.*
11. Mol, *Logic of Care,* 1.
12. Mol, Moser, and Pols, *Care in Practice,* 9–13.

13. Tsing, "Monster Stories."

14. Mason, "Blenders, Hammers, Knives."

15. Douglas and Michaels, *Mommy Myth,* 4.

16. Mardorossian, "Laboring Women."

17. Kukla, *Mass Hysteria.*

18. Pateman, *Sexual Contract.*

19. Pateman, *Sexual Contract,* 14.

20. Ehrenreich and English, *For Her Own Good,* 102.

21. Also called "feminist" and "domestic" (or "chauvinist"). Ehrenreich and English, *For Her Own Good,* 22–23.

22. Ehrenreich and English, *For Her Own Good,* 201. See also Zelizer, *Priceless Child.*

23. Schiebinger, "Why Mammals."

24. Beauvoir, *Second Sex,* 35; Young, *Female Body Experience,* 46.

25. Kristeva, *Powers of Horror,* 6.

26. Casper, *Unborn Patient.*

27. Lancy, "Babies Aren't Persons."

28. Cromer, *Conceiving Christian America.*

29. Dumont, *Essays on Individualism,* 76.

30. Dumont, Essays on Individualism, 266, 267.

31. Illich, *Gender.*

32. Halberstam, *Trans.*

33. Halberstam, *Trans,* 129.

34. Dumm, *Loneliness,* 22.

35. Arendt, *On Origins.*

36. Dumm, *Loneliness,* 25.

37. Hochschild, "Time Bind," 22.

38. TallBear, "Making Love and Relations."

39. Toupin, *Wages for Housework;* Lewis, *Full Surrogacy Now.*

40. Krueger, "Takes a Village."

41. Birdsong, *How We Show Up.*

42. Boal et al., *West of Eden.*

43. Waldman, "Truly, Madly, Guiltily"; Jones, "Only Two Choices."

44. Rich, *Of Woman Born.*

45. Pollock, *Telling Bodies,* 11–18.

5. AUTHENTICITY

1. Gerosa, *Hipster Economy.*

2. Cronon, "Trouble with Wilderness"; Solnit, *Savage Dreams.*

3. Currid-Halkett, *Small Things;* Messeri, *Land of Unreal;* Franklin, *Biological Relatives.*

4. Menke, "Inner Nature."

5. Critiques of obstetrics include Wendland, "Vanishing Mother"; Morris, *Cut It Out*. For critiques of the natural, see MacDonald, "Gender Expectations"; Bobel, "Resisting"; Faircloth, "'Natural' Breastfeeding."

6. Ruddick, "Maternal Thinking."

7. Ortner, "Is Female to Male." See also MacCormack and Strathern, *Nature, Culture, Gender*.

8. Haraway, *Simians, Cyborgs, Women*, 2.

9. "Three Kinds of Knowing," Birthing from Within blog, accessed May 18, 2018. Updated 2019 as "Three Ways of Knowing."

10. Foucault, *History of Sexuality;* Menke, "Inner Nature."

11. Sanabria, *Plastic Bodies,* 191.

12. See, for example, Franklin, *Biological Relatives.*

13. Sanabria, *Plastic Bodies.*

14. Ford, "Birthing from Within," building on Davis-Floyd, *American Rite.*

15. Gammeltoft, *Haunting Images.*

16. Lyerly, "Shame, Gender, Birth."

17. Davis-Floyd, *American Rite.*

18. Yoder, *Nightbitch,* 196.

19. Yoder, *Nightbitch,* 196.

20. Taylor, *Dark Green Religion.*

21. Starhawk, *Dreaming the Dark,* xxv.

22. Abel and Browner, "Selective Compliance."

23. Biss, *On Immunity,* 50

24. Enright, *Making Babies,* 21.

25. Faircloth, *Militant Lactivism.*

26. Boyer and Boswell-Penc, "Breast Pumps."

27. Paxson, *Making Modern Mothers.*

28. Foucault, "Technologies of the Self."

29. Bordo, "Are Mothers Persons?"

30. Villalobos, *Motherload.*

31. Abel and Browner, "Selective Compliance," 310.

32. Masco, *Nuclear Borderlands.*

33. Bowlby, *Attachment.*

34. Otto and Keller, *Different Faces.*

35. Panel at the 2014 American Anthropological Association meeting.

36. McKenna and Gettler, "No Such Thing," 17.

37. Tucker, *Mom Genes,* cover copy.

38. Haraway, *Simians, Cyborgs, Women,* 21.

39. Haraway, *Simians, Cyborgs, Women,* 1.

40. LeVine, "Attachment Theory"; Zuk, *Paleofantasy.*

41. Odent, *Childbirth and the Evolution,* 18.

42. "Midwife Myth 1," *Indie Birth* podcast, www.indiebirth.com/the-midwife-myth-how-to-hire-an-expert-who-isnt-an-agent-of-the-state/.

43. Seremetakis, *Senses Still,* 4.

44. Starhawk, *Dreaming the Dark,* xxvii.

6. IMMUNITY

1. Ford, "Triple Toxicity."

2. Cohen, *Body Worth Defending, 29.*

3. Ford and Swallow, "Immune System."

4. This is called the Arctic paradox; Cone, *Silent Snow.*

5. For all statistics and facts cited in this opening anecdote, see Steingraber, *Having Faith.*

6. Nixon, *Slow Violence.*

7. Murphy, "Chemical Regimes."

8. Neale, "PFAS."

9. Adams, *Glyphosate.*

10. Neale, "PFAS."

11. Many scholars emphasize this: Murphy, "Alterlife;" Shotwell, *Against Purity;* Adams, *Glyphosate;* Liboiron, Tironi, and Calvillo, "Toxic Politics."

12. Kupfer, "Good Earth."

13. Masco, "Side Effect."

14. Martin and Holloway, "Something."

15. Buntin, "Speaking Truth."

16. MacKendrick, *Better Safe Than Sorry,* 4.

17. See, for example, Waggoner, *Zero Trimester;* Valdez, "Redistribution."

18. Lamoreaux, *Infertile Environments.*

19. Almeling, *GUYnecology.*

20. Dow and Chaparro-Buitrago, "Toward." See also Hoover, *River Is in Us.*

21. Lock, "Recovering the Body," 5.

22. Murphy, "Alterlife."

23. Kupfer, "Good Earth."

24. Jain, *Malignant.*

25. Ford, "Purity," 4.

26. More recently, see Yong, *Multitudes.*

27. Yates-Doerr, "Placenta," 170.

28. Illich, *Tools for Conviviality,* x.

29. Heidegger, "Question Concerning," 9.

30. Simms, "Eating One's Mother," 276.

31. See, for example, Paxson, "Post-pasteurian Cultures"; Paxson, *Eating Beside Ourselves;* Scaramelli, "Making Sense"; Lorimer, "Hookworms Make Us."

32. Takeshita, "Mother/fetus to Holobiont(s)."

33. Land, "Learning to Walk."

34. See Lewis, *General Theory of Love.*

35. Young, "Discourse on Stress," 136.

36. Young, "Discourse on Stress," 133.

37. Young, "Discourse on Stress," 133.

38. Center on the Developing Child, "Excessive Stress."

39. Pincott, "When Stress."

40. Kristof, "Poverty Solution."

41. Geronimus, *Weathering.*

42. Schuster, *Neurasthenic Nation.*

43. Dumont, *Essays on Individualism,* 11.

44. Biss, *On Immunity,* 73.

45. Biss, *On Immunity,* 125.

46. Biss, *On Immunity,* 128.

47. Biss, *On Immunity,* 40.

48. Quoted in Biss, *On Immunity,* 133–34.

49. Biss, *On Immunity,* 140

50. Napier, "Nonself Help."

51. Napier, "Nonself Help," 125.

52. Napier, "Nonself Help," 128.

53. Biss, *On Immunity,* 151.

54. Yates-Doerr, "Placenta," 166.

55. Yates-Doerr, "Placenta," 169, 177.

56. Paxson, *Eating Beside Ourselves,* 5.

57. Yates-Doerr, "Placenta," 169.

58. Lawrence, "What Is a Monster?"

59. Ford, "Purity."

7. REDEMPTION

1. Ross and Solinger, *Reproductive Justice.*

2. SisterSong's webpage, www.sistersong.net/reproductive-justice

3. Robinson, *What Are We Doing,* 138.

4. Facebook's slogan before it became Meta, which inspired a wider ethos of careless "disruption."

5. See the work of Kim TallBear and Michelle Murphy, for example.

6. On sociology, see Smith, *Sacred Project;* on anthropology, see Cromer, Hardin, and Nyssa, "Reckoning."

7. Cromer, Hardin, and Nyssa, "Reckoning," 67; Cromer, "Be Wary."

8. Burton, "How to Escape."

9. Benson, "Crime of Innocence."

10. In Commonwealth settler colonies like Canada and Australia, the term used is "reconciliation," which is more moderate than an American all-or-nothing view on guilt and innocence.

11. Haraway, *Staying with the Trouble.*

12. Mazzarella, "Affect," 292.

13. McClintock, *Imperial Leather.*

14. Davis-Floyd and Premkumar, *Obstetricians Speak.*

15. Olson, "Before the Creative Class"; Olson, "Blood and Soil Bohemianism."

16. Reagan, "Creative Society."

17. Rose, *Politics of Life.*

18. Berlant, *Queen of America.*

19. Berlant, *Queen of America,* 2.

20. Gilmore, *Golden Gulag,* 5.

21. Sufrin, *Jailcare.*

22. Craven, "Consumer's Right."

23. NACPM, "Recognizing MANA."

24. Fixmer-Oraiz, "Contemplating Homeland Maternity."

25. Fixmer-Oraiz, "Contemplating Homeland Maternity," 131–32.

26. Kwon, "Mothers' Hopes."

27. Petersen, "Pretty White Moms"; see also Ginsburg, *Contested Lives.*

28. Inhorn, *Motherhood on Ice.*

29. Sasser, *Infertile Ground.*

30. Roberts et al., *Bushfire Babies;* Sasser, *Climate Anxiety.*

31. Haraway, *Staying with the Trouble;* Clarke and Haraway, *Making Kin, Not Population.*

32. Murphy, *Seizing the Means;* Murphy, *Economization of Life;* see also Moore, "Postures of Empowerment."

33. Murphy, "Alterlife."

34. Gumbs, *Revolutionary Mothering.*

35. This quote was taken from a version of the BADP website that is no longer active. Since being founded in 2011, BADP "has changed over time based on the skills and capacity of the collective members," as quoted at https://bayareadoula project.org/who-we-are.html (accessed September 5, 2024), and the group now exclusively focuses on abortion support.

36. Pérez, "Remarks."

37. ACOG, "Opinion No. 687."

38. Nash, "National Embarrassment."

39. Bey et al., "Advancing Birth Justice."

40. The Momnibus Act webpage, published by the Black Maternal Health Caucus of the U.S. Legislature, https://blackmaternalhealthcaucus-underwood .house.gov/Momnibus.

41. Nash, "Birthing Black Mothers," 31.

42. Nash, "Birthing Black Mothers," 101.

43. See the Birth Justice Project's website (http://birthjusticeproject.org/east-bay-community-birth-support-project) and Stanley et al., "Evaluation."

44. Nguyen et al., "Supporting Birthing People"; Marshall et al., "Barriers and Facilitators"; Arcara et al., "What, When, How Long?"

45. Gómez et al., "Sisterweb"; Marshall et al., *Partnering with Community Doulas;* Gómez, "9 to 5 Job."

46. As independent contractors doulas were paid $1,600 per birth, as a City JOBS program participant it was minimum wage, and as a SisterWeb employee they are currently paid a starting salary of $25 an hour. Chen, Robles-Fradet, and National Health Law Program, "Summaries."

47. Sakala, "Listening to Mothers."

48. The #DeliverBirthJustice webpage, a partnership with five Bay Area counties and part of the statewide Perinatal Equity Initiative, https://deliverbirthjustice.org.

49. See the DHCS website, www.dhcs.ca.gov/provgovpart/Pages/Doula-Services .aspx, and Marshall, Yang, and Gómez "Understanding Barriers."

50. Chen, Robles-Fradet, and Arega, "Building a Successful Program." See all the project materials at https://healthlaw.org/cadoulapilots.

51. Chen, Robles-Fradet, and National Health Law Program, "Lessons Learned," 5.

52. Chen, Robles-Fradet, and Arega, "Building a Successful Program," 17.

53. Gómez, "9 to 5 Job," 1.

54. Young, "Professional Ambivalence."

55. Cancelmo, "Protecting Black Mothers."

56. Simpson, "Consent's Revenge"; Sojoyner, "Another Life Is Possible."

57. Weiss, "Refusal as Act," 351–52.

CONCLUSION

1. Some prominent voices run in the opposite direction, asserting that perfect contextual attunement is always successful at forestalling death and injury. Davis-Floyd asserts this in her "wholistic" model of American birth; *American Rite of Passage*, 157.

BIBLIOGRAPHY

Abel, Emily, and Carole Browner. "Selective Compliance with Biomedical Authority and the Uses of Experiential Knowledge." In *Pragmatic Women and Body Politics,* edited by Margaret Lock and Patricia Kaufert, 310–26. Cambridge: Cambridge University Press, 1998.

ACOG. "Committee Opinion No. 687: Approaches to Limit Intervention during Labor and Birth." *Obstetrics and Gynecology* 129, no. 2 (2017): e20–28.

Adams, Vincanne. *Glyphosate and the Swirl: An Agroindustrial Chemical on the Move.* Durham, NC: Duke University Press, 2022.

Addams, Èské. "Why I Don't Use The Word 'Doula.'" *Medium.* 2020. https://eskeaddams.medium.com/why-i-dont-use-the-word-doula-9d42d9e4a241.

Almeling, Rene. *GUYnecology: The Missing Science of Men's Reproductive Health.* Oakland: University of California Press, 2020.

American Medical Association. "Statement of the AMA to the US House of Representatives' Committee on Oversight and Reform Re: Birthing While Black." 2021.

Amnesty International. "Deadly Delivery: The Maternal Health Care Crisis in the USA." 2010.

Aoki, Keith. "No Right to Own? The Early Twentieth-Century 'Alien Land Laws' as a Prelude to Internment." *Boston College Third World Law Journal* 19, no. 1 (1998): 37–72.

Appiah, Kwame Anthony. "The Case for Capitalizing the B in Black." *Atlantic,* June 18, 2020.

Apple, Rima. *Mothers and Medicine: A Social History of Infant Feeding, 1890–1950.* Madison: University of Wisconsin Press, 1987.

———. *Perfect Motherhood: Science and Childrearing in America.* New Brunswick, NJ: Rutgers University Press, 2006.

Arcara, Jennet, Alli Cuentos, Obaida Abdallah, Marna Armstead, Andrea Jackson, Cassondra Marshall, and Anu Manchikanti Gomez. "What, When, and How Long? Doula Time Use in a Community Doula Program in San Francisco, California." *Women's Health* 19 (2023): 1–10.

Arendt, Hannah. *On the Origins of Totalitarianism.* New York: Schocken Books, 1951.

Armstrong, N., and S. Kenyon. "When Choice Becomes Limited: Women's Experiences of Delay in Labour." *Health* 21, no. 2 (2017): 223–38.

Badger, Emily. "Immigrant Shock: Can California Predict the Nation's Future?" *New York Times,* February 1, 2017.

Barbrook, Richard, and Andy Cameron. "The Californian Ideology." *Science as Culture* 6, no. 1 (1996): 44–72.

Barthes, Roland. *Mythologies.* New York: Hill & Wang, 2013.

Basso, Keith. *Wisdom Sits in Places: Landscape and Language among the Western Apaches.* Albuquerque: University of New Mexico Press, 1996.

Beauvoir, Simone de. *The Second Sex.* Translated by Constance Borde and Sheila Malovany-Chevallier. New York: Vintage, 1997.

Belkin, Lisa. "The Opt-Out Revolution." *New York Times,* October 26, 2003.

Bell, Aleeca, Elise Erickson, and Sue Carter. "Beyond Labor: The Role of Natural and Synthetic Oxytocin in the Transition to Motherhood." *Journal of Midwifery & Women's Health* 59, no. 1 (2014): 35–42.

Benson, Peter. "The Crime of Innocence and the Depths of Sorriness: Notes on Apologies and Reparations in the United States." *Cultural Dynamics* 28, no. 2 (2016): 121–41.

Berlant, Lauren. *Cruel Optimism.* Durham, NC: Duke University Press, 2011.

———. *The Female Complaint: The Unfinished Business of Sentimentality in American Culture.* Durham, NC: Duke University Press, 2008.

———. *The Queen of America Goes to Washington City: Essays on Sex and Citizenship.* Durham, NC: Duke University Press, 1997.

Bey, Asteir, Aimee Brill, Chanel Porchia-Albert, Melissa Gradilla, and Nan Strauss. "Advancing Birth Justice: Community-Based Doula Models as a Standard of Care for Ending Racial Disparities." 2019. https://everymothercounts.org/wp-content/uploads/2019/03/Advancing-Birth-Justice-CBD-Models-as-Std-of-Care-3–25–19.pdf.

Birdsong, Mia. *How We Show Up: Reclaiming Family, Friendship, and Community.* New York: Hachette, 2020.

Biss, Eula. *On Immunity: An Inoculation.* Minneapolis, MN: Graywolf Press, 2015.

Boal, Iain, Janferie Stone, Michael Watts, and Cal Winslow, eds. *West of Eden: Communes and Utopia in Northern California.* Oakland, CA: PM Press, 2012.

Bobel, Chris. "Resisting, But Not Too Much: Interrogating the Paradox of Natural Mothering." In *Maternal Theory,* edited by Andrea O'Reilly. Bradford: Demeter Press, 2021.

Bordo, Susan. "Are Mothers Persons? Reproductive Rights and the Politics of Subject-ivity." In *Unbearable Weight: Feminism, Western Culture, and the Body,* 71–97. Berkeley: University of California Press, 2004.

Bowlby, John. *Attachment.* New York: Basic Books, 1969.

Boyer, Kate, and Maia Boswell-Penc. "Breast Pumps: A Feminist Technology, or (Yet) 'More Work for Mother'?" In *Feminist Technology,* edited by Linda Layne, Sharra Vostral, and Kate Boyer. Urbana: University of Illinois Press, 2010.

Buckley, Sarah. "Ecstatic Birth: Nature's Hormonal Blueprint for Labor." 2010. http://protectingnormalbirth.org/images/EsctaticBirth.docx.

Buntin, Simmons. "Speaking Truth to Power: An Interview with Sandra Steingraber." *Terrain,* September 22, 2007.

Burton, Tara Isabella. "How to Escape 'the Worst Possible Timeline.'" *Atlantic,* June 27, 2023.

Cancelmo, Cara. "Protecting Black Mothers: How the History of Midwifery Can Inform Doula Activism." *Sociology Compass* 15, no. 4 (2021): 1–11.

Casper, Monica. *The Making of the Unborn Patient: A Social Anatomy of Fetal Surgery.* New Brunswick, NJ: Rutgers University Press, 1998.

Cattelino, Jessica. "Anthropologies of the United States." *Annual Review of Anthropology* 39 (2010): 275–92.

Center on the Developing Child, Harvard University, and National Scientific Council on the Developing Child. "Working Paper 3: Excessive Stress Disrupts the Architecture of the Developing Brain." 2014.

Chen, A., A. Robles-Fradet, and Helen Arega. "Building a Successful Program for Medi-Cal Coverage for Doula Care: Findings from a Survey of Doulas in California." National Health Law Program. 2022.

Chen, A., A. Robles-Fradet, and National Health Law Program. "Lessons Learned from Panel Discussion on California Doula Pilot Programs." National Health Law Program, 2022.

———. "Summaries of California Doula Pilot Programs." National Health Law Program, 2022.

Chodorow, Nancy. *The Reproduction of Mothering.* Berkeley: University of California Press, 1978.

Clarke, Adele, and Donna Haraway, eds. *Making Kin Not Population: Reconceiving Generations.* Chicago: Prickly Paradigm, 2018.

Clifford, James, and George Marcus. *Writing Culture: The Poetics and Politics of Ethnography.* Berkeley: University of California Press, 1986.

Cohen, Ed. *A Body Worth Defending: Immunity, Biopolitics, and the Apotheosis of the Modern Body.* Durham, NC: Duke University Press, 2009.

Collins, Patricia Hill. "Shifting the Center: Race, Class, and Feminist Theorizing about Motherhood." In *Mothering: Ideology, Experience, and Agency*, edited by Evelyn Nakano Glenn, Grace Change, and Linda Rennie Forcey, 45–65. New York: Routledge, 2016.

Cone, Martha. *Silent Snow: The Sow Poisoning of the Arctic.* New York: Grove, 2005.

Cook, Katsi. "Reproductive Rights and Native Peoples." *Akwesasne Notes* 14, no. 5 (1982): 1–6.

———. "Women Are the First Environment: An Interview with Mohawk Elder Katsi Cook." *The Moon Magazine* (no date).

Cooper, Davina. *Everyday Utopias: The Conceptual Life of Promising Spaces.* Durham, NC: Duke University Press, 2014.

Craven, Christa. "A Consumer's Right to Choose a Midwife: Shifting Meanings for Reproductive Rights under Neoliberalism." *American Anthropologist* 109, no. 4 (2007): 701–12.

Crenshaw, Kimberle. "Mapping the Margins: Intersectionality, Identity Politics, and Violence Against Women of Color." *Stanford Law Review* 43, no. 6 (1991): 1241–99.

Cromer, Risa. "Be Wary of White Saviorism in Post-Roe Politics." NYU Press Blog, June 23, 2023.

———. *Conceiving Christian America: Embryo Adoption and Reproductive Politics.* New York: NYU Press, 2023.

Cromer, Risa, Jessica Hardin, and Zoe Nyssa. "Reckoning with Saving." *Journal for the Anthropology of North America* 23, no. 1 (2020): 67–69.

Cronon, William. "The Trouble with Wilderness: Or, Getting Back to the Wrong Nature." *Environmental History* 1 (1996): 7–28.

Csordas, Thomas. "Somatic Modes of Attention." *Cultural Anthropology* 8, no. 2 (1993): 135–56.

Currid-Halkett, Elizabeth. *The Sum of Small Things : A Theory of the Aspirational Class.* Princeton, NJ: Princeton University Press, 2017.

Daston, Lorraine, and Peter Galison. *Objectivity.* New York: Zone Books, 2007.

Davis, Dána-Ain. *Reproductive Injustice: Racism, Pregnancy, and Premature Birth.* New York: NYU Press, 2019.

Davis-Floyd, Robbie. *Birth as an American Rite of Passage.* Berkeley: University of California Press, 2004.

Davis-Floyd, Robbie, and Elizabeth Davis. "Intuition as Authoritative Knowledge in Midwifery and Home Birth." In *Childbirth and Authoritative Knowledge,* edited by Carolyn Fishel Sargent and Robbie Davis-Floyd. Berkeley: University of California Press, 1997.

Davis-Floyd, Robbie, and Ashish Premkumar. *Obstetricians Speak: On Training, Practice, Fear, and Transformation.* New York: Berghahn Books, 2023.

de Certeau, Michel. *The Practice of Everyday Life.* Berkeley: University of California Press, 1984.

Didion, Joan. *Slouching Towards Bethlehem.* New York: Farrar, Straus and Giroux, 1968.

Douglas, Susan, and Meredith Michaels. *The Mommy Myth: The Idealization of Motherhood and How It Has Undermined All Women.* New York: Free Press, 2004.

Dow, Katharine. *Making a Good Life: An Ethnography of Nature, Ethics, and Reproduction.* Princeton, NJ: Princeton University Press, 2016.

Dow, Katharine, and Julieta Chaparro-Buitrago. "Toward Environmental Reproductive Justice." In *A Companion to the Anthropology of Reproductive Medicine and Technology,* edited by Cecilia Coale Van Hollen and Nayantara Sheoran Appleton, 266–81. London: Wiley, 2023.

Dowling, Emma. "Love's Labour's Cost: The Political Economy of Intimacy." Verso Blog, February 13, 2016.

Dumm, Thomas. *Loneliness as a Way of Life.* Cambridge, MA: Harvard University Press, 2008.

Dumont, Louis. *Essays on Individualism: Modern Ideology in Anthropological Perspective.* Chicago: University of Chicago Press, 1986.

Ehrenreich, Barbara, and Deirdre English. *For Her Own Good: Two Centuries of the Experts' Advice to Women.* New York: Anchor, 2013.

———. *Witches, Midwives, and Nurses: A History of Women Healers.* Old Westbury, NY: Feminist Press, 1973.

English-Lueck, J. A. *Cultures@SiliconValley.* Stanford, CA: Stanford University Press, 2017.

Enright, Anne. *Making Babies: Stumbling into Motherhood.* London: W. W. Norton, 2004.

Faircloth, Charlotte. *Militant Lactivism? Attachment Parenting and Intensive Motherhood in the UK and France.* New York: Berghahn, 2013.

———. "'Natural' Breastfeeding in Comparative Perspective: Feminism, Morality, and Adaptive Accountability." *Ethnos* 82, no. 1 (2017): 19–43.

Farber, David, and Beth Bailey. "Afterword: The Counterculture's Looking Glass." In *Groovy Science: Knowledge, Innovation, and American Counterculture,* edited by David Kaiser and W. Patrick McCray. Chicago: University of Chicago Press, 2016.

Federici, Silvia. *Caliban and the Witch: Women, the Body and Primitive Accumulation.* Brooklyn, NY: Autonomedia, 2014.

Fisher, Mark. *Capitalist Realism: Is There No Alternative?* London: John Hunt Publishing, 2009.

Fixmer-Oraiz, Natalie. "Contemplating Homeland Maternity." *Women's Studies in Communication* 38, no. 2 (2015): 129–34.

Ford, Andrea. "Advocating for Evidence in Birth: Proving Cause, Effecting Outcomes, and Making the Case for 'Curers.'" *Medicine Anthropology Theory* 6, no. 2 (2019): 25–48.

———. "Attuned Consent: Birth Doulas, Care, and the Politics of Consent." *Frontiers: A Journal of Women Studies* 42, no. 2 (2021): 111–32.

———. "Birthing from Within: Nature, Technology, and Self-Making in Silicon Valley Childbearing." *Cultural Anthropology* 35, no. 4 (2020): 602–30.

———. "Purity Is Not the Point: Chemical Toxicity, Childbearing, and Consumer Politics as Care." *Catalyst: Feminism, Theory, Technoscience* 6, no. 1 (2020): 1–25.

———. "Triple Toxicity." *Theorizing the Contemporary, Fieldsights,* April 25, 2019.

Ford, Andrea, Roslyn Malcolm, Sonja Erikainen, Lisa Raeder, and Celia Roberts, eds. *Hormonal Theory: A Rebellious Glossary.* London: Bloomsbury, 2024.

Ford, Andrea, and Julia Swallow. "The Immune System, Immunity and Immune Logics: Troubling Fixed Boundaries and (Re) Conceptualizing Relations." *Medicine Anthropology Theory* 11, no. 1 (2024): 1–12.

Foucault, Michel. *History of Sexuality, Vol. 1.* New York: Vintage, 1990.

———. "Of Other Spaces, Heterotopias." *Architecture, Mouvement, Continuité* 5 (1985): 46–49.

———. "Technologies of the Self." In *Ethics: Subjectivity and Truth,* edited by Paul Rabinow. New York: The New Press, 1982.

Franklin, Sarah. *Biological Relatives: IVF, Stem Cells, and the Future of Kinship.* Durham, NC: Duke University Press, 2013.

———. *Embodied Progress: A Cultural Account of Assisted Reproduction.* London: Routledge, 1997.

Fraser, Gertrude. "Modern Bodies, Modern Minds: Midwifery and Reproductive Change in an African American Community." In *Conceiving the New World Order: The Global Politics of Reproduction,* edited by Faye D. Ginsburg and Rayna R. Reiter. Berkeley: University of California Press, 1995.

Furedi, Frank. *How Fear Works: Culture of Fear in the Twenty-First Century.* London: Bloomsbury, 2018.

Gammeltoft, Tine. *Haunting Images: A Cultural Account of Selective Reproduction in Vietnam.* Berkeley: University of California Press, 2014.

Gaskin, Ina May. *Ina May's Guide to Childbirth.* New York: Bantam Books, 2003.

———. *Spiritual Midwifery.* Summertown, TN: Book Publishing Company, 2002.

Geronimus, Arline. *Weathering: The Extraordinary Stress of Ordinary Life in an Unjust Society.* London: Virago, 2023.

Gerosa, Alessandro. *The Hipster Economy: Taste and Authenticity in Late Modern Capitalism.* London: UCL Press, 2024.

Gilmore, Ruth Wilson. *Golden Gulag: Prisons, Surplus, Crisis, and Opposition in Globalizing California.* Oakland: University of California Press, 2007.

Ginsburg, Faye. *Contested Lives: The Abortion Debate in an American Community.* Berkeley: University of California Press, 1998.

Gómez, A. M., S. Arteaga, J. Arcara, A. Cuentos, M. Armstead, R. Mehra, R. G. Logan, A. V. Jackson, and C. J. Marshall. "'My 9 to 5 Job Is Birth Work': A Case Study of Two Compensation Approaches for Community Doula Care." *International Journal of Environmental Research and Public Health* 18, no. 20 (2021): 10817.

Gómez, A. M., S. Arteaga, C. Marshall, J. Arcara, A. Cuentos, M. Armstead, and A. Jackson. *Sisterweb: San Francisco Community Doula Network: Process Evaluation Report.* Berkeley: SHARE (Sexual Health and Reproductive Equity Program), University of California, Berkeley, 2020.

Gonzalez, Maya, and Irene Lusztig. "The Birth of Motherhood: Interview with Irene Lusztig." *New Inquiry,* July 10, 2013.

Goodman, Amy. "Midwives at Dakota Access Resistance Camps: We Can Decolonize, Respect Women & Mother Earth." *Democracy Now,* October 18, 2016.

Gordon, Avery F. *The Hawthorn Archive: Letters from the Utopian Margins.* New York: Fordham University Press, 2017.

Grusauskas, Maria. "Labor of Love." *Santa Cruz Good Times,* September 24, 2014.

Gumbs, Alexis Pauline, China Martens, and Mai'a Williams, eds. *Revolutionary Mothering: Love on the Front Lines.* Binghamton, NY: PM Press, 2016.

Halberstam, J. *Trans: A Quick and Quirky Account of Gender Variability.* Oakland: University of California Press, 2017.

Haraway, Donna. *Primate Visions: Gender, Race, and Nature in the World of Modern Science.* New York: Routledge, 1989.

———. *Simians, Cyborgs, and Women: The Reinvention of Nature.* New York: Routledge, 1991.

———. "Situated Knowledges: The Science Question in Feminism and the Privilege of Partial Perspective." *Feminist Studies* 14, no. 3 (1988): 575–99.

———. *Staying with the Trouble.* Durham, NC: Duke University Press, 2016.

Harjo, Joy. "Three Generations of Native American Women's Birth Experience." In *Imagine What It's Like : A Literature and Medicine Anthology,* edited by Victoria Bonebakker and Ruth L. Nadelhaft, Honolulu: University of Hawai'i Press, 2008.

Hays, Sharon. "Why Can't a Mother Be More Like a Businessman?" In *Maternal Theory,* edited by Andrea O'Reilly. Toronto: Demeter Press, 2022.

Heidegger, Martin. "The Age of the World Picture." In *The Question Concerning Technology, and Other Essay,* 115–54. New York: Harper and Row, 1977.

———. "The Question Concerning Technology." In *The Question Concerning Technology and Other Essays.* New York: Garland Publishing, 1977.

Heti, Sheila. *Motherhood.* New York: Vintage, 2018.

Hochschild, Arlie. "The Time Bind." *WorkingUSA* 1, no. 2 (1997): 21–29.

Hoover, Elizabeth. *The River Is in Us: Fighting Toxics in a Mohawk Community.* Minneapolis: University of Minnesota Press, 2017.

Illich, Ivan. *Gender.* New York: Pantheon, 1982.

———. *Limits to Medicine: Medical Nemesis, the Expropriation of Health.* New York: Marion Boyars, 1976.

———. *Tools for Conviviality.* London: Marion Boyars, 1973.

Inhorn, Marcia C. *Motherhood on Ice: The Mating Gap and Why Women Freeze Their Eggs.* New York: NYU Press, 2023.

Irigaray, Luce. *This Sex Which Is Not One.* Ithaca, NY: Cornell University Press, 1985.

Jain, Lochlann. *Malignant: How Cancer Becomes Us.* Berkeley: University of California Press, 2013.

Jay, Martin. "Experience Without a Subject: Walter Benjamin and the Novel." In *The Actuality of Walter Benjamin,* edited by Lynda Nead and Laura Marcus. London: Lawrence and Wishart, 1998.

———. *Songs of Experience: Modern American and European Variations on a Universal Theme.* Berkeley: University of California Press, 2006.

Joas, Hans, and Klaus Wiegandt, eds. *The Cultural Values of Europe* Liverpool: Liverpool University Press, 2008.

Jobson, Ryan Cecil. "The Case for Letting Anthropology Burn: Sociocultural Anthropology in 2019." *American Anthropologist* 122, no. 2 (2020): 259–71.

Johnson, Greg. "The Situated Self and Utopian Thinking." *Hypatia* 17, no. 3 (2002): 20–44.

Jones, Bernie, ed. *Women Who Opt Out: The Debate Over Working Mothers and Work-Family Balance.* New York: NYU Press, 2012.

Jones, Honor. "The Only Two Choices I've Ever Made: Motherhood and Divorce." *Atlantic,* October 20, 2022.

Jordan, Brigitte. *Birth in Four Cultures: A Crosscultural Investigation of Childbirth in Yucatan, Holland, Sweden, and the United States.* Salem, WI: Waveland Press, 1993.

Kapsalis, Terri. *Public Privates: Performing Gynecology from Both Ends of the Speculum.* Durham, NC: Duke University Press, 1997.

Kirmayer, Laurence. "Mind and Body as Metaphors: Hidden Values in Biomedicine." In *Biomedicine Examined,* edited by Margaret Lock and D. R. Gordon, 57–93. Berlin: Kluwer Academic Publishers, 1988.

Kline, Wendy. *Building a Better Race: Gender, Sexuality, and Eugenics from the Turn of the Century to the Baby Boom.* Berkeley: University of California Press, 2001.

———. "The Little Manual That Started a Revolution: How Hippie Midwifery Became Mainstream." In *Groovy Science: Knowledge, Innovation, and American Counterculture,* edited by David Kaiser and W. Patrick McCray. Chicago: University of Chicago Press, 2016.

Knight, Kelly Ray. *addicted.pregnant.poor.* Durham, NC: Duke University Press, 2015.

Kristeva, Julia. *Powers of Horror: An Essay on Abjection.* Translated by Leon S. Roudiez. New York: Columbia University Press, 1982.

Kristof, Nicholas. "A Poverty Solution That Starts with a Hug." *New York Times,* January 7, 2012.

Krueger, Alyson. "It Takes a Village to Care for a Baby. And, for a Lucky Few, a Luxury Hotel." *New York Times,* June 1, 2022.

Kukla, Rebecca. *Mass Hysteria: Medicine, Culture, and Women's Bodies.* Lanham, MD: Rowman and Littlefield, 2005.

Kupfer, David, and Sandra Steingraber. "The Good Earth: Sandra Steingraber on How We've Made the Environment Dangerous to Our Health." *The Sun Magazine,* 2010.

Kwon, Jong Bum. "Mothers' Hopes and Domestic Magic: White Racial Habitus and Fantasies of White Suburban Childhood." *Journal for the Anthropology of North America* 25, no. 2 (2022): 74–93.

Lamoreaux, Janelle. *Infertile Environments: Epigenetic Toxicology and the Reproductive Health of Chinese Men.* Durham, NC: Duke University Press, 2022.

Lancy, David F. "'Babies Aren't Persons': A Survey of Delayed Personhood." In *Different Faces of Attachment,* edited by H. Otto and H. Keller, 66–110. Cambridge: Cambridge University Press, 2014.

Land, Stephanie. "Learning to Walk in a Homeless Shelter." *New York Times,* February 7, 2016.

Lang, Raven. *Birth Book.* Itasca, IL: Genesis Press, 1972.

Latour, Bruno. *We Have Never Been Modern*. Cambridge, MA: Harvard University Press, 2012.

Lawrence, Natalie. "What Is a Monster?" 2015. www.cam.ac.uk/research/discussion /what-is-a-monster.

Le Guin, Ursula K. "A Non-Euclidean View of California as a Cold Place to Be." In *Dancing at the Edge of the World: Thoughts on Words, Women, Places*, 80–100. New York: Grove Press, 1989.

LeVine, Robert. "Attachment Theory as Cultural Ideology." In *Different Faces of Attachment*, 50–65. Cambridge: Cambridge University Press, 2014.

Lewis, Sophie. *Full Surrogacy Now: Feminism Against Family*. London: Verso, 2021.

Lewis, Thomas, Fari Amini, and Richard Lannon. *A General Theory of Love*. New York: Random House, 2000.

Liboiron, Max, Manuel Tironi, and Nerea Calvillo. "Toxic Politics: Acting in a Permanently Polluted World." *Social Studies of Science* 48, no. 3 (2018): 331–49.

Liedloff, Jean. *The Continuum Concept: In Search of Happiness Lost*. Cambridge, MA: Perseus, 1977.

Lira, Natalie. *Laboratory of Deficiency: Sterilization and Confinement in California, 1900–1950s*. Oakland: University of California Press, 2021.

Lock, Margaret. "Recovering the Body." *Annual Review of Anthropology* 46, no. 1 (2017): 1–14.

Lock, Margaret, and Judith Farquhar, eds. *Beyond the Body Proper: Reading the Anthropology of Material Life* Durham, NC: Duke University Press, 2007.

Lorimer, Jamie. "Hookworms Make Us Human: The Microbiome, Eco-Immunology, and a Probiotic Turn in Western Health Care." *Medical Anthropology Quarterly* 33, no. 1 (2019): 60–79.

Löwy, Ilana. "Prenatal Diagnosis: The Irresistible Rise of the 'Visible Fetus.'" *Studies in History and Philosophy of Biological and Biomedical Sciences* 47 (2014): 290–99.

Lyerly, Anne Drapkin. "Shame, Gender, Birth." *Hypatia* 21, no. 1 (2006): 101–18.

MacCormack, Patricia, and Marilyn Strathern, eds. *Nature, Culture, and Gender*. Cambridge: Cambridge University Press, 1980.

MacDonald, Margaret. "Gender Expectations: Natural Bodies and Natural Births in the New Midwifery in Canada." *Medical Anthropology Quarterly* 20, no. 2 (2006): 235–56.

MacKendrick, Norah. *Better Safe Than Sorry: How Consumers Navigate Exposure to Everyday Toxics*. Oakland: University of California Press, 2018.

Madley, Benjamin. *An American Genocide: The United States and the California Indian Catastrophe, 1846–1873*. New Haven, CT: Yale University Press, 2016.

————. "California's First Mass Incarceration System." *Pacific Historical Review* 88, no. 1 (2019): 14–47.

Maharidge, Dale. *The Coming White Minority: California's Eruptions and America's Future*. New York: Random House, 1996.

Marcus, George. "Experimental Forms for the Expression of Norms in the Ethnography of the Contemporary." *HAU: Journal of Ethnographic Theory* 3, no. 2 (2013): 197–217.

Mardorossian, Carine. "Laboring Women, Coaching Men: Masculinity and Childbirth Education in the Contemporary United States." *Hypatia* 18, no. 3 (2003): 113–34.

Marshall, C., S. Arteaga, J. Arcara, A. Cuentos, M. Armstead, A. Jackson, and A. Manchikanti Gómez. "Barriers and Facilitators to the Implementation of a Community Doula Program for Black and Pacific Islander Pregnant People in San Francisco: Findings from a Partnered Process Evaluation." *Maternal and Child Health Journal* 26, no. 4 (2022): 872–81.

Marshall, C., A. Nguyen, S. Arteaga, M. Armstead, N. Berbick, S. Britt, A. Chen, M. Cohen, A. Darch, K. Durdin, S. Davies-Balch, E. Hubbard, M. Kudumu, P. Mittal, C. Palmer, S. Peprah-Wilson, A. Selassie, T. Tang, K. Thomas, C. Yang, M. McLemore, and A. M. Gómez. *Partnering with Community Doulas to Improve Maternal and Infant Health Equity in California.* Berkeley: School of Public Health, University of California, Berkeley, 2022.

Marshall, C., A. Nguyen, C. Yang, and A. M. Gómez. "Understanding Barriers and Facilitators to Payer Investment in Doula Care in California." Berkeley Public Health Report, 2023.

Martin, Aryn, and Kelly Holloway. "'Something There Is That Doesn't Love a Wall': Histories of the Placental Barrier." *Studies in History and Philosophy of Biological and Biomedical Sciences* 47 (2014): 300–310.

Martin, Emily. *The Woman in the Body: A Cultural Analysis of Reproduction.* Boston: Beacon Press, 2001.

Martin, Nina, ProPublica, Emma Cillekens, and Alessandra Freitas. "Lost Mothers." ProPublica, July 17, 2017.

Masco, Joseph. *The Nuclear Borderlands: The Manhattan Project in Post–Cold War New Mexico.* Princeton, NJ: Princeton University Press, 2006.

———. "Side Effect." *Somatosphere,* December 2, 2013.

———. *The Theater of Operations: National Security Affect from the Cold War to the War on Terror.* Durham, NC: Duke University Press, 2014.

Mason, Katherine A. "Blenders, Hammers, and Knives: Postpartum Intrusive Thoughts and Unthinkable Motherhood." *Anthropology and Humanism* 47, no. 1 (2022): 117–32.

Mazzarella, William. "Affect: What Is It Good For?" In *Enchantments of Modernity: Empire, Nation, Globalization,* edited by Saurabh Dube, 291–309. New York: Routledge, 2009.

McClintock, Anne. *Imperial Leather: Race, Gender, and Sexuality in the Colonial Contest.* New York: Routledge, 1995.

McKenna, James, and Lee Gettler. "There Is No Such Thing as Infant Sleep, There Is No Such Thing as Breastfeeding, There Is Only Breastsleeping." *Acta Paediatrica* 105, no. 1 (2016): 17–21.

Melich, Tanya. *The Republican War against Women: An Insider's Report from Behind the Lines.* New York: Random House, 2000.

Menke, Christoph. "Inner Nature and Social Normativity: The Idea of Self-Realization." In *The Cultural Values of Europe,* edited by Hans Joas and Klaus Wiegandt. Liverpool: Liverpool University Press, 2008.

Messeri, Lisa. *In the Land of the Unreal: Virtual and Other Realities in Los Angeles.* Durham, NC: Duke University Press, 2024.

Miller, Kristin. "Mapping Our Disconnect." *Boom: A Journal of California* 4, no. 2 (2014): 62–67.

Mills, C. Wright. *The Sociological Imagination.* Oxford: Oxford University Press, 2000.

Mol, Annemarie. *The Logic of Care: Health and the Problem of Patient Choice.* New York: Routledge, 2008.

Mol, Annemarie, Ingunn Moser, and Jeannette Pols, eds. *Care in Practice: On Tinkering in Clinics, Homes and Farms.* Bielefeld: transcript Verlag, 2010.

Moore, Erin V. "Postures of Empowerment: Cultivating Aspirant Feminism in a Ugandan NGO." *Ethos* 44, no. 3 (2016): 375–96.

Morris, Theresa. *Cut It Out: The C-Section Epidemic in America.* New York: NYU Press, 2016.

Morris, Theresa, Joan H. Robinson, Keridwyn Spiller, and Amanda Gomez. "'Screaming, "No! No!" It Was Literally Like Being Raped': Connecting Sexual Assault Trauma and Coerced Obstetric Procedures." *Social Problems* 70, no. 1 (2021): 55–70.

Morton, Christine. *Birth Ambassadors: Doulas and the Re-Emergence of Woman-Supported Birth in America.* Amarillo, TX: Praeclarus Press, 2014.

———. "Where Are the Ethnographies of US Hospital Birth?" *Anthropology News* 50, no. 3 (2009): 10–11.

Murphy, Michelle. "Alterlife and Decolonial Chemical Relations." *Cultural Anthropology* 32, no. 4 (2017): 494–503.

———. "Chemical Regimes of Living." *Environmental History* 13, no. 4 (2008): 695–703.

———. *The Economization of Life.* Durham, NC: Duke University Press, 2017.

———. *Seizing the Means of Reproduction: Entanglements of Feminism, Health, and Technoscience.* Durham, NC: Duke University Press, 2012.

NACPM. "Recognizing Mana." 2024. www.nacpm.org/news/recognizing-mana.

Napier, David. "Nonself Help: How Immunology Might Reframe the Enlightenment." *Cultural Anthropology* 27, no. 1 (2012): 122–37.

Nash, Jennifer. *Birthing Black Mothers.* Durham, NC: Duke University Press, 2021.

———. "Black Maternal Mortality Rates Are a National Embarrassment. Doulas Can Help." *San Francisco Chronicle,* October 18, 2021.

———. "Re-Thinking Intersectionality." *Feminist Review* 89, no. 1 (2008): 1–15.

Neale, Timothy. "Poly- and Perfluorinated Alkyl Substances (PFAS)." *Theorizing the Contemporary: Fieldsights,* June 27, 2019.

Nelson, Maggie. *The Argonauts*. Minneapolis, MN: Greywolf Press, 2015.

Nguyen, A., S. Arteaga, M. I. Mystic, A. Cuentos, M. Armstead, J. Arcara, A. V. Jackson, C. Marshall, and A. M. Gomez. "Supporting Birthing People and Supporting Doulas: The Impact of the Covid-19 Pandemic on a Community-Based Doula Organization in San Francisco." *Health Equity* 7, no. 1 (2023): 356–63.

Nissim, Rina. *Une sorcière des temps modernes: Le self-help et le mouvement femmes et santé*. Vineuil, France: MAMAMELIS, 2014.

Nixon, Rob. *Slow Violence and the Environmentalism of the Poor*. Cambridge, MA: Harvard University Press, 2011.

Nori, Mehera. "Asian/american/alien: Birth Tourism, the Racialization of Asians, and the Identity of the American Citizen." *Hastings Women's Law Journal* 27, no. 1 (2016): 87–108.

Odent, Michel. *Childbirth and the Evolution of Homo Sapiens*. London: Pinter and Martin, 2014.

Olmsted, Kathryn. *Right Out of California: The 1930s and the Big Business Roots of Modern Conservatism*. New York: The New Press, 2010.

Olson, Alexander. "Before the Creative Class: Recruiting Artists to Berkeley in the 1920s." Creative Cities Symposium, Stanford University, 2018.

———. "Blood and Soil Bohemianism: Mary Austin's Racial Imaginary." Talk at the Modern Language Association Conference, 2019.

Olza, Ibone, Kerstin Uvnas-Moberg, Anette Ekström-Bergström, Patricia Leahy-Warren, Sigfridur Inga Karlsdottir, Marianne Nieuwenhuijze, Stella Villarmea, Eleni Hadjigeorgiou, Maria Kazmierczak, and Andria Spyridou. "Birth as a Neuro-Psycho-Social Event: An Integrative Model of Maternal Experiences and Their Relation to Neurohormonal Events during Childbirth." *Plos one* 15, no. 7 (2020): e0230992.

Oparah, Julia Chinyere, Helen Arega, Dantia Hudson, Linda Jones, and Talita Oseguera. *Battling Over Birth: Black Women and the Maternal Health Care Crisis in California*. Amarillo, TX: Praeclarus Press, 2016.

Orfalea, Gregory. "The Exceptional State: What Made California Stand Out and Then Stand Up to a Sitting President." *Pacific Standard,* September 13, 2018.

Ortner, Sherry. "Dark Anthropology and Its Others Theory Since the Eighties." *HAU: Journal of Ethnographic Theory* 6, no. 1 (2016): 47–73.

———. "Is Female to Male as Nature Is to Culture?" In *Woman, Culture, and Society,* edited by Michelle Zimbalist Rosaldo, Louise Lamphere, and Joan Bamberger. Stanford, CA: Stanford University Press, 1974.

Osnos, Evan. "Doomsday Prep for the Super-Rich." *New Yorker,* January 22, 2017.

Otto, Hiltrud, and Heidi Keller, eds. *Different Faces of Attachment: Cultural Variations on a Universal Human Need* Cambridge: Cambridge University Press, 2014.

Oudshoorn, Nelly. *Beyond the Natural Body: An Archaeology of Sex Hormones*. New York: Routledge, 1994.

Owens, Deirdre Cooper. *Medical Bondage: Race, Gender, and the Origins of American Gynecology*. Athens: University of Georgia Press, 2017.

Owens, Kellie. "Too Much of a Good Thing? American Childbirth, Intentional Ignorance, and the Boundaries of Responsible Knowledge." *Science, Technology, & Human Values* 42, no. 5 (2017): 848–71.

Pastor, Manuel. *State of Resistance: What California's Dizzying Descent and Remarkable Resurgence Mean for America's Future.* New York: The New Press, 2018.

Pateman, Carole. *The Sexual Contract.* Stanford, CA: Stanford University Press, 1988.

Patterson, Amy Suzanne. "'We Ought Not to Be Inactive Spectators': Physicians and Childbirth in America, 1780–1840." PhD diss., University of California, Davis, 1999.

Paxson, Heather. *Eating Beside Ourselves: Thresholds of Foods and Bodies.* Durham, NC: Duke University Press, 2023.

———. *Making Modern Mothers: Ethics and Family Planning in Urban Greece.* Berkeley: University of California Press, 2004.

———. "Post-Pasteurian Cultures: The Microbiopolitics of Raw-Milk Cheese in the United States." *Cultural Anthropology* 23, no. 1 (2008): 15–47.

Pellow, David, and Lisa Sun-Hee Park. *The Silicon Valley of Dreams: Environmental Injustice, Immigrant Workers, and the High-Tech Global Economy.* New York: NYU Press, 2002.

Pérez, Miriam Zoila. *The Radical Doula Guide.* Self-published, 2012.

———. "Remarks from Squatfest: Birth Activism as Part of the Movement for Reproductive Justice." 2013. https://radicaldoula.com/2013/09/03/remarks-from-squatfest-birth-activism-as-part-of-the-movement-for-reproductive-justice/.

Petersen, Anne Helen. "Pretty White Moms in Their Pretty White Houses: An Interview with Sara Petersen." 2023. https://annehelen.substack.com/p/pretty-white-moms-in-their-pretty.

Petersen, Emily, et al. "Vital Signs: Pregnancy-Related Deaths, United States, 2011–2015, and Strategies for Prevention, 13 States, 2013–2017." *Morbidity and Mortality Weekly Report, Centers for Disease Control and Prevention* 68, no. 18 (2019): 423–29.

Petersen, Sara. *Momfluenced: Inside the Maddening, Picture-Perfect World of Mommy Influencer Culture.* Boston: Beacon, 2023.

Pincott, Jena. "When Stress Comes with Your Mother's Milk." *Nautilus,* November 23, 2015.

Pollock, Della. *Telling Bodies, Performing Birth: Everyday Narratives of Childbirth.* New York: Columbia University Press, 1999.

Ramirez, Renya. *Native Hubs: Culture, Community, and Belonging in Silicon Valley and Beyond.* Durham, NC: Duke University Press, 2007.

Rapp, Rayna. *Testing Women, Testing the Fetus: The Social Impact of Amniocentesis in America.* New York: Routledge, 2004.

Reagan, Ronald. "The Creative Society Speech." 1966. https://freerepublic.com/focus/news/742041/posts.

Rees, Tobias. *After Ethnos.* Durham, NC: Duke University Press, 2018.

Relman, Arnold. "The Health Care Industry: Where Is It Taking Us." *New England Journal of Medicine* 325, no. 12 (1991): 854–59.

Reyes, Barbara. *Private Women, Public Lives: Gender and the Missions of the Californias.* Austin: University of Texas Press, 2009.

Reyes-Foster, Beatriz. "'No Justice in Birth': Maternal Vanishing, VBAC, and Reconstitutive Practice in Central Florida." *American Anthropologist* 125, no. 1 (2023): 49–62.

Rich, Adrienne. *Of Woman Born: Motherhood as Experience and Institution.* New York: W. W. Norton, 1996.

Roberts, Celia. *Messengers of Sex: Hormones, Biomedicine, and Feminism.* Cambridge: Cambridge University Press, 2007.

Roberts, Celia, Mary Lou Rasmussen, Louisa Allen, and Rebecca Williamson. *Reproduction, Kin and Climate Crisis: Making Bushfire Babies.* Bristol: Bristol University Press, 2023.

Roberts, Dorothy. *Killing the Black Body: Race, Reproduction, and the Meaning of Liberty.* New York: Pantheon Books, 1997.

———. "Race, Gender, and Genetic Technologies: A New Reproductive Dystopia?" *Signs* 34, no. 4 (2009): 783–803.

Robinson, Marilynne. *What Are We Doing Here?* London: Virago, 2018.

Rose, Nikolas. *The Politics of Life Itself: Biomedicine, Power, and Subjectivity in the Twenty-First Century.* Princeton, NJ: Princeton University Press, 2007.

Ross, Loretta, and Rickie Solinger. *Reproductive Justice: An Introduction.* Oakland: University of California Press, 2017.

Rothman, Barbara Katz. *In Labor: Women and Power in the Birthplace.* New York: W. W. Norton, 1991.

Rothman, Barbara Katz, and Wendy Simonds. "The Birthplace." In *Motherhood and Space: Configurations of the Maternal through Politics, Home, and the Body,* edited by Sarah Boykin Hardy and Caroline Alice Wiedmer. New York: Palgrave Macmillan, 2005.

Rountree, Kathryn. "The New Witch of the West: Feminists Reclaim the Crone." *Journal of Popular Culture* 30, no. 4 (1997): 211–29.

Ruddick, Sara. "Maternal Thinking." In *Maternal Theory,* edited by Andrea O'Reilly. Toronto: Demeter, 2021.

Sahlins, Marshall. *The Western Illusion of Human Nature: With Reflections on the Long History of Hierarchy, Equality and the Sublimation of Anarchy in the West, and Comparative Notes on Other Conceptions of the Human Condition.* Chicago: Prickly Paradigm Press, 2008.

Sakala, Carol, E. Declercq, J. Turon, and M. Corry. "Listening to Mothers in California: Full Survey Report." California Health Care Foundation, 2018.

Sakala, C., A. M. Romano, and S. J. Buckley. "Hormonal Physiology of Childbearing, an Essential Framework for Maternal-Newborn Nursing." *Journal of Obstetrics, Gynecology & Neonatal Nursing* 45, no. 2 (2016): 264–75.

Sanabria, Emilia. *Plastic Bodies: Sex Hormones and Menstrual Suppression in Brazil.* Durham, NC: Duke University Press, 2016.

Sánchez, Rosaura. *Telling Identities: The Californio Testimonios.* Minneapolis: University of Minnesota Press, 1995.

Sandelowski, Margarete. *Devices and Desires: Gender, Technology, and American Nursing.* Chapel Hill: University of North Carolina Press, 2000.

Sasser, Jade. *Climate Anxiety and the Kid Question: Deciding Whether to Have Children in an Uncertain Future.* Oakland: University of California Press, 2024.

———. *On Infertile Ground: Population Control and Women's Rights in the Era of Climate Change.* New York: NYU Press, 2018.

Scaramelli, Caterina. "Making Sense of Water Quality: Multispecies Encounters on the Mystic River." *Worldviews* 17 (2013): 150–60.

Schiebinger, Londa. "Why Mammals Are Called Mammals." In *Nature's Body: Gender in the Making of Modern Science,* 40–74. New Brunswick, NJ: Rutgers University Press, 1993.

Schuster, David G. *Neurasthenic Nation: America's Search for Health, Happiness, and Comfort, 1869–1920.* New Brunswick, NJ: Rutgers University Press, 2020.

Scott, Karen A., and Dána-Ain Davis. "Obstetric Racism: Naming and Identifying a Way Out of Black Women's Adverse Medical Experiences." *American Anthropologist* 123, no. 3 (2021): 681–84.

Sempruch, Justyna. "Feminist Constructions of the 'Witch' as a Fantasmatic Other." *Body & Society* 10, no. 4 (2004): 113–33.

Seremetakis, Nadia. *The Senses Still: Perception and Memory as Material Culture in Modernity.* Chicago: University of Chicago Press, 1994.

Shapiro, Samantha. "Mommy Wars: The Prequel." *New York Times Magazine,* May 23, 2012.

Shotwell, Alexis. *Against Purity: Living Ethically in Compromised Times.* Minneapolis: University of Minnesota Press, 2016.

Simeon, Wade. *Foucault in California.* Berkeley, CA: Heyday, 2019.

Simms, Eva-Maria. "Eating One's Mother." *Environmental Ethics* 31, no. 3 (2009): 263–77.

Simpson, Audra. "Consent's Revenge." *Cultural Anthropology* 31, no. 3 (2016): 326–33.

Singh, Maanvi. "California Wildfires: Thousands Evacuate as 'Siege' of Flames Overwhelms State." *Guardian,* August 20, 2020.

Sloterdijk, Peter. *Stress and Freedom.* Translated by Wieland Hoban. Cambridge: Polity, 2016.

Small, Meredith. *Our Babies, Ourselves: How Biology and Culture Shape the Way We Parent.* New York: Anchor, 1999.

Smith, Christian. *The Sacred Project of American Sociology.* Oxford: Oxford University Press, 2014.

Sojoyner, Damien M. "Another Life Is Possible: Black Fugitivity and Enclosed Places." *Cultural Anthropology* 32, no. 4 (2017): 514–36.

Solnit, Rebecca. *A Paradise Built in Hell.* New York: Penguin Random House, 2010.

———. *Savage Dreams: A Journey into the Hidden Wars of the American West.* Berkeley: University of California Press, 2014.

Spretnak, Charlene. *Resurgence of the Real: Body, Nature, and Place in a Hypermodern World*. New York: Routledge, 1999.

Stanley, Darcy, Nicole Sata, Julia Chinyere Oparah, and Monica R. McLemore. "Evaluation of the East Bay Community Birth Support Project, a Community-Based Program to Decrease Recidivism in Previously Incarcerated Women." *Journal of Obstetrics, Gynecology &Neonatal Nursing* 44, no. 6 (2015): 743–50.

Star, Susan Leigh. "This Is Not a Boundary Object: Reflections on the Origin of a Concept." *Science, Technology & Human Values* 35, no. 5 (2010): 601–17.

Starhawk. *Dreaming the Dark: Sex, Magic, and Politics*. Boston: Beacon, 1997.

Starr, Kevin. *Americans and the California Dream, 1850–1915*. Oxford: Oxford University Press, 1973.

———. *California: A History*. New York: Modern Library, 2005.

———. *Coast of Dreams: California on the Edge, 1990-2003*. Oxford: Oxford University Press, 2004.

———. *The Dream Endures: California Enters the 1940s*. Oxford: Oxford University Press, 1997.

———. *Embattled Dreams: California in War and Peace, 1940-1950*. Oxford: Oxford University Press, 2002.

———. *Endangered Dreams: The Great Depression in California*. Oxford: Oxford University Press, 1996.

———. *Inventing the Dream: California Through the Progressive Era*. Oxford: Oxford University Press, 1985.

———. *Material Dreams: Southern California Through the 1920s*. Oxford: Oxford University Press, 1990.

Steingraber, Sandra. *Having Faith: An Ecologist's Journey to Motherhood*. Cambridge, MA: Perseus, 2001.

Stengers, Isabelle. "The Doctor and the Charlatan." *Cultural Studies Review* 9, no. 2 (2003): 11–36.

Strathern, Marilyn. "The Nice Thing about Culture Is That Everyone Has it." In *Shifting Contexts,* edited by Marilyn Strathern. New York: Routledge, 1995.

Sufrin, Carolyn. *Jailcare: Finding the Safety Net for Women Behind Bars*. Oakland: University of California Press, 2017.

Summers, A. K. *Pregnant Butch: Nine Long Months Spent in Drag*. Berkeley: Soft Skull Press, 2014.

Swanson, K. W. "Human Milk as Technology and Technologies of Human Milk: Medical Imaginings in the Early Twentieth-Century United States." *Women's Studies Quarterly* 37, no. 1/2 (2009): 21–37.

Takeshita, Chikako. "From Mother/fetus to Holobiont(s): A Material Feminist Ontology of the Pregnant Body." *Catalyst: Feminism, Theory, Technoscience* 3, no. 1 (2021): 1–28.

TallBear, Kim. "Making Love and Relations Beyond Settler Sex and Family." In *Making Kin Not Population: Reconceiving Generations,* edited by Adele Clarke and Donna Haraway, 145–66. Chicago: Prickly Paradigm, 2018.

Taylor, Bron Raymond. *Dark Green Religion: Nature Spirituality and the Planetary Future.* Berkeley: University of California Press, 2010.

Taylor, Janelle. *The Public Life of the Fetal Sonogram: Technology, Consumption, and the Politics of Reproduction.* New Brunswick, NJ: Rutgers University Press, 2008.

Teran, Jackie. "The Violent Legacies of the California Missions: Mapping the Origins of Native Women's Mass Incarceration." *American Indian Culture and Research Journal* 40, no. 1 (2016): 19–32.

Toupin, Louise. *Wages for Housework: A History of an International Feminist Movement, 1972–77.* London: Pluto Press, 2018.

Tsing, Anna. "Monster Stories: Women Charged with Perinatal Endangerment." In *Uncertain Terms: Negotiating Gender in American Culture,* edited by Faye Ginsburg and Anna Tsing. Boston: Beacon Press, 1990.

Tucker, Abigail. *Mom Genes: Inside the New Science of Our Ancient Maternal Instinct.* Oldcastle, Ireland: The Gallery Press, 2021.

Turner, Fred. *From Counterculture to Cyberculture: Stewart Brand, the Whole Earth Network, and the Rise of Digital Utopianism.* Chicago: University of Chicago Press, 2008.

Uvnäs-Moberg, Kerstin. *Oxytocin: The Biological Guide to Motherhood.* Amarillo, TX: Praeclarus Press, 2016.

Valdez, Natali. "The Redistribution of Reproductive Responsibility: On the Epigenetics of "Environment" in Prenatal Interventions." *Medical Anthropology Quarterly* 32, no. 3 (2018): 425–42.

Villalobos, Ana. *Motherload: Making It All Better in Insecure Times.* Berkeley: University of California Press, 2014.

Villarosa, Linda. "Why America's Black Mothers and Babies Are in a Life-or-Death Crisis." *New York Times Magazine,* April 11, 2018.

Vincent, Peggy. *Baby Catcher: Chronicles of a Modern Midwife.* New York: Scribner, 2001.

Waggoner, Miranda. *Zero Trimester: Pre-Pregnancy Care and the Politics of Reproductive Risk.* Oakland: University of California Press, 2017.

Wagner, Marsden. *Born in the USA: How a Broken Maternity System Must Be Fixed to Put Women and Children First.* Berkeley: University of California Press, 2008.

Waldman, Ayelet. "Truly, Madly, Guiltily." *New York Times,* March 27, 2005.

Warren, Louis. "The California Dream: History of a Myth." *Pacific Historical Review* 92, no. 2 (2023): 260–98.

Washington, Harriet. *Medical Apartheid: The Dark History of Medical Experimentation on Black Americans From Colonial Times to the Present.* New York: Harlem Moon, 2007.

Weiss, Erica. "Refusal as Act, Refusal as Abstention." *Cultural Anthropology* 31, no. 3 (2016): 351–58.

Wendland, Claire. "The Vanishing Mother: Cesarean Section and Evidence-Based Obstetrics." *Medical Anthropology Quarterly* 21, no. 2 (2007): 218–33.

Weston, Kath. *Families We Choose: Lesbians, Gays, Kinship.* New York: Columbia University Press, 1997.

Williamson, Rachel. *21st-Century Narratives of Maternal Ambivalence.* Cham, Switzerland: Springer International Publishing, 2023.

Wilson, Jane. "Immaculate Deception." *New York Times,* June 22, 1975.

Womersley, Kate. "Why Giving Birth Is Safer in Britain Than in the US." ProPublica, Aug. 31, 2017.

Wright, Susan. "The Politicization of 'Culture.'" *Anthropology Today* 14, no. 1 (1998): 7–15.

Yates-Doerr, Emily. "The Placenta: An Ethnographic Account of Feeding Relations." In *Eating Beside Ourselves,* edited by Heather Paxson. Durham, NC: Duke University Press, 2023.

Yoder, Rachel. *Nightbitch.* New York: Doubleday, 2021.

Yong, Ed. *I Contain Multitudes: The Microbes Within Us and a Grander View of Life.* London: Vintage, 2017.

Young, Allan. "The Discourse on Stress and the Reproduction of Conventional Knowledge." *Social Science and Medicine* 14B (1980): 133–46.

Young, Christina. "Professional Ambivalence among Care Workers: The Case of Doula Practice." *Health* 25, no. 3 (2021): 306–21.

Young, Iris Marion. *On Female Body Experience: "Throwing Like a Girl" and Other Essays.* Oxford: Oxford University Press, 2005.

Zelizer, Viviana. *Pricing the Priceless Child: The Changing Social Value of Children.* New York: Basic Books, 1994.

Zuk, Marlene. *Paleofantasy : What Evolution Really Tells Us about Sex, Diet, and How We Live.* New York: W. W. Norton, 2013.

INDEX

conception, why not discussed, 11n20

consent, 192, 203; circumcision as nonconsensual, 197; versus refusal, 214

contextual. *See* regular versus contextual

Cook, Katsi, 161

Cooper, Davina, 24

COVID-19, 34, 181, 212

Craven, Christa, 91

Creative Society, 199

crisis: Black maternal bodies as site of, 210;
Battling Over Birth, 32; U.S. maternal
health, 31, 34, 205, 209–10. *See also*
maternal mortality

Cromer, Risa, 188; saviorism, 188

Csordas, Thomas, 60

cultural congruence, versus competence
versus humility, 213

culture: American, 5; car, 17; defined, 4–5,
221; versus nature, 129–30

Cummings, Roxanne, 15–16, 33, 69, 169;
Mindfulness-Based Childbirth Education, 47, 69, 105, 128, 169

cybernetics, 27, 181

cyborg, 130, 140, 142

Davis, Dána-Ain, 32, 89, 214; on obstetric
racism, 32, 89

Davis-Floyd, Robbie, 32, 44, 60

death, 219; doulas, 33; infant, 49; maternal,
10, 31–32, 34, 151, 209; and medical
progress, 52, 93; and technology, 151

de Certeau, Michel, 57–58, 62; *The Practice
of Everyday Life,* 57

Descartes, René, 55; Cartesian self, 182

Developmental Origins of Health and
Disease (DOHaD), 175

Dick-Read, Grantly, 85

Didion, Joan, 22

disenchantment, 62, 115

Douglas, Susan, 107

doula: community-based, 209, 211–13; cost,
33; defined, 1–2, 33; full-spectrum, 16;
history and controversy of term, 12, 33,
208–9; as mothering the mother, 107; as
paid family member, 116–18; payment,
117–18, 122, 213–4; as political activism,
209; professionalization, 121; volunteer-
ism, 9

Doulas of North America (DONA), 33, 117,
204

Doulas Telar, 211

Dowling, Emma, 28

dualism, 55, 129–31, 139

Dumm, Thomas, 116

Dumont, Louis, 6, 114, 115, 177

ecofeminism, 138, 145, 189

ectogenesis, 111, 151

Ehrenreich, Barbara, 110, 174; *Bright-Sided,*
174; and Deirdre English, 53; *For Her
Own Good,* 111; *Witches, Midwives, and
Nurses,* 53

Ehrlich, Karen, 201

emergency, 39–40, 49–51, 57, 72, 74

empowerment. *See* power

enchantment. *See* disenchantment

endocrine disrupting chemicals (EDCs), 158,
159, 178, 217. *See also* chemicals; hormones

Enlightenment, the, 62–63, 64, 109, 111,
125, 151, 180, 203, 218

Enright, Anne, 43, 140

environment, versus ecology, 154–55, 177

environmental justice, 161; overlap with
reproductive justice, 161, 179

Environmental Protection Agency, 162

epistemology, 40; experience and, 59; and
ontology, 40. *See also* knowledge

Epstein, Abby, 34; *The Business of Being
Born,* 34

equality: versus equity, 109; impossibility of,
100–101, 114, 123; incompatibility with
difference, 112, 115; in social contract, 109

eugenics, 22–23, 100, 180, 197–98, 201, 206,
218; and creativity, 198–9; and prisons,
201, 205

evidence, 57–58, 62–66, 74, 91, 147, 166,
217; as boundary object, 63; of cause
versus outcomes, 64; merged with
politics, 195–96

evidence-based medicine, 63; doulas as, 212

evolution, 22, 145, 146–52

experience, 40, 44, 50, 52–66, 69

Faircloth, Charlotte, 142

family: Black, 100; chosen, 120; doulas
as, 117–18; as exploitative, 119;

family *(continued)*
    heteronormative nuclear, 118–23, 200;
        Indigenous critique of, 100, 118; love
        versus money undergirding the, 123; as
        private, 199–200; queer, 22, 118; as
        reproductive justice, 209
fathers and partners: and doulas, 121;
    involved in birth, 107–8, 120–21
fear: and/versus fantasy, 216; healing, 192;
    and immunity, 179–80, 182, 184; and
    knowledge, 132; navigating, 72, 77–84,
    89–90; and physiology, 43, 48–49;
    refusal of, 27, 204, 208
Federici, Silvia, 53, 62, 151; *Caliban and the
    Witch,* 53
feminism: contests over, 201–3; ecofemi-
    nism, 138–39, 145; having it all, 86, 120,
    132, 142, 206; libertarian, 200; neolib-
    eral, 133; and pain relief, 54, 138; post-
    feminism, 206; and science, 56, 111,
    147–48; waves of, 114
FemTech, 27, 34; breast pump startup, 141;
    limits of, 142
Fisher, Mark, 35
Fixmer-Oraiz, Natalie, 206
Food and Drug Administration (FDA), 99,
    162
Foucault, Michel, 24, 143; heterotopia, 24;
    technologies of the self, 143
Frankfurt School, 62
Franklin, Sarah, 21
Fraser, Gertrude, 56
free birth, 69, 214
freedom, 17, 126, 142
frontier: California as, 7, 13, 19, 22, 217;
    mythology, 13, 18, 21, 187, 197; and
    nature, 125; religious, 187
full-spectrum doulas. *See under* abortion;
    doula

Gaskin, Ina May, 26, 49; The Farm Mid-
    wifery Center, 204; Gaskin maneuver,
    39; *Ina May's Guide to Childbirth,* 43;
    sphincter law, 43, 47; *Spiritual Mid-
    wifery,* 26, 78, 93
genes: as biological truth, 148; epigenetic
    influences, 165, 168, 179; genetic testing,
    73, 74, 100; microbial, 154, 165

genocide, 7, 19, 20, 185, 192, 197, 223
germ theory of disease, 166–67
Geronimus, Arline, 176
Gettler, Lee, 147
Gilman, Charlotte Perkins, 110–11; "The
    Yellow Wallpaper," 110
Gilmore, Ruth Wilson, 201; *Golden Gulag,*
    201
Griffin, Susan, 138
gynecology, 35–36, 89

Halberstam, Jack, 116; *Trans,* 116
Haraway, Donna, 11, 130, 142, 148, 190, 207;
    make kin, not babies, 207; "Simians,
    Cyborgs, and Women," 11, 130, 148;
    staying with the trouble, 190
Harjo, Joy, 54; "Three Generations of
    Native American Women's Birth Expe-
    rience," 54
Hays, Sharon, 106; "Why Can't a Mother
    Be More Like a Businessman?," 106
hegemony, 10, 29, 53, 71, 107, 220
Heidegger, Martin, 62, 167; technological
    enframing, 167
heterotopia, 24, 195, 215
Heti, Sheila, 96
Hippocrates, 109
history: of birth care, 52–54, 217; of birth-
    ing bodies, 56; forgetting/whitewash-
    ing, 197–8; and nostalgia, 150, 199;
    whose is recognized, 199, 202
home: anthropology of, 2, 20; and
    nostalgia, 150; schooling/steading/
    birth, 20
homeland maternity, 206
hormones: in birth, 47–49, 131–32; and
    cascade of interventions, 47–48; cas-
    cades of, 104, 149; oxytocin, 47, 104,
    149; Pitocin, 38, 48, 165; of stress/
    trauma, adrenaline/cortisol, 149, 170,
    173, 175
human: versus animal/spiritual, 135; versus
    environment, 155; species, 149–50. *See
    also* personhood
Human Betterment Foundation, 23

iatrogenic illness, 74
Illich, Ivan, 74, 115, 167

immune system, 178, 181; labor and, 165; mother and baby's shared, 104, 164

immunity, 179–80; defined, 154–55; temporal, 187

inclusion, 12, 55, 112, 190, 203, 217–18; diversity and, 204; inclusivity, 54

Indie Birth (podcast), 150

Indigenous communities: critique of nuclear family, 100, 118–19; environmental reproductive justice, 161; midwifery and activism, 34; Mohawk, 161; Navajo, 144; Nisenan and Miwok, 19

individual, the, 6, 114; and childbearing, 6; and contracts, 110; edges of, 183; and loneliness, 116, 143–45; versus relations, 177

individualism, 6, 55; finding truth and authenticity within, 126; as inadequate, 216; rejection of, 24

innovation: and California, 24, 28, 35, 144, 198, 217; as non-solution, 31, 36; as solution/progress, 18, 24, 187–88

intersectionality, 10, 34, 100

intuition, 57–62, 76, 92, 151, 217; defined, 59; versus instinct, 132, 145; intuiting care, 106; as tacit knowledge, 60; technological, 141

In Utero (film), 153, 170

in-vitro fertilization (IVF), 3, 11, 22, 29, 100, 118

Jain, Lochlann, 162

Japanese American midwifery license, 34

Jay, Martin, 58, 59

Jones, Honor, 120

Jones, Linda, 190, 193–94, 211

Just a Mom League, 196

Kaiser Permanente, 31

Kirmayer, Lawrence, 40

Knight, Kelly Ray, 35; *addicted.pregnant. poor.*, 35

knowledge: authoritative, 60, 64–65, 143; as co-constituted with being, 40, 51–52, 220; conventional /tacit, 174–75; cultural, 4; evidence and empiricism as, 62–66; and experience, 50, 54–55, 57–58; experiential, 143; gut, 74, 132;

hormonal, 47–48; intentional non-knowledge, 50; intuitive, 58–62; as mastery/progress, 52, 188; and objectivity, 64; and power, 57, 91–92; primal/animal, 135–37, 138; primordial, modern, and self, 127; privatization of, 53–54; regular and contextual, 44, 61; as risk management, 68–74; self-actualization through, 129, 143; self-knowledge, 83, 132–34, 139, 145; situated, 9n17; traditional versus innovative, 144; and witches, 53; women's, 148. *See also* epistemology; science

Kristeva, Julia, 112

Kukla, Rebecca, 109

Kwon, Jong Bum, 206

labor land, 131–32, 135–37

lactivism, militant, 142

Lake, Ricki, 34; *The Business of Being Born*, 34

Lang, Raven, 25; *Birth Book*, 25

Latour, Bruno, 6

leave, parental/maternal, 6, 29, 101, 106–8, 119, 142

Le Guin, Ursula, 24

Lewis, Sophie, 119

liability, 2, 33, 44, 69, 73, 196

Liedloff, Jean, 102, 151; *The Continuum Concept,* 102, 151

"Listening to Mothers in California" survey, 32, 33, 212

local and situated biologies, 161–62

Lock, Margaret, 161–62

logic of care, 106

Lucy, 36

Lusztig, Irene, 85; *The Motherhood Archives,* 85

MacKendrick, Norah, 160

magic, 62, 65, 139; neopaganism, 138–9

mammals, 112, 142, 172

Manifest Destiny, 18, 125

Martin, Emily, 42, 45, 50, 73, 181; *The Woman in the Body,* 42; *Flexible Bodies,* 181

Masco, Joseph, 145

Massumi, Brian, 61

neoliberalism: and California, 28, 197, 199, 217; dominance of, 220; and doulas, 33, 122–23; as feedback loop, 174; and feminism, 133, 142, 206

new momism, 107

Nixon, Rob, 157

nostalgia, 150–51, 215, 218; and scandal of ex-privilege, 199–200

Oakeshott, Michael, 52; *Experience and Its Modes,* 52

obstetrics, 40, 53–54, 60, 63, 65, 112; and human rights, 203; law of three Ps, 43, 47; obstetricians, 2n3, 196–97; partogram, 42; racism/violence, 32, 89, 203

Odent, Michel, 149; *Childbirth and the Evolution of Homo Sapiens,* 149

ontology, 40, 183; and/as epistemology, 40

optimism, 174, 188, 214

optimization, 23, 91, 133–34, 145, 187, 198–99

opt-out revolution, 98, 206. *See also* Mommy Wars

origins, 171, 175, 183, 187; fetishized, 191, 193, 218

Ortner, Sherry, 5, 129–30; "Is Female to Male as Nature Is to Culture?," 129

Outlaw Midwife (blog/zine), 204

Owens, Kellie, 75

pain, 84–90; relief, 53–54, 138; versus suffering, 84, 87

paleofantasies, 149

paleo parenting, 146, 148, 151

parturition, 112, 126

Pasteur, Louis, 166

Pateman, Carol, 110

Paxson, Heather, 183

Perez, Laura, 196

Pérez, Miriam Zoila, 59, 209; *The Radical Doula Guide,* 209

perinatal psychology, 170, 195. *See also* Association for Prenatal and Perinatal Psychology and Health

Perinatal Substance Abuse Task Force, 191

personhood: birth and, 8; of fetus/infants/children, 113–14; as formed in early life, 175; processual and flexible, 114, 116; of woman/mother, 12, 104, 112, 114

Peskowitz, Miriam, 98; *The Truth Behind the Mommy Wars,* 98

Petersen, Sara, 206

Pfaffl, Nasima, 204

physiology, 40, 50, 217; physiological birth, 40

Pitocin. *See under* hormones

placenta, 32, 159, 176, 182–83

Planned Parenthood, 22

Pollan, Michael, 163–64, 168; "Some of My Best Friends Are Germs," 163

pollution: and Bay Area, 154; effects on fertility, 151; and environmental justice, 161; ubiquity of, 194. *See also* chemicals; toxins

population, 100, 161, 206–7; population-wide disease, 149, 175

postpartum period, 104, 170–71; breast-feeding anxiety, 140; glossing over, 105; suffering, 87. *See also* motherbaby

power: and alienation, 145–46; animal/spiritual, 136–40, 142; in birth, 69–70, 90–94, 124; and birth movements, 25–27, 57; dynamics during birth, 56, 57, 63, 81, 123; and equality, 101, 110; feminist empowerment, 27, 91, 133, 206, 220; hegemonic, 10; immanence as, 92–93, 139; and knowledge, 57, 63; and nature, 130, 149; pain as, 85–86; and vulnerability, 180–81; and witches, 53, 55

precautionary consumption, 160–61

primal, the: primal continuum, 191; primal period, 149–50; valorization of, 125–26, 136, 149, 152; and women, 137, 148

primates, 130, 147–49

professionalization, 32–33, 53, 54, 214

progress, 18–20, 187, 217, 219; and California, 13, 19, 24; and capitalism, 35; and the frontier, 21; individual growth as, 28–29; in labor, 42, 45, 57, 58, 83; "light of," historical fantasy, 52–54, 73; protest against, 125, 62, 187, 197; and/versus redemption, 36, 187–88, 214–15; reversal

progress (continued)
of, 149, 152; "sideways" orientation toward, 24, 215; and utopia, 23–24; and the "woman question," 111

public versus private: doing away with, 119; and love versus money, 118, 123; origins of, 110

purity, 180, 194; bodies as not having, 159; fetus/newborn/children as having, 154, 183; frontier as having, 187; past, 151

race: and animality, 132, 137; California and, 21–22, 29; of Californians, 198; and childbearing disparities/activism, 10, 31, 32 (see also reproductive justice); and childhood, 111; and class, 29; and discrimination, 92, 96; and domestic work, 117; and eugenics, 22–23; and pollution, 161; White people grappling with, 186, 191, 194; and witches/midwives, 53, 151

Raphael, Dana, 33

Rapp, Rayna, 74

Reagan, Ronald, 100, 199

redemption, 36, 186–88, 196, 199, 207, 214–15

refusal, 214

regular versus contextual: physiology, 39–47, 51, 55, 57, 61, 68; subjects, 115

relational autonomy, 96

religion, 62, 152, 186–88; America at frontiers of, 187; versus science, 152, 58, 62. See also redemption; salvation; spirituality

religion, types of: Catholics, Buddhists, Quakers and atheists, 139; Christianity, 85, 152, 211; neopaganism, 139, 138–9; Peoples Temple Agricultural Project, 187; Protestant, 86, 198; Puritans, Mormons, and Adventists, 187

reproductive justice, 34, 91–92, 185–86, 193, 201; and doulas, 208–9; and environmental justice, 161, 179; and feminism, 201–2; versus rights or choice, 186, 202–3

Reyes-Foster, Beatriz, 32

Rich, Adrienne, 120

rights, 202–4, 219; consumer, 202; human, in childbirth, 203; versus right relations, 204

risk: in birth, 10, 46, 68–69, 70–77, 127, 150; counterculture, 75; and fear, 79–80, 82, 84; and modern overwhelm, 146, 205; and power, 91, 93; and selfhood, 182

rite of passage, 77, 134–40

ritual, 135, 137, 139, 144

Robinson, Marilynne, 187; "How America Talks about Itself," 187

Roe v. Wade, 99, 200. See also abortion

Rose, Nikolas, 199

Ross, Loretta, 185–86, 190, 203, 207

Rothman, Barbara Katz, 43, 60, 90

Rousseau, Jean-Jacques, 111; Emile, 111

Ruddick, Sara, 129

salvation, 156, 186, 188, 191–92, 200, 211

Sandberg, Sheryl, 200

Sandelowski, Margarete, 73

Sanger, Margaret, 22, 110

Santa Cruz, 15–17; versus Bay Area, 17

Santa Cruz Doula Salon, 58

saviorism, 188; doctors as saviors, 80; doulas as saviors, 210–11, 213

scapegoat, 188, 196; doulas as, 210–11, 213

Schiebinger, Londa, 112

science: of attachment, 146–47; authority of, 148, 151; and California, 35; ecological, 156; empiricism and objectivity as, 58, 61, 64; and evidence, 62–66, 166; feminist studies, 147, 148; immunological, 181–82; as liberation, 111; of microbiome, 164; and midwifery, 26; of/and motherhood, 73, 99, 112, 148, 161; neuroscience, 131, 140, 145; of productivity, 42; and/as religion or ideology, 56, 62, 76, 152, 187–88; of stress, 175–76

scopolamine, 53–54. See also pain

Scott, Karen, 32, 89, 214

Seremetakis, Nadia, 150

sexual contract, 110

side effects, 159; instances of, 18, 82, 93, 151

Silicon Valley, 17, 21–29, 35, 141, 143, 187

Simms, Eva-Maria, 167

Simpkin, Peggy, 107; The Birth Partner, 107–8

www.ingramcontent.com/pod-product-compliance
Lightning Source LLC
Chambersburg PA
CBHW020845270326
41928CB00006B/554